ATLAS OF THE
DIFFICULT AIRWAY

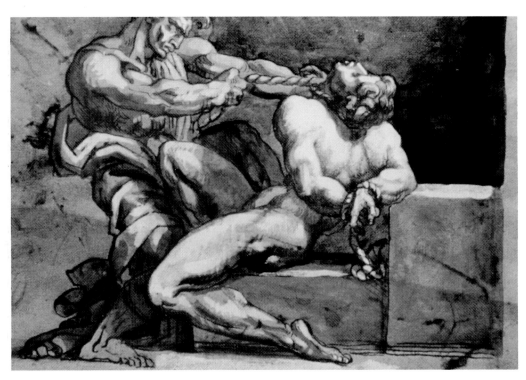

Homme Supplicié,
watercolor by Theodore Gericault (1791-1824),
painted between 1815 and 1820.
Used with permission of Musée Bonnat,
Ville de Bayonne, 5 rue Jacques-Laffitte, Bayonne, France.

ATLAS OF THE
DIFFICULT AIRWAY

MARTIN L. NORTON,
M.S.P.H. (San. Eng.), M.D., D.An., J.D.

Emeritus Professor,
Department of Anesthesiology;
Emeritus Associate Professor (Anesthesia)
Department of Otorhinolaryngology;
Active Emeritus Professor,
Department of Postgraduate Medicine and
Health Sciences Education,
University of Michigan Medical School,
Ann Arbor, Michigan

Editorial Associate
Jeanne T. Fitzgerald, M.A., D.A.

Medical Artist
Claudia Bernardi, M.F.A.

Second Edition

with **300** *illustrations*

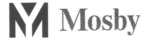 Mosby

St. Louis Baltimore Boston Carlsbad Chicago Naples New York Philadelphia Portland
London Madrid Mexico City Singapore Sydney Tokyo Toronto Wiesbaden

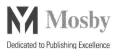

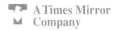

Vice President and Publisher: Anne S. Patterson
Editor: Laurel Craven
Developmental Editor: Sandra Clark Brown
Associate Developmental Editor: Wendy Buckwalter
Project Manager: Patricia Tannian
Senior Production Editor: Suzanne C. Fannin
Manufacturing Manager: David Graybill
Book Design Manager: Gail Morey Hudson
Cover Designer: Teresa Breckwoldt

SECOND EDITION

Printed in the United States of America
Composition by Top Graphics
Printing/binding by Walsworth Press

Mosby–Year Book, Inc.
11830 Westline Industrial Drive
St. Louis, MO 63146

Library of Congress Cataloging in Publication Data

Atlas of the difficult airway / [edited by] Martin L. Norton:
    editorial associate, Jeanne T. Fitzgerald; medical artist, Claudia
Bernardi. — 2nd ed.
        p. cm.
    Includes bibliographical references and index.
    ISBN 0-8151-6433-5 (alk. paper)
        1. Trachea—Intubation—Atlases.   2. Laryngoscopy—Atlases.
I. Norton, Martin L.   II. Fitzgerald, Jeanne Tashian.
III. Bernardi, Claudia.
        [DNLM: 1. Intubation, Intratracheal—methods—atlases.
    2. Anesthesia—methods—atlases.   3. Respiration, Artificial—
instrumentation—atlases.   4. Airway Obstruction—therapy—atlases.
WO 517 A8817 1996]
RF517.A87   1996
616.2—dc20
DNLM/DLC
    for Library of Congress   96-3205
                                                                CIP

96 97 98 99   00 / 9 8 7 6 5 4 3 2 1

"He who does not increase his knowledge, decreases it."
Pirke Aboth, *Chapter 1, 13*

Contributors

STEPHEN BUCHMAN, M.D.

Assistant Professor of Plastic and Reconstructive Surgery;
Director, Craniofacial Surgery;
Chief of Pediatric Plastic Surgery;
University of Michigan Medical School,
Ann Arbor, Michigan

ALLAN C. D. BROWN, M.B., Ch.B., FFARCS

Associate Professor, Department of Anesthesiology,
University of Michigan Medical School,
Ann Arbor, Michigan

FRANK LONDY, R.R.T.

Research Associate, Department of Radiology,
University of Michigan Medical School,
Ann Arbor, Michigan

LYNETTE J. MARK, M.D.

Assistant Professor, Departments of Anesthesiology and Critical Care Medicine
and Otolaryngology—Head and Neck Surgery,
The Johns Hopkins Medical Institutions,
Baltimore, Maryland

BERNARD R. MARSH, M.D.

Professor and Chairman, Department of Otolaryngology—Head and Neck Surgery,
The Johns Hopkins Medical Institutions,
Baltimore, Maryland

FERNANDO J. MARTINEZ, M.D.

Assistant Professor; Medical Director; Pulmonary Diagnostic Laboratory,
Division of Pulmonary and Critical Care Medicine,
University of Michigan Medical School,
Ann Arbor, Michigan

VILDAN MULLIN, M.D.

Assistant Professor of Anesthesiology;
Director, Neurosurgical Anesthesia,
University of Michigan Medical School,
Ann Arbor, Michigan

MARTIN L. NORTON, M.S.P.H. (San. Eng.), M.D., D.An., J.D.

Emeritus Professor, Department of Anesthesiology;
Emeritus Associate Professor (Anesthesia),
Department of Otorhinolaryngology;
Active Emeritus Professor,
Department of Postgraduate Medicine and Health Sciences Education,
University of Michigan Medical School,
Ann Arbor, Michigan

ANDRANIK OVASSAPIAN, M.D.

Professor of Clinical Anesthesia,
Northwestern University Medical School;
Chief of Service, VA Lakeside Medical Center,
Chicago, Illinois

VIJAYALAKSHMI U. PATIL, M.D.

Associate Professor of Anesthesiology,
State University of New York Health Science Center,
Syracuse, New York

CHARLES POLLACK, M.D.

Director of Research and Education,
Department of Emergency Medicine,
Maricopa Medical Center,
Phoenix, Arizona

R. BARRY POWELL, B.S.N., M.N., C.R.N.A.

Instructor, Department of Anesthesiology;
University of Michigan Medical School,
Ann Arbor, Michigan

PAUL REYNOLDS, M.D.

Clinical Associate Professor of Anesthesiology;
Head of Pediatric Anesthesiology,
University of Michigan Medical School,
Ann Arbor, Michigan

RICHARD SCOTT, D.D.S., M.S.

Private Practitioner,
Ann Arbor, Michigan

Foreword

"First, the patient, second, the patient, third, the patient, fourth, the patient, fifth, the patient, and then maybe comes science. We first do everything for the patient; science can wait, research can wait!"

BÉLA SCHICK (1877-1967)

Aphorisms and Facetiae of Béla Schick

My first experience in the area of airway management came when I was a child undergoing a tonsillectomy. I was on the receiving end of an open-drop ether anesthetic, and my most vivid memories are of a distinct choking sensation during induction. The experience was so bad that, when I needed an appendectomy several years later, I begged to be put to sleep before a mask was placed on my face. I still feel grateful to the anesthesiologist who complied with my wishes and administered pentothal per vein.

I can only imagine, then, the terror that a patient with a difficult airway must feel when told, preoperatively, that certain uncomfortable manipulations must be performed before going to sleep. Indeed, anesthesiologists who can safely anesthetize such a patient with little or no discomfort are among the most respected among our specialty. Dr. Martin L. Norton is one of them.

Dr. Norton has devoted a significant portion of his medical career to the study of the difficult airway. He pioneered and popularized many of the techniques that are taken for granted today. He has been widely regarded as both a teacher and researcher. Thus it is no surprise that, some years ago, he recognized that the increasingly complex surgeries being performed on higher risk patients had created a population of individuals with airways so difficult that simply dealing with them in the operating room morning of surgery would not suffice. For this reason, in 1987 at the University of Michigan he established the first dedicated Difficult Airway Clinic in the world.

The results of his effort were immediate and profound. Patients referred to the clinic were assessed by experts using the most sophisticated equipment and techniques available. The consultative resources of a major medical center were used to provide a multidisciplinary approach to evaluate and care; a large patient population was identified to be used for teaching and research; medical students, resident physicians, and practitioners were educated in advanced airway management techniques; and, finally, the first edition of *Atlas of the Difficult Airway* was published.

I first saw *Atlas of the Difficult Airway* at a national meeting of anesthesiologists, and I immediately ordered a copy for our departmental library. Within a week of its arrival, the book was accorded the greatest accolade that can be bestowed upon a medical text. It was stolen. The replacement edition has since been kept in my locked office and only loaned out in my presence.

Atlas of the Difficult Airway is an excellent book because it is based on the enormous fund of clinical experience possessed by Dr. Norton and his colleagues. The second edition is even better. Once again, Dr. Norton has collected a cadre of local and national experts who have written an excellent road map for traveling a safe route to establishing an airway under the most challenging circumstances.

The reader is carefully guided through all aspects of dealing with the difficult airway. The scope of topics covered ranges from those as simple as intubation of a normal patient to those as complex as organizing a difficult airway clinic. Numerous photographs and drawings make clear even the most difficult concepts. The multidisciplinary focus allows the book to be useful to a variety of specialists outside of anesthesiology, including otolaryngologists, radiologists, emergency physicians, oral surgeons, plastic surgeons, intensivists, and respiratory therapists.

The organization of the new edition has been improved, and several areas of management have been added, reflecting the results of new insights gained from ongoing research in the area, along with improvements in technology. The result is a thoroughly up-to-date atlas that retains the strengths of the first edition: readability, practicality, completeness, clarity, and superb illustrations. This is the book to reach for when confronted with an impossible airway.

I congratulate Dr. Norton and his colleagues on their achievement. To you, the reader, I offer a bit of advice. Keep this book in a locked office.

Michael L. Nahrwold, M.D.

Preface

The material contained herein is the result of many years of interest and experience with the problem of the difficult airway. To this has been added the collective presentations of the annual seminars on *The Difficult Airway* presented at the Towsley Center for Continuing Medical Education, University of Michigan Medical Center, Ann Arbor from 1988 to the present and the results of an ongoing study of these patients at the Difficult Airway Clinic of The Department of Anesthesiology, University of Michigan Hospitals. We have, at all times, had a continued participatory interaction with the Departments of Radiology, the Pulmonary Function Testing Service, the Sleep Apnea Clinic, and the Division of Otorhinolaryngology.

This new edition of the *Atlas of the Difficult Airway* has been expanded to make it more practical and to cover areas such as fiberoptic views, communication, and Le Fort facial trauma, among others, that were not fully addressed in the first edition. Contributing authors have been chosen for their expertise and national or international recognition in various specialties such as emergency medicine, plastic surgery, oral and maxillofacial surgery, and pulmonary medicine, as well as the various subspecialties of anesthesiology. Although a salient reference list is presented with each chapter, the writers' have emphasized their own experience drawn from their special interests in clinical practice. The bibliographies are by no means meant to be exhaustive.

Visual presentations are emphasized in this work. It is, after all, an atlas. The visual presentations include a collection of teaching materials from past years and from the archives of the Difficult Airway Clinic. The subjects of this presentation have, after extensive discussion and explanation, graciously granted permission for their pictures and cases to be reproduced herein for the education of health professionals and resultant benefit of future patients we are so honored and privileged to serve.

Points of singular importance are drawn out from the text as highlighted axioms. I recommend the reader to read these significant axioms.

ACKNOWLEDGMENTS

Special recognition in the preparation of this volume is given to my secretary, Mrs. Tina Szegda; artist, Claudia Bernardi; and editorial associate, Jeanne T. Fitzgerald. I would like to extend my appreciation to Suzanne Fannin, Wendy Buckwalter, and Sandra Clark Brown, Mosby. Perhaps most important of all was the encouragement of my wife, Shirley Harrison Norton; my parents, Julia Kaufer Norton and Edward Victor Norton; and my former teachers who initiated my interest in medicine. Last, but by no means least, I wish to acknowledge Dr. Jay Finch, former Chairman of the University of Michigan Department of Anesthesiology, whose first priority was always patient care; Dr. Allan C. D. Brown; and, especially, R. Barry Powell, CRNA, who has worked so hard supporting my efforts in the Difficult Airway Clinic.

Martin L. Norton

Contents

BACKGROUND

"Errors are not in the art but in the artificiers."

SIR ISAAC NEWTON, 1687

Philosophiae Naturalis Principia Mathematica

CHAPTER 1

The Difficult Airway

PART A *The Problem*

MARTIN L. NORTON

PHYSIOLOGY AND VARIATIONS OF THE DIFFICULT AIRWAY

Any anatomic obstruction of the upper airway may contribute to the difficult airway syndrome. Conditions such as nasal septal deviation, adenoid-tonsillar hypertrophy, craniovertebral anomalies, vocal fold paresis or paralysis, and glottic web have been reported to impede access to the airway.

Physiologic Variations

Lesser known and less well understood are the physiologic variations that should be considered. During sleep and while under anesthesia the tongue and the velopharyngeal sphincter musculature reduce tone. Excellent descriptions of the controlling mechanisms and their related biomechanics are discussed in the texts by Fink[1] and Fink and Demarest.[2]

Sukerman and Healy[3] discuss the controlling mechanisms somewhat differently. They believe that the patency of the upper airway is partially controlled by the central nervous system and that spontaneous adjustment of the shape and volume of the upper respiratory tract can be demonstrated. Tactile and proprioceptive messages from the pharyngeal mucosa and musculature supply higher centers with information important for involuntary adjustments. Patency of the pharyngeal airway is maintained by adjustments in its muscular tone.

The pharyngeal muscles must increase their tone to overcome the tendency to collapse during inspiration. The forces contributing to upper airway collapse during inspiration include the following:
1. Surrounding atmospheric pressure and weight of the nuchal tissue
2. Local compliance of the airway walls
3. Negative pressure inside the lumen of airway during inspiration

Anatomic Variations and Resulting Biomechanical Changes

To the previously mentioned forces and conditions must be added others, such as anatomic variations and the resulting biomechanical changes they impose and superimposed positioning effects with abnormal biomechanics induced by use of endoscopic instruments and approaches, as well as the effects of sedatives, analgesics, and anesthetics. Similarly, airway wall compliance may be affected by fatty infiltration, fluid from edema and exudates, and localized lesions.

Fink[1] and Sukerman and Healy[3] discuss the complex relationship between airflow and upper airway resistance, noting the following: **Airflow varies inversely with the resistance and directly with pressure developed between the alveoli and the airway opening.** The greater the resistance to airflow, the greater the driving force that is needed to maintain a normal tidal volume. Consequently, if resistance is high, a larger negative pressure must be created during inspiration. This increased negative pressure is transmitted along the airway, and it, in turn, increases the tendency of the airway to collapse.

The Bernoulli effect, similarly, contributes to collapse. If the volume of airflow is constant, the velocity of air at a constriction decreases. The lower pressure at the site of narrowing increases the tendency to collapse. Understanding these phenomena is paramount to an appreciation of the biomechanics of upper airway ventilation, but they certainly should not be new concepts to the anesthesiologist, otolaryngologist, pulmonologist, and thoracic surgeon. For example, the Bernoulli principle specifies that flow energy is partitioned into potential energy (pressure) and kinetic energy (velocity). If the total energy is constant, acceleration of streamlined flow at a constriction is indicated by a gain in kinetic energy and a corresponding loss of potential energy. The loss of potential energy, in the context of the airway, results in a dynamic fall in pressure at the glottic constriction, which then tends to constrict further.

During inspiration the glottic aperture increases as the posterior cricoarytenoid muscle contracts and opens the vocal fold aperture. During expiration the activity of the cricoarytenoid muscle decreases, and the vocal folds return to their "passive" position. The respiratory motion of the vocal folds is of obvious importance in decreasing airway resistance during inspiration and in regulating the rate of airflow during expiration.

The epiglottis, which may occlude the glottic chink, is retracted ventrally by its attachment to the hyoid bone through the hyoepiglottic ligament, thereby opening the hypopharynx. The hyoid bone lies ventral to the genioglossus muscle and serves as a point of attachment for several muscles, most notably the geniohyoid, the digastric, and the thyrohyoid muscles. Contraction of the geniohyoid and the digastric muscles pulls the hyoid ventrally, thereby pulling the base of the tongue and the epiglottis ventrally.

The main muscle of the tongue is the fan-shaped genioglossus muscle, with its fibers inserting laterally on the internal surface of the mandible. When the genioglossus muscle contracts during inspiration, it pulls the ventral wall of the oropharynx further ventrally. Thus the tongue enlarges the lumen of the oropharynx, resulting in a collapsible pharynx stemming from the dorsal movement of the ventral pharyngeal wall. The motion of the tongue is resisted by contraction of muscles attached to the mandible, including the genioglossus, geniohyoid, and digastric muscles.

Early and convincing clinical evidence for this proposition derives from experience with anesthetized humans, presented in the landmark paper by Dr. Peter Safar and others.[4] It was subsequently demonstrated that closure of the mouth and extension of the neck establish a patent oropharynx by stretching the muscles attached to the mandible and thereby increasing the force exerted by the genioglossus, geniohyoid, and digastric muscles. This pulls the ventral wall of the pharynx away from its dorsal wall.[5,6]

PROFESSIONAL LIABILITY IN DIFFICULT AIRWAY INTUBATIONS

The dramatic results of a failed airway intubation have been evaluated in studies by the American Society of Anesthesiologists' Committee on Professional Liability Closed Claims Project.[7,8] The original analysis (1975 to 1979) of approximately 1541 closed malpractice insurance claims for all types of surgical procedures revealed that respiratory mishaps are the most common cause of brain damage and death during anesthesia, accounting for 34% of the claims. Three mechanisms of injury accounted for three-fourths of all adverse respiratory events: inadequate ventilation, 38%; unintentional esophageal intubation, 18%; and "difficult intubation," 17%. Of all the respiratory mishaps studied, 66% died and 9% suffered from permanent brain damage.

Subsequent trend analysis (1980 to 1984) following much publicity and many courses on the difficult airway revealed that claims decreased to 28%, then to 17% after 1990. This trend is proof positive that efforts on the part of anesthesiologists can result in better patient outcomes. The balance of injuries were grouped as "other" (e.g., airway obstruction, bronchospasm, aspiration, premature or unintentional extubation, inadequate inspired oxygen delivery, and endobronchial intubation).

The contribution of the difficult airway to adverse outcomes is more apparent now than in the past because other causes of morbidity and mortality are being lessened by monitoring patients and using pharmaceutic techniques.[9-11] Although 90% of difficult intubations should be anticipated with careful, routine examination of the airway, unexpected problems with difficult airway or intubation continue to occur.[12] Reports of the unanticipated incidence of difficult airway events range from 1% to 3.5% for all patients requiring intubation of the trachea.[13-15] Based on the number of anesthetics administered annually, there are more than 100,000 potential difficult airway patients per year in the United States.[16]

Recent studies have concluded that failure to secure a patent airway was the predominant cause of anesthesia-related maternal deaths (Table 1-1).[17-19] When obstetric cases alone were analyzed, and despite the fact that regional anesthesia was the predominant technique for cesarean sections (with epidural anesthesia frequently administered for routine deliveries), respiratory-related problems were still the most common critical incident reported (14% involved difficult or esophageal intubations). Other authors[20,21] have found similar, related problems.

The obstetric patient is of particular concern. First the processes of pregnancy, labor, and delivery (i.e., weight gain, fluid retention, and ventilatory embarrassment) predispose the patient to airway problems. Diaphragmatic and thoracic excursions are progressively limited. Edema and increased central venous pressure causes laryngeal tissue thickening with a tendency to vestibular and vocal fold swelling, both predelivery and postdelivery. Further, as the fetus enlarges, the abdominal contents push against the diaphragm. Resultant pressure limits the expansion of the lungs, while the trachea is pushed somewhat cephalad, particularly in the supine position. This reduces the mandibulohyothyroid distances.

The combination of all of the previously mentioned problems leads to greater intubation difficulties, even when regional anesthesia is chosen for labor and delivery. **The obligation to guarantee airway control is not obviated by epidural, spinal, or other regional approaches.** In fact, that obligation is enhanced if failure or complications from regional anesthesia occur.

Recent statistics on the occurrence of anesthesia-related maternal deaths indicate that at least 12% were related to airway management or intubation. Coupling this with an aspiration mortality rate of 23%, the rate is now 35%. Furthermore, of the maternal deaths related to regional anesthesia, respiratory events are reported at 22%, whereas the figure for general anesthesia is approximately 48%. Regional anesthesia poses significant risk, requiring constant concern for airway management. The conclusion is that anesthesiologists must be just as vigilant about assuring airway access when administering regional anesthesia to parturients as they are when administering general anesthesia.

The American Society of Anesthesiologists (ASA) report clearly demonstrates that respiratory problems are the most common cause of brain damage and death under anesthesia, with unintentional intubation of the esophagus being a major cause. This excellent study involved only closed insurance claims that actually led to a lawsuit, and thus research findings are skewed. The data did not include other cases of morbidity that never reached the point of legal action or manifest insurance claim.

Table 1-1   Anesthesia-Related Deaths Associated with Obstetric Delivery, United States, 1979-1990*

Cause of death	Number	Percent
Airway problems		
Aspiration	29	23
Failed intubation	15	12
Inadequate ventilation	16	12
Respiratory failure	2	1
Intraoperative cardiac arrest	30	23
Local anesthetic toxicity	17	13
High spinal or epidural anesthesia	12	9
Overdose	1	1
Anaphylaxis	1	1
TOTAL	123	95

Data from Joy Hawkins, M.D., Director of Obstetric Anesthesia, University of Colorado Health Sciences Center, Denver, Colo 80602.

*This represents a reanalysis of the data, which excludes abortion and ectopic pregnancy deaths.

Contrary to the categorization of the ASA committee, the authors are convinced that esophageal intubations rightfully belong in the category of difficult intubations—or what rationale can we give for the rate of improper placement? (If they are not in the difficult airway grouping, the level of teaching and practice of endotracheal intubation must be deplorable!)

This position is supported by the International Committee for Prevention of Anesthesia Mortality and Morbidity 1988 summary report by Dr. Gaisford Harrison.[21a] Harrison came to the conclusion over the years, that, although there has been improvement in responding to problems associated with monitoring vital signs and using the intellect, problems associated with manual skills have not substantially improved.

Let us take a moment to examine the contributions by the "medical giants" of the past. Sir William Macewen, a Scottish surgeon, is often reported to have been the first to perform endotracheal intubation in 1880.[22] In fact, endotracheal intubation, more or less, as we know it was first accomplished by Kirstein[23] with the aid of a laryngoscope in 1895. However, even this accomplishment was preceded by blind nasal intubation (originally described by Desault,[24] Surgeon-in-Chief of the Great Hospital of Humanity in Paris in 1814 and popularized by Magill and Rowbotham[25] in the 1920s) and tactile intubation practiced by Kite in the 18th century as described by Herholdt and Rafn[26] in 1796. They mentioned passing a catheter blindly over their fingers, which were placed behind the epiglottis into the windpipe.

Above all, we are indebted to the father of clinical endoscopy, Chevalier Jackson, for his teaching, instrumentation, and clinical textual material. Although the modern endoscopist can no longer be considered as practicing state-of-the-art intubation if he or she is unfamiliar with flexible fiberoptic techniques, it is no less important that facility with both straight and curved rigid laryngoscopes and rigid bronchoscopic instrumentation be part of the armamentarium.

Moving into the 21st century does not mean discarding the knowledge and skills of those who preceded us. The use of a stylet, light-reflective and retrograde techniques, as well as a laryngeal mask should also be learned and applied where suitable. The box below gives a listing of older intubation techniques and contemporary techniques which are their "heirs."

Despite all of the previously mentioned advances, no reliable study of the clinical practitioner's experience with difficult intubations has been done in recent times, nor has the true incidence of unintentional esophageal intubations been determined. Also, information on delayed recognition of unintentional esophageal intubations that did not go on to catastrophe is not available. The few studies of note suffer from the problems of varying definitions of the difficult airway, the most glaring omission being a lack of clear, prospective, reproducible criteria for identification of a difficult airway situation.[27,28]

The question is who is responsible for what arises among surgeons, anesthesiologists, and other specialists requiring access to the airway. Experience has shown that the problem does not reside in the hands of one specialty. Of course, we want to hear about problem cases in advance—and at our convenience—and then the surgeon and the anesthesiologist fail to give the problem the med-

---

HISTORIC AND CONTEMPORARY INTUBATION TECHNIQUES

Older	Newer
Intubation guides	Magnetic
Cricothyroidotomy	Flexible stylette
Digital	Flexible laryngoscope
Fiberoptic bronchoscope	Mirror or prism
Endotrol tube	Bullard laryngoscope
Oral hook	Laryngeal mask or airway
Retrograde	Guidewire
Whistle catheter	Fiberoptic stylette laryngoscope
Rigid brochoscope	Jet catheter or stylette

ical consideration it deserves. Physicians act as technicians. This is where a professional attitude, manifesting itself through thorough examination and evaluation based on an understanding of anatomy and biomechanics, can contribute the most.

The profession and, above all, the patient, cannot accept ego-driven statements like "I can handle airway problems," "I don't need someone else to tell me...," or "I know a difficult airway when I see it." It must be recognized that airway problems are of primary concern and usually precede other considerations of surgery. Let us remember the A for *airway* of the ABCs of cardiorespiratory management.*

It has come to recognition that a wide disparity in airway management skills and abilities exists among modern anesthesiologists, otolaryngologists, and other endoscopists. The notion that anyone can insert a tube in any airway demonstrates that many of our colleagues have shifted their focus from the ABCs of resuscitation to the esoteric world of calculated doses (which are often given to the patient, whether or not the patient's response shows a need), microspheric cardiac studies, and end tidal Pco_2 values seen on a screen, without consideration of the meaning of the pattern visualized, among other examples.

Endotracheal intubation is a matter of particular sensitivity for the anesthesiologist and the otolaryngologist, compounded by the fact that not real criteria exist for defining endoscopic and intubation skills. Of equal importance is the failure of surgeons to recognize the problem except in the most obvious situations. The surgeon often assumes that access to the airway is a simple mechanical problem solved by a simple, mechanically minded "gas passer" of lesser stature sitting at the head of the table. Of course, if things do not work out, "we can always do a tracheostomy," potential complications of tracheostomies notwithstanding (see box below).[29]

In certain cases an anesthesiologist may find it impossible to introduce an endotracheal tube after the patient has been induced for anesthesia. There may be no immediate life, limb, or organ-saving emergency making it necessary to proceed with the surgery, but the surgeon may still insist on doing a tracheostomy (which of course is his prerogative). Often the *reason* for the problem appears to carry no weight in surgical considerations. Worse still, the fact that the same patient may, in the future, be faced with the same airway access dilemma, does not appear to give the surgeon cause to consider a proper evaluation of the reasons for the intubation difficulty. This mentality represents an emphasis on factors of convenience rather than concern for the patient's future welfare.

It is time for the medical profession to reassess goals with patient care considerations uppermost, so that physicians can come to terms and recognize that management of the difficult airway pre-

---

*A, Airway; *B*, breathing; *C*, circulation.

SOME TRACHEOSTOMY COMPLICATIONS

1. Infection
2. Opening of fascial planes (infection; aerodissection around the larynx, trachea, or mediastinum)
3. Tracheal stenosis
4. Pneumothorax (especially on right)
5. Hemorrhage, hematoma, tracheoinnominate (brachiocephalic) artery fistula
6. Difficulties of access (tumors, obesity)
7. Cosmesis (keloid and other scar formation)
8. Injury to structures adjacent to the trachea (damage to recurrent laryngeal nerves, entrance into major vessels, rare but possible laceration of the esophagus or tracheoesophageal fistula)
9. Failure to cannulate the airway
10. Long-term complications from the use of endotracheal or tracheostomy tubes (pressure necrosis, tracheomalacia, ball valve obstruction, granulation tissue)

From Kirstein A: *Berl Klin Wochenschr* 32:475, 1895.

sents special problems and solutions. That time is *not* the night before surgery or the moment the patient is put on the operating table. It must be done in advance through a consultancy service like that in the Difficult Airway Clinic (DAC). **Preanesthesia assessment of the airway is more important than a preoperative electrocardiogram (ECG).** This can only be achieved by providing sufficient time for proper and considered evaluation and planning for the final objective. **Evaluation and management of potential airway problems must be addressed before the patient is brought to the operating room.**

With this information, the growing availability of flexible fiberoptic instruments, and attention to the problem as exemplified by the development of a Difficult Airway Evaluation Clinic,[30,31] catastrophic events can be reduced.

PART B *One Solution: The Difficult Airway Clinic*

R. BARRY POWELL

The DAC was established at the University of Michigan in May 1987 to evaluate known and potential airway problems. A prime goal was to identify prognostic signs (Table 1-2) that lead to patient morbidity and mortality, including failed intubations, traumatic intubations, need for emergent or emergency tracheostomy, case cancellations, and anesthesia risk management cases.

The objectives of the clinic include the following:
1. To provide presurgical evaluation of potential or known intubation problems
2. To identify and evaluate patients at risk
3. To present recommendations for airway management
4. To expedite, through the development of a comprehensive plan, operating room management of the difficult airway patient
5. To provide experience-based reassurance to the patient and the physician of available methods for airway problem identification and management
6. To accumulate research data on prospective, reproducible criteria for detecting the difficult airway syndrome

Table 1-2 Projected Difficult Endoscopy Prognostic Signs*

Sign	Score
Skill of the intubationist	±5
Intubationist's ego	±5
Planning for endoscopy	±5
Micrognathia with acute mandibular angles	±5
Glossoptosis or basal macroglossia	4
Temporomandibular joint limitation	4
Müller's sign	(3-4)
Difficulty with prior laryngoscopy	3
Limited motion of lower cervical vertebrae	3
Pathologic signs of airway obstruction	3
Decreased distance of epiglottis from posterior wall of pharynx	3
Adverse sign (3+ or 4+)	2
Long, high-arched palate associated with long, narrow dental arc	2
Short muscular neck with full dentition	2
Protruding maxillary dentition with premaxillary overgrowth	2
Limited extension of the upper cervical vertebrae	2
Decreased distance between hyoid and thyroid cartilages	2
Increased alveolomental depth	1

*Scale ranges from 1 to 5, with 1 being best and 5 being worst.

7. To encourage teaching of less common intubation techniques, with particular emphasis on flexible fiberoptic skills

The accomplishment of these goals has been successful. When comparing quality assurance data before and after the inception of the DAC, the number of undiagnosed difficult airways has decreased. The key to this success is the fact that anesthesiologists insist on seeing these patients in the DAC at the time they are first considered for elective surgery. This strategy usually avoids the pitfall of having to wait until the night before or the morning of surgery to evaluate the airway.

The majority of departmental anesthesia care providers should have specific courses in the management of the difficult airway to include fiberoptic intubation and other techniques, including programs for the identification and management of the patient with a difficult airway that are con-

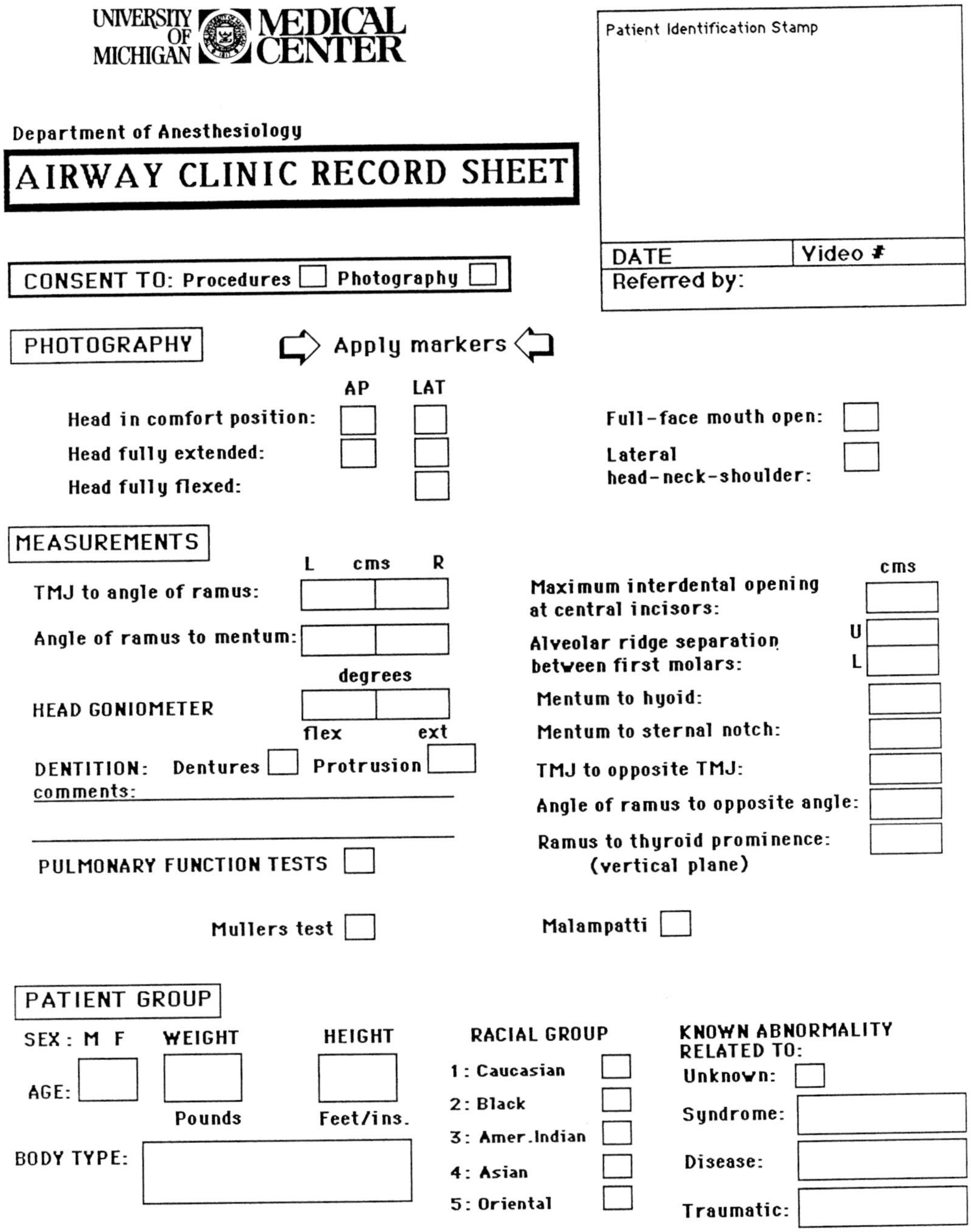
UNIVERSITY OF MICHIGAN MEDICAL CENTER

Patient Identification Stamp

Department of Anesthesiology

AIRWAY CLINIC RECORD SHEET

DATE | Video #

Referred by:

CONSENT TO: Procedures ☐ Photography ☐

PHOTOGRAPHY — Apply markers

	AP	LAT
Head in comfort position:	☐	☐
Head fully extended:	☐	☐
Head fully flexed:		☐

Full-face mouth open: ☐

Lateral head-neck-shoulder: ☐

MEASUREMENTS

	L cms R
TMJ to angle of ramus:	☐ ☐
Angle of ramus to mentum:	☐ ☐

HEAD GONIOMETER — degrees: flex ☐ ext ☐

DENTITION: Dentures ☐ Protrusion ☐

comments:

PULMONARY FUNCTION TESTS ☐

Mullers test ☐

	cms
Maximum interdental opening at central incisors:	☐
Alveolar ridge separation between first molars:	U ☐ L ☐
Mentum to hyoid:	☐
Mentum to sternal notch:	☐
TMJ to opposite TMJ:	☐
Angle of ramus to opposite angle:	☐
Ramus to thyroid prominence: (vertical plane)	☐

Malampatti ☐

PATIENT GROUP

SEX: M F

AGE: ☐

WEIGHT ☐ Pounds

HEIGHT ☐ Feet/ins.

BODY TYPE: ☐

RACIAL GROUP
1: Caucasian ☐
2: Black ☐
3: Amer.Indian ☐
4: Asian ☐
5: Oriental ☐

KNOWN ABNORMALITY RELATED TO:
Unknown: ☐
Syndrome: ☐
Disease: ☐
Traumatic: ☐

FIG. 1-1 Difficult Airway Clinic record sheet.

PATIENT REFERRAL

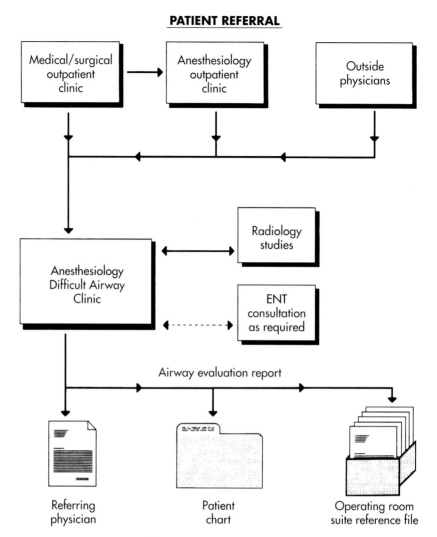

FIG. 1-2 Patient referral process.

ducted at various locations throughout the country. The parameters that are studied in the DAC are indicated in Fig. 1-1. Fig. 1-2 depicts the patient referral process. A decision tree for guiding clinical evaluation is depicted in Fig. 1-3. The box on p. 13 indicates the categories of patients. The examination procedure is detailed in the box on p. 14.

When using screening pulmonary function tests (PFTs), the emphasis is on reviewing airflow loops for signs of upper airway obstruction in the sitting and supine positions. Significant value is placed on the practice of using a video cassette recorder (VCR) connected to the C-arm for the VCR reproduction of dynamic fluoroscopy studies with a camera attached to the fiberscope for the VCR reproduction of the fiberoptic examination. Also, several clinicians can watch the actual fiberoptic examination on the adjacent television color monitor. These techniques serve as teaching methods and make it possible for consulting colleagues to review unusual findings or confirm endoscopic impressions. For the latter it is possible to reproduce the VCR tape on VHS format with a voice dub giving a detailed description of the examination and findings, which can then be forwarded to the referring physician.

APPLICATION FOR DAILY PRACTICE

More than 625 patients had been seen in the DAC between 1988 and January 1993. Even though this is a specialized clinic for patients with a wide variety of airway problems, the majority of these prob-

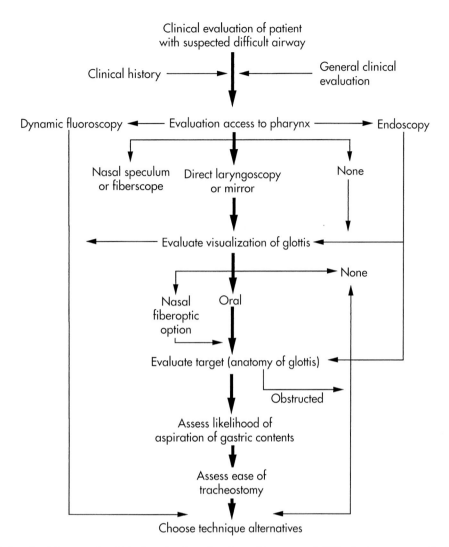

FIG. 1-3   Decision tree for clinical evaluation of patient with suspected difficult airway. NOTE: Evaluation should be done with patient both in sitting and in supine positions.

lems are encountered by most anesthesia providers at some time. Reviewing the diagnosis of these patients and eliminating return visits for normal follow-up or intubation or both before surgery leaves 402 patients with varying major diagnoses of airway abnormalities. Many of these patients have several concurrent problems, for example, obesity with obstructive sleep apnea or arthritis with temporomandibular joint involvement.

Counting the number of major disease diagnoses that comprise 10 or more patients (Table 1-3), it was noted that 333 (83%) of the 402 patients had a difficult airway diagnosis that most physicians see at least once during their careers.

Techniques that are employed in the DAC can be readily applied to everyday clinical practice for the identification and anesthetic management of patients with potential or real difficult airways. The endoscopist performs the primary examination, and an assistant operates the VCR, makes entry notes, and assists with the endoscopy. During the examination, the DAC record sheet is completed.

Initially, the patient and family are introduced to the staff and are given a detailed explanation of the reason for referral to the clinic. Both patient and family are questioned as to their knowledge of airway history, including the patient's past airway problems.

Next the patient is given an explanation of the clinic referral and the need for airway examination. Emphasis is placed on the need to ascertain the ability to intubate the patient's trachea by ei-

Table 1-3   Major Diagnoses of Difficult Airway Patients (as of February 15, 1993)

Diagnosis	Number
Cancers, lesions, masses, tumors of the airway	132
Intubations, difficult or failed	37
Rheumatoid arthritis	29
Thyroid nodule or goiter	28
Obstructive sleep apnea	24
Juvenile rheumatoid arthritis	23
Obesity	20
Temporomandibular joint abnormalities	15
Ankylosing spondylitis	13
Mucopolysaccharidosis	12
Klippel-Feil syndrome	8
Motor vehicle accident	8
Retrognathia	7
Goldenhar's syndrome	5
Gunshot wounds with facial trauma	5
True vocal cord paralysis	5
Hallermann-Streiff-François syndrome	4
Macroglossia	4
Maxillofacial dysostosis	4
Micrognathia	4
Pierre Robin syndrome	4
Trismus	4
Glossoptosis	3
Treacher Collins syndrome	3
Arthrogryposis	1
TOTAL	402

ther the oral or nasal route for upcoming surgery. **It must be pointed out that the use of regional anesthesia for the surgical procedure does *not* rule out the possible need for tracheal intubation to maintain an airway or the potential to convert to a general anesthesia.**

Each step of airway examination is explained in detail. The patient is assured that the examination will be concluded when it is believed that the airway can be maintained and that the trachea can be safely intubated. Thus the examination may end after dynamic fluoroscopy, after a direct examination of the oral pharynx with a laryngoscopy, or after successful tracheal intubation with the fiberscope. Once the patient and family understand the procedure and possible complications and all of their questions have been answered to their satisfaction, an informed consent is obtained. If a 35-mm camera will be used; the patient is assured that the photographs will be used only for patient records and for educational purposes. A separate consent form for photographing all procedures is obtained.

The first step of the examination involves obtaining basic data for the clinic record: age, weight, sex, disease process, etc. This is followed by a standard airway examination and evaluation that is used on all patients with the patient *in the sitting position.*

The patient is questioned about nasal breathing patterns. Is there a history of nasal trauma or surgery? A cotton applicator, soaked with local anesthesia, is used to palpate the nasal passages for patency, obstruction, direction, and depth to the posterior nasopharyngeal wall (8 to 10 cm for the normal adult).

Next, the oral examination is performed. The maximum oral opening at the central incisors is measured. This opening should be at least 2.5 cm. The Mallampati classification, both unassisted and assisted with a rigid laryngoscope, is noted and recorded. Visualization of the epiglottis and

CATEGORIES OF PATIENTS WITH DIFFICULT AIRWAY PROBLEMS*

1. Primarily soft tissue
   a. Glossoptosis or macroglossia: acromegaly, achondroplasia, obesity, amyloidosis, Beckwith-Wiedemann syndrome, lymphangioma, hemangioma, Hurler's syndrome (gargoylism; also Hunter's syndrome, including all mucopolysaccharidoses), some cases of Pierre Robin and Treacher Collins' syndrome
   b. Superior larynx: normal pediatric patients, achondroplasia, micrognathia
   c. Pharyngeal anatomic distortions: postradical neck dissection, glossectomy, laryngectomy, flaps, most inflammatory pharyngeal diseases including tumor formations (e.g., Sturge-Weber syndrome)
   d. Inflammatory diseases: quinsy, retropharyngeal abscess, epiglottitis, leprosy, diphtheria, Epstein-Barr virus, croup, pharyngouveitis
   e. Miscellaneous: sleep apnea, burns, trauma
2. Primarily hard tissue
   a. Chondrocalcinosis (larynx), acromegaly
   b. Cervical vertebral limitation: Engelmann's disease (osteopathia hyperostotica scleroticus multiplex), osteoarthritis, fibrofascial myositis ossificans progressiva, Marie-Strümpbell disease, Klippel-Feil syndrome, postcervical spinal fusion, Hurler's and Hunter's syndromes, ankylosing spondylitis of either osteoarthritic or other etiology
   c. Micrognathia: Pierre Robin syndrome, Crouzon's disease, Treacher Collins' syndrome, Hallermann-Streiff syndrome, hypoplastic bony development secondary to rheumatoid arthritis
   d. Temporomandibular joint limitation: osteoarthritis, Treacher Collins' syndrome, some rheumatoid syndromes
   e. Odontoid-peg disease: atlantoaxial instability, osteoporosis, Paget's disease, Morquio's syndrome
   f. Radiation treatment

*This listing is only partial and representative of the most frequent conditions. Almost all conditions mentioned are mixed in nature. Therefore regardless of category, the patient should be examined and managed with the understanding that it is rare to find one purely causative factor for a given difficult airway problem.

other laryngeal structures with a straight-blade rigid laryngoscope is attempted. Note that visualization of the epiglottis does not indicate that the patient can be successfully intubated in the normal fashion. Neither does a Mallampati score of one. The oropharynx is noted with particular attention to the intermolar spread, a high-arched palate, and any other abnormality. Dentition is noted as well as appearance of the tongue, lips, mucous membrane, masses, swelling, and inflammation.

The degree of flexion and extension of the neck is noted. The locations of the larynx in relation to the mentum and the hyoid cartilage in relation to the mentum and thyroid cartilage are noted and measured. The location of the cricothyroid membrane should be identified in case of the need of an emergent cricothyrotomy.

Indications for further examination of the facies include patients with macrognathia, micrognathia, rheumatoid arthritis, trauma, postradical head or neck surgery, and congenital anomalies (see the box on p. 14). Measurements include, but are not limited to, the temporomandibular notch to angle of ramus, angle of ramus to mentum, mentum to hyoid, and mentum to thyroid notch.

Based on the findings of this first part of the examination, it may be concluded that the patient will not present a difficult airway at the time of anesthesia. If so, the examination is now completed. If it is determined that further examination of the patient's airway is needed, dynamic C-arm fluoroscopy is initiated. This technique is discussed in detail in Chapter 8.

At the conclusion of the dynamic fluoroscopy examination, if the decision is to continue

---

EXAMINATION PROCEDURE AT THE DIFFICULT AIRWAY CLINIC

1. Review the referral chart.
2. Stamp consultation and other forms with the patient identification card.
3. Discuss with the patients the reasons for their being referred to the clinic. What does the patient know about his or her airway problem? What procedures will be done during the patient's visit? What do we expect to accomplish?
   a. Obtain procedure consent.
   b. Obtain photographic consent.
4. Perform a visual and tactile examination of the oral and nasal structures.
5. Perform a dynamic fluoroscopy sequence.
6. If indicated by either the patient's anatomy or history, take measurements, to include the following:
   a. Temporomandibular joint to angle of ramus
   b. Angle of ramus to mentum
   c. Interdental opening at central incisors
   d. Mentum to hyoid
   e. Mentum to thyroid notch
7. Examine the nose: patency of nasopharyngeal pathway, right and left, and depth from nares to nasopharynx.
8. Check oral patency:
   a. Mirror laryngoscopy: results and possible limits
   b. Direct laryngoscopy: results and possible limits
9. Perform fiberoptic examination: nasopharyngolaryngoscopy and possible limits.
10. If indicated, give the patient an airway alert tag. Tell the patient to take nothing by mouth.
11. Complete the consultation sheets. Make recommendations.
12. Put the originals of consultation on the patient's chart. Copies of all forms are filed alphabetically in anesthesia holding room open file.

---

with the airway evaluation procedures, fiberoptic intubation through the oral or nasal route is accomplished.

When the examination phase concludes, the patient is asked if he or she would like to review the VCR tape of the examination, with the findings and ramifications explained to the patient.

The patient is informed that a written consultation form will be forwarded to his or her referring physician and that a copy of the consultation form will be kept in the DAC files. A copy is available in an open file 24 hours a day. This copy can be used by the anesthesia team that will be anesthetizing the patient for surgery. It is also available in case the patient has need of surgery under emergent or nonemergent surgery at another institution. In cases identified as a severe intubation problem, an Airway Alert bracelet or necklace is given to the patient. This identification includes the telephone number at the Operating Room control desk so that the consultation is available over the telephone.

If topical anesthesia has been used, the patient is instructed to take nothing by mouth (NPO) for 2 hours. Questions are answered and the patient is permitted to go either to the next clinic visit or home.

The consultation form is completed with a summary of the findings and recommendations of techniques that could be used for intubation on the day of surgery. If the patient is to have surgery within a day or two of the DAC examination, an immediate report to the referring physician is given over the telephone, with the option of reviewing a voiced-over VCR tape.

Several individuals are involved in a smooth-running clinic. They include the following:
1. A secretary averages 4 hours of work for each patient clinic visit. This person is responsible for scheduling the appointment time with a specific member of the DAC. He or she orders patients' medical records for review by the individual who will examine the patient. Unless there are central dictating services, he or she types up the evaluation on the consultation form and forwards it to the referring physician.
2. An anesthesia technician is assigned each day to help with the setup and cleaning of equipment, especially the cleaning and sterilization of the fiberoptic bronchoscope.
3. The examiner or endoscopist performs the examination and dictates the findings. The examination averages 2 hours per patient seen.
4. Another member of the clinic acts as an assistant. This individual helps chart findings of the examination and assists the fiberoptic endoscopy. Additionally, this person operates the camera and VCR, thus freeing the primary examiner to focus on the fiberoptic examination.

REFERENCES

1. Fink BR: *The human larynx,* New York, 1975, Raven Press.
2. Fink BR, Demarest RJ: *Laryngeal biomechanics,* Cambridge, Mass, 1978, Harvard University Press.
3. Sukerman S, Healy GB: Sleep apnea syndrome associated with upper airway obstruction, *Laryngoscope* 6:878-884, 1979.
4. Safar P, Escarraga LA, Chang F: Upper airway obstruction in the unconscious patient, *J Appl Physiol* 14:760-764, 1959.
5. Sauerland EK, Mitchel SP: Electromyographic activity of intrinsic and extrinsic muscles of the human tongue, *Tex Rep Biol Med* 33:445-455, 1975.
6. Sauerland EK, Mitchel SP: Electromyographic activity of human genioglossus muscle in response to respiration and to positional changes of the head, *Bull Los Angeles Neurol Soc* 35:69-73, 1970.
7. American Society of Anesthesiologists, Committee on Professional Liability: Preliminary study of closed claims, *ASA Newsletter* 52(4):8-10, 1988.
8. Caplan RA, Posner K, Ward WJ et al: Adverse respiratory events in anesthesia: a closed claims analysis, *Anesthesiology* 72:828-833, 1990.
9. Keats AS: Anesthesia mortality in perspective, *Anesth Analg* 71:113-119, 1990.
10. Eichhorn JH: Documenting improved anesthesia outcome, *J Clin Anesth* 3:351-353, 1991.
11. Orkin FK: Practice standards: the Midas touch or the emperor's new clothes? *Anesthesiology* 70:567-571, 1989.
12. Norton ML, Brown ACD: *Atlas of the difficult airway: a source book,* St Louis, 1991, Mosby.
13. Wilson ME, Spiegelhalter D, Robertson JA et al: Predicting difficult intubation, *Br J Anaesth* 61:211-216, 1988.
14. Mallampati SR, Gatt SP, Gugino LD et al: A clinical sign to predict difficult intubation: a prospective study, *Can Anaesth Soc J* 32:429-434, 1985.
15. Caplan RA, Posner K, Ward RJ et al: Adverse respiratory events in anesthesia: a closed claims analysis, *Anesthesiology* 72:828-833, 1990.
16. Mark LJ: *The consultant anesthesiologist: a new profile for the profession of the anesthesiologist,* Baltimore, 1991, The Foundation for Anesthesia Education and Research (unpublished grant).
17. Endler GC, Mariona FG, Sokol RJ et al: Maternal death as a result of anesthesia—the Michigan experience, *Am J Obstet Gynecol* 159:187-193, 1988.
18. Chadwick HS, Posner K, Ward RJ et al: A review of anesthesia malpractice claims (abstract), *Anesthesiology* 71(3A):A942, 1989.
19. Caplan RA, Ward RJ, Posner K et al: Unexpected cardiac arrest during spinal anesthesia: closed claims analysis of predisposing factors, *Anesthesiology* 68:5-11, 1988.
20. Holland R: Anesthesia related mortality in Australia. In Pierce EC, Cooper JB (eds): *International anesthesiology clinics,* Boston, 1984, Little, Brown.
21. Caplan RA, Todd DP: Respiratory mishaps: principal anesthetic of risk and implications for anesthesia, *Anesthesiology* 67:A469, 1987.
21a. Harrison G: Personal communication, Dec, 1988.
22. Macewen W: Clinical observations on the introduction of tracheal tubes by the mouth instead of performing tracheotomy or laryngotomy, *Br Med J* 2:163, 1880.
23. Kirstein A: Autoskopie des larynx und der trachea, *Berl Klin Wochenschr* 32:475, 1895.
24. Bichat X: *The surgical works, or statement of doctrine and practice of P. J. Desault,* Philadelphia, 1814, T. Dobson.
25. Magill JW, Rowbotham S: Technique in endotracheal anesthesia, *Br Med J* 1:817-819, 1930.
26. Herholdt JD, Rafn CG: *An Attempt at an historical survey of life-saving measures for drowning persons and information of the best means by which they can again be brought back to life,*

Copenhagen, 1796, H. Tikiobs. Reprinted by the Scandinavian Society of Anesthesiology, Aarhus, Denmark, Stiftsbogtrykkerie, 1960.

27. Sia RL, Edens ET: How to avoid problems when using the fiberoptic bronchscope for difficult intubations, *Anesthesia* 36:74, 1981.

28. Aro L, Takki S, Aromaa U: Technique for difficult intubation, *Br J Anesth* 43:1081, 1974.

29. Stauffer JL, Olson DE, Petty TL: Complications and consequences of endotracheal intubation and tracheostomy: a prospective study of 150 critically ill adult patients, *Am J Med* 70:65-76, 1981.

30. Norton ML, Wilton N, Brown AC: The difficult airway clinic, *Anesth Rev* 15:25-28, 1988.

31. Norton ML, Brown ACD: Evaluating the patient with a difficult airway for anesthesia, *Otorhinolaryngol Clin North Am* 23(4):771-785, 1990.

CHAPTER 2

Medic Alert, Communication, Confidentiality, and Other Medicolegal Considerations

LYNETTE J. MARK AND BERNARD R. MARSH

"Words are very rascals since bonds disgraced them" *

WILLIAM SHAKESPEARE

Twelfth Night, Act III, Scene 1

The importance of documentation to the medical profession has long been recognized. There has been, however, a significant amount of discussion concerning the methods by which documented information may be effectively disseminated. This chapter addresses various mechanisms for the dissemination of critical anesthetic information and aspects of the provider-patient relationship as related to communication and inherent medicolegal issues.

The medical record is the cornerstone in which patient information is entered and archived and from which it is retrieved. It sets forth the particulars of a patient's symptoms, diagnosis, therapy, clinical course, and outcomes during hospitalization. Information about the patient is entered by all professional caregivers. The medical record is a confidential document that conforms to institutional, governmental, and legal requirements.[1]

Historically, when medical practice was defined by the patient-primary practitioner relationship, the medical record, as conceived, was a satisfactory tool for documentation. However, the evolution of modern medicine has fostered an environment of specialization and intricate treatment strategies. Thus there is a need for a comprehensive reexploration of the content and intent of the medical record.

The process and purpose of dissemination of information must be critically reevaluated. Even when the information in the medical record is comprehensive, release of that information may be limited or delayed. Practices for disposing of the record can include purging hard copy from the main file after 2 years of inactivity, with conversion to microfilm after 10 years. The medical records may be stored off-site.[1] In the event that critical information is required immediately, in geographically separate locations, or by health care providers who may be unfamiliar with a patient's complex therapy, retrieval of the record may be untimely or impossible.

Patients acting on their own behalf as educated consumers now insist on access to information from caregivers. Patients may request (in writing) access to their records or may approach the physician directly for information. This request may be denied in cases of psychiatric illness or if the attending physician deems it medically contraindicated.[1] However, in the majority of cases, patients should be educated as to their medical conditions and should be encouraged to become active participants in decisions concerning their own care.

From a legal point of view the need for appropriate documentation and effective communication of information has become critical, particularly when lack of knowledge regarding specific disease processes may expose the patient to an increased risk of morbidity or mortality. However, com-

---

*Bonds refer to contracts and more broadly to lawyers' work.

We wish to acknowledge James F. Schauble, M.D., and the Medic Alert Foundation Anesthesia Advisory Council for their inspiration and dedication to this project.

plex issues of patient and disease process confidentiality, quality assurance, and, at times, conflicting agendas for dissemination of information cloud information exchange.

Effective documentation and dissemination of critical information must address the following fundamental questions:

1. Once a patient event occurs, is there a consistent format for recording relevant information?
2. Is the information recorded understood by all health care providers?
3. Is there a consistent way in which patients and health care personnel can be informed of critical information?
4. Is the documentation readily accessible regardless of geographic location or time of day?
5. Have issues of confidentiality and liability been addressed?
6. What component reports are necessary to establish quality assurance or quality improvement and effective health care?

When these issues are addressed and dissemination of information is effective, a resulting improvement in patient care, outcomes, and quality of life will occur.

MEDICAL COMMUNICATION AND THE LAW

The confidence of the patient that his or her privacy will be maintained is at the basis of traditional medical practice. When discussing any aspect of medical information, considerations of privacy, confidentiality, and implied consent, at the least, must be addressed. These concepts are defined as follows:

1. *Privacy* is the right to be left alone. It is a generic term, quite broad, and exists only so far as its assertion is consistent with the law or public policy. Public disclosure of private facts is a cause of action in publicity of a highly objectionable type. The term used is *invasion of privacy.*
2. *Confidentiality* relates to confidential communication in the medical sense. This includes the entire scope of written medical records as well as verbal communications. It refers to information created under circumstances indicating that the speaker or writer intended the information to be known and used by the health care professional in the care of the patient. In essence it must be released only on a *need-to-know basis* and only for the benefit of the patient.*
3. By the very act of listing the physician's name, address, and telephone number, an explicit (or at the least, implied) consent is given for release of this information. Thus the patient tells the physician to release all information as a *need-to-know* situation arises. By extension, therefore, the patient consents to having this information released by an organization such as the Medic Alert Foundation on a *need-to-know* basis for his or her benefit.

COMMUNICATION AND AIRWAY MANAGEMENT

Specifically related to airway management, precise documentation and information exchange are critical. Complex airway management necessitates a team approach that involves the integration of multispecialty treatments and the cross-referencing of information from numerous locations in the medical record. Effective dissemination of information related to complex airway management is a significant missing link in decreasing patient adverse outcomes and increasing patient safety.[2,3] The consequences of unsuccessful airway management continue to be a potentially disastrous problem from both a medical and legal point of view (see Chapter 1).[4-12]

Documenting the presence and nature of airway difficulty in conjunction with successful and unsuccessful airway techniques and disseminating that information to the medical record, to the patient, and to future health care providers not only decreases the incidence of difficult airway situations, but also undoubtedly facilitates the delivery of quality anesthetic care.

---

*This is different from the legal concept of privileged communications not admissible into evidence in a court of law. Note that, in this sense, the physician may occasionally evoke the principle when testifying.

In spite of the best efforts to document and communicate information, emergency conditions can arise in which the single most important mechanism for dissemination of information is a visible emblem that, in essence, speaks for itself. This emblem should provide a minimum level of essential information that may mean the difference between successful and unsuccessful airway management or even life and death.

Thus to adequately meet the multifaceted demands of difficult airway management, innovative strategies of documentation that use multiple mechanisms for dissemination of information are needed. In response to this need and in the name of patient safety, the following steps have been taken:

1. The American Society of Anesthesiologists Task Force on Management of the Difficult Airway addressed patient safety issues during airway management and developed practice guidelines to assist practitioners and patients in making decisions about health care. Specifically, these guidelines cite the following recommendations:
   - Examining previous anesthetic records, if available
   - Documenting in the medical record the presence and nature of the airway difficulty to facilitate future care
   - Informing the patient of the difficulty encountered
   - Evaluating and following the patient for potential adverse events related to the airway difficulty[13]

2. Quality assurance or quality improvement data acquisition tools are being widely implemented in clinical practice. Ongoing analysis using these tools enables practitioners to assess pertinent airway-related problems. These tools function as the means to demonstrate competence, assess performance, improve patient outcome, further patient education, and define quality patient care.[14]

3. *The Anesthesiology Consultant Report (ACR)* (Fig. 2-1), a brief summary document, provides an interpretation of anesthetic information and events. The traditional time-based intraoperative data record may be selectively accompanied by an ACR describing preoperative evaluation and preparation, intraoperative techniques and management, and recommendations for future anesthetics. Critical information is uniformly reported and communicated in nonsymbolized terminology to primary care providers, specialists, and other health care professionals, as well as future anesthesiologists.[15]

4. Airway photodocumentation technology has been pioneered by otolaryngology head and neck surgeons and anesthesiologists (see also Chapter 8). Videotapes and hardcopy images of airway pathophysiology support the adage, "A picture is worth 1000 words." These photodocuments enable physicians to review the patient's pathology and make appropriate recommendations. They become an integral part of the permanent medical record and can easily be disseminated to physicians, patients, families, and lawyers.

Certain comprehensive systems for documentation and dissemination of critical information have already been implemented (see box on p. 22).

It becomes increasingly apparent that merging selected components of Medic Alert and the Difficult Airway Clinic (DAC) could create a more efficient and effective system that maximizes resources while improving quality of care. In September 1992 The Difficult Airway/Intubation Alert (which later became The National Difficult Airway/Intubation Registry) was established by a task force representing anesthesiologists, otolaryngology head and neck surgeons, and the Medic Alert Foundation. The major objectives of the task force were to develop a uniform recording system for the difficult airway and to maintain a central registry of patients who have difficult airways. This project complemented work done by the American Society of Anesthesiologists (ASA) Task Force on Management of the Difficult Airway and the work of Dr. Martin L. Norton of the University of Michigan Difficult Airway Clinic.

The National Difficult Airway/Intubation Registry is a natural expansion of the Medic Alert concept, maintaining the same quality assurance and medicolegal standards and disseminating critical information about airway management to health care providers. In 1993 The National Registry was officially endorsed by the World Federation Societies of Anaesthesiologists and by the Ameri-

Johns Hopkins
Anesthesiology and
Critical Care Medicine
600 North Wolfe Street, Baltimore, MD 21287-8711
(410) 955-6482

ANESTHESIOLOGY CONSULTANT REPORT

Patient Name: Smith, John
Medical Record #: 000-00-000
Anesthesiology Attending: Lynette J. Mark, M.D.
Surgery Attending: William R. Jones, M.D.
Operative Procedure: Whipple procedure
Date: 02/25/9-

ANESTHETIC CONSIDERATIONS

1. ASA Class III.*
2. Pancreatic cancer.
3. Pulmonary: Chronic obstructive pulmonary disease, bronchogenic carcinoma.
   Status post right upper lobe lobectomy (12/90) with postoperative radiation therapy.
4. Frequent premature ventricular contractions (PVCs).
5. History of general anesthesia without difficulty (patient report).

ANESTHETIC PROCEDURES

1. Standard monitoring* and intravenous access.
2. General endotracheal anesthesia.
3. Invasive: Radial arterial line, right external jugular central venous pressure (CVP) line.
4. DIFFICULT AIRWAY\INTUBATION.
5. Consultation: Evaluation of dental trauma.

Dear Doctor:

Mr. Smith, on 02/25/9-, underwent a Whipple procedure for a preoperative diagnosis of pancreatic cancer. Anesthetic considerations and procedures are identified above.

Significant preoperative evaluation included a pulmonary consultation (FEV_1 1.25, FVC 2.56, room air arterial blood gas 7.45/39/85--no change with bronchodilators) with recommendations for postoperative bronchodilators; cardiac consultation for frequent PVCs with recommendation of benign nature; review of General Hospital surgery operative note and discharge summary which noted endotracheal anesthesia without problems.

Mr. Smith underwent a general endotracheal anesthetic. He was identified as having a DIFFICULT AIRWAY/INTUBATION. Specific technical information appears at the end of this report. The remainder of

Note: The Anesthesiology Consultant Report provides summary information. A more detailed anesthetic history is available in the medical record.

FIG. 2-1   Anesthesia Consultant Report with its 10 components.

his anesthetic course was uneventful with oxygenation of 99-100%, end-tidal CO_2 30-40 mmHg, blood pressure range 110-150/70-80, heart rate in the 80s with a normal sinus rhythm, and CVP 7-15. He had an estimated blood loss of 1,000 ml, urine output of 700 ml, and received a volume replacement of 7,000 ml of crystalloid solution. The operating room time was 7 hours. He was transported, intubated and asleep, in stable condition to the SICU.

Mr. Smith was extubated awake within 4 hours in the SICU and transferred after 24 hours to the ward without complication.

The anesthetic record from General Hospital was obtained and relayed a history of difficult airway/intubation. Mr. Smith was informed of the intraoperative events here and his prior history of difficult intubation. He identified possible dental trauma. Consultation with Patient Relations was obtained regarding follow-up dental care.

I appreciated the opportunity to care for Mr. Smith. If you have any questions regarding the anesthetic management or about any anesthesia-related issues in general, please feel free to contact me.

COMMENTS AND RECOMMENDATIONS FOR FUTURE ANESTHETICS

1. Awake fiberoptic intubation techniques.
2. Enrollment into Medic Alert Foundation International: DIFFICULT AIRWAY/INTUBATION ALERT.

Sincerely,

Lynette J. Mark, M.D.

cc: William R. Jones, M.D., Johns Hopkins University
  Medic Alert Foundation International; ATTENTION: Joyce Drake
   840 N. Lakeshore Drive, 6 East, Chicago, IL 60611
  Jane S. Carson, M.D., General Hospital, Baltimore, Maryland

---

Anesthesia technical information
Clinical airway algorithm: Mask airway okay. Glottic opening not visualized with MacIntosh (MAC) #4, Miller #2. Asleep nasal fiberoptic: Glottic opening anterior with deviation to left; vocal cords visualized; unable to advance ET tube; #7.5 ET tube placed orally with Miller #2 with extreme positioning, cricoid pressure.

---

* Explanation of ASA (American Society of Anesthesiologists) CLASSIFICATION OF HEALTH STATUS:
I   Healthy patient
II   Mild systemic disease; no functional limitation
III   Severe systemic disease; definite functional limitation
IV   Severe systemic disease that is a constant threat to life
V   Moribund patient; unlikely to survive 24 hours without operation
E   Modifier indicating emergency surgery

STANDARD INTRAOPERATIVE MONITORING
Automated blood pressure cuff, continuous wave-form capnography, intravenous catheter, temperature, oxygen saturation, oxygen analyzer

---

c. 1992 The Johns Hopkins University
Note: The Anesthesiology Consultant Report provides summary information. A more detailed anesthetic history is available in the medical record.

FIG. 2-1, cont'd.   For legend see opposite page.

DIFFICULT AIRWAY DOCUMENTATION AND INFORMATION SYSTEMS

1. The Medic Alert Foundation was created in 1956 by Dr. Marion C. Collins. It is a charitable, nonprofit organization that provides a comprehensive emergency medical identification service for over 4 million members worldwide. Three components of this service include a metal alerting emblem, a 24-hour-a-day emergency response center, and a wallet card. In 1979 the American Society of Anesthesiologists' House of Delegates officially endorsed Medic Alert. Medic Alert addresses issues of confidentiality and quality assurance as well as medicolegal concerns through the use of membership identification numbers instead of patient names, restricted access to medical information, and the use of a legal statement signed by patients who enroll.

2. The University of Michigan Difficult Airway Clinic was established at the University of Michigan in 1987 by Martin L. Norton. It is believed to be the first formally established clinic for comprehensive evaluation of patients with upper airway problems. Clinical documentation included an airway clinic record sheet, photodocumentation, and an information response center.[9]

---

can Academy of Otolaryngology-Head and Neck Surgery Foundation, Inc. By 1997 hopefully there will be international implementation of this Registry.

This chapter seeks to raise the level of awareness of communication issues in those who are charged with responsibility for airway management. Reflective of the multispecialty nature of airway management, multidisciplinary and multimedia strategies of documenting and sharing information about difficult airway management is discussed through the use of case studies.

CASE STUDIES OF AIRWAY MANAGEMENT EVENTS*

Nine case studies that represent common airway management events as well as controversial scenarios are presented on the following pages. These underscore the importance of precise documentation and information exchange. Common themes intrinsic to these cases include the following:

1. Documentation must be precise, succinct, and archived in a uniform location within the medical record. Written documentation should be phrased in language commonly understood by all health care providers, avoiding the use of specialty-specific jargon and abbreviations. Appropriate graphics or photodocumentation should be used.

2. Communication regarding patient events should be available to the patient, family, immediate health care personnel, and referring health care personnel and should enhance education, patient safety, and awareness of future anesthetic implications.

3. Increased awareness of issues of confidentiality and the adherence to medicolegal guidelines regarding documentation and communication of patient events facilitate continuous quality improvement within the profession, promote better medical practice, and increase patient safety.

4. Critical information must be immediately accessible, independent of geographic location or time, and must provide a minimum but sufficient amount of information, while maintaining patient confidentiality.

5. In the event of an airway emergency, information must be immediately accessible via a visible emblem worn by the patient at all times.

---

*Details of the case studies have been changed to ensure patient confidentiality.

CASE 2-1 *"WHY DIDN'T MY OTHER ANESTHESIOLOGIST TELL ME?"**

A 67-year-old man with a history of pancreatic adenocarcinoma was scheduled for a Whipple procedure. His medical history was significant for a right thoracotomy with right upper lobectomy for bronchogenic carcinoma 14 months before this admission with postoperative radiation therapy. The patient denied any history of difficulty with anesthesia. Examination of his airway revealed poor dentition with multiple crowns, good oral excursion, and full visualization of the uvula (Mallampati Class 1).

Review of the operative report and discharge summary did not reveal any information about difficult airway management. The anesthesia team was satisfied with this documentation, and no attempts were made to retrieve the anesthesia record.

Anesthesia was induced with thiopental and fentanyl. Mask ventilation was established, and intubation of the trachea was attempted after achieving muscle relaxation with pancuronium. Numerous attempts at direct laryngoscopy with rigid laryngoscopes failed to expose the glottic opening. Mask ventilation was reestablished. Nasal fiberoptic intubation of the trachea on the sleeping patient was unsuccessful. Ultimately the trachea was successfully intubated by direct laryngoscopy with a Miller #2 blade, extreme cricoid pressure, and lateral displacement of the trachea toward the midline. Endotracheal position was confirmed with bronchoscopy, continuous waveform capnography, and bilateral breath sounds. Oxygen saturation was greater than 95% throughout the procedure. The patient had uncomplicated surgery and had his trachea extubated without complications within 24 hours in the intensive care unit. No airway management complications were reported by the anesthesia team.

Communication Issues. The anesthesia team retrieved the prior intraoperative anesthesia record. The phrase *difficult intubation* was noted on the record. Personal communication with that anesthesiologist revealed that there had been active involvement by the thoracic surgeon to assist in securing the airway, first with a single-lumen endotracheal tube and then ultimately with a double-lumen endotracheal tube. It was communicated that the patient had been informed of the events of anesthesia during the postoperative visit.

On this postoperative visit, the patient was informed of the events that had transpired and that there had again been significant difficulty in intubating his trachea. He promptly informed the anesthesia team of dental trauma. He was given a copy of his Anesthesiology Consultant Report (ACR). When informed of difficulty during prior surgery, he adamantly denied any prior knowledge of difficulty and demanded documentation from the other hospital, which was reviewed with him. He asked, "Why didn't my other anesthesiologist tell me?"

Discussion. This case illustrates the following issues of documentation and dissemination of information:

1. Operative reports and discharge summaries traditionally record only the type of anesthesia administered (for example, general endotracheal versus regional) without qualification. On one hand the anesthesiologists faulted the operative report for misinforming them; however, it is not the responsibility of the surgeons to report anesthetic events in their documents, unless they are adverse.
2. The ACR (see Fig. 2-1) provided summary information about the perioperative events, communicating events about present and prior difficulties encountered in an understandable manner. It contained technical anesthesia information to assist in *future* management.
3. It was not until there was an adverse patient outcome that these documentation and communication issues came to the forefront. It is interesting to note that most complaints against physicians are unrelated to the physician's technical skill, but arise from poor communication or inadequate records.[16] In cases of potential litigation, more complete documentation and communication may be the practitioner's best defense and may actually play a deterring role by preventing claims from being initiated.

*Contributed by Dr. Christine Sang, Department of Anesthesiology and Critical Care Medicine, The Johns Hopkins Medical Institutions.

CASE 2-2   "WHAT DO YOU MEAN YOU WON'T LIST 'DIFFICULT INTUBATION' ON MY MEDICAL RECORD PROBLEM LIST?"

A 40-year-old nurse presented to the operating room for emergency incision and drainage of an abscess on her right forearm. She reported a history of being "impossible to intubate," arising 3 months earlier during an outpatient gynecologic procedure. Examination of her airway revealed a small mouth, good oral excursion and dentition, partial visualization of the uvula (Mallampati Class 2), and full range of motion of the neck.

The patient received monitored anesthesia, intravenous sedation, and local anesthesia infiltration of the surgical site. Surgery was uncomplicated and she required no airway management.

Communication Issues. During the postoperative visit, the patient related details of her prior airway difficulty and anesthetic management. At that time, she had been discharged from the gynecology outpatient surgical center with routine discharge planning instructions by an anesthesiologist other than her primary one. No mention of airway management difficulty was made to her at that time. The next day she experienced significant facial and throat pain and called the anesthesiologist. He explained that there had been difficulty with intubation of her trachea, but because mask ventilation had been reestablished and the procedure was short, he had not persisted in intubation attempts.

He had documented his actions in the anesthesia record but had not seen her at the time of her discharge to communicate the information to her. He informed her that she needed to tell health care personnel that she was "impossible to intubate." She inquired if any kind of bracelet or wallet card existed so that she could carry the information around in the event that she was unable to communicate it; she was told "No."

During the postoperative visit, she further stated that, when admitted to this institution, she informed the admitting office and admitting medical house staff of her condition of "difficult intubation" and requested that it be entered into her medical record as a medical problem. When the request was denied, she asked, "What do you mean you won't list 'difficult intubation' on my medical record problem list?" She expressed concerns that she might experience respiratory difficulty while on the ward, and she was told not to worry. Following the postoperative visit, her anesthesia record was subsequently retrieved from the prior outpatient center to verify documentation and she was enrolled in an in-house airway registry.

Discussion. The following points should be noted:

1. The in-house airway registry at The Johns Hopkins Medical Institutions was modeled after the Medic Alert concept and includes a visible alert armband, chart label (Fig. 2-2), and ACR.*

2. An optical scanning card was implemented as a quality assurance or quality improvement data acquisition tool. Use of this card facilitates both data entry and generation of reports from a computer database. In this case, because airway management was not required, formal documentation from the gynecology outpatient center was retrieved and verified.

3. Although the ASA has recognized *difficult airway* as a medical condition, until other health care providers are aware of this designation, it will be difficult to rely on its being consistently entered into the medical record.

---

*The Joint Committee on Clinical Investigations has issued a waiver to written informed consent to place wristbands on identified patients. Health care personnel *and* patients recognize the tremendous implications of patient safety (versus breach of confidentiality) as modeled in existing in-hospital "allergy alert" temporary wristbands and out-of-hospital permanent medical alert bracelets.[2]

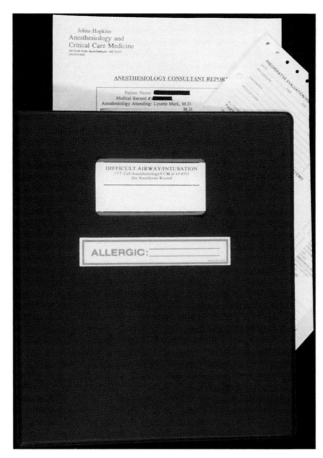

FIG. 2-2   In-house Airway Registry Medical Record Chart Label and Anesthesia Consultant Report used at The Johns Hopkins Medical Institutions.

CASE 2-3   *DIFFICULT AIRWAY/INTUBATION ALERT IN THE EMERGENCY DEPARTMENT*

A 64-year-old man with a history of ascending aortic aneurysm was admitted to the hospital for aortic valve replacement and composite graft of the aorta. His significant medical history included a subtotal thyroidectomy 12 years earlier. The patient related dental trauma with the surgery but denied any specific knowledge of difficult intubation of his trachea. Examination of his airway revealed full range of neck motion (with scar from thyroid surgery), good oral excursion and mandibular profile, and good dentition. Faucial pillars and a soft palate were seen, and the uvula was partially visualized (Mallampati Class 2). Attempts to obtain the prior anesthesia record were unsuccessful; the records were on microfilm and would take 2 weeks to retrieve. Oral rigid laryngoscopy while the patient is asleep with intubation of the trachea was planned.

Anesthesia was induced with fentanyl and midazolam. Muscle relaxation was achieved with pancuronium. Mask ventilation was established. Attempts at oral laryngoscopy with numerous Macintosh and Miller blades failed to expose the glottic opening. Nasal fiberoptic intubation of the trachea while the patient was asleep was successful with visualization of the complete glottic opening. Airway management complications included minimal soft tissue damage to his oropharynx and dental trauma. The patient had uncomplicated surgery and had his trachea extubated within 24 hours in the intensive care unit without complications.

Communication Issues. The patient was enrolled into an in-house airway registry and received consultation for his dental trauma. He was given a copy of his ACR. He consented for enrollment into

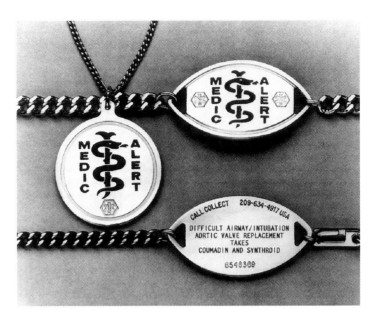

FIG. 2-3   Medic Alert Foundation bracelets and necklace emblem.

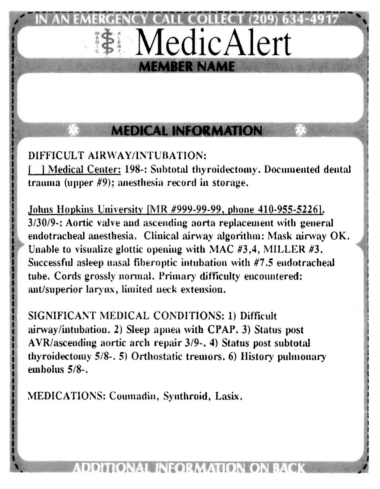

FIG. 2-4   Medic Alert Foundation wallet card. Specific documentation includes category: difficult airway/intubation, institution registry, clinical airway algorithm, and surgical procedure and date.

The National Difficult Airway/Intubation Registry, Medic Alert Foundation, and enrollment was initiated at the time of discharge.

Weeks later the patient presented to a distant emergency department with increasing respiratory distress and hemodynamic compromise. The emergency department physicians were informed about the difficulty with prior airway management. The patient was transported to the radiology suite for further evaluation. There he suffered a respiratory arrest at which time "stat anesthesia" was called for and mask ventilation attempted. Upon arrival the anesthesiologist was notified of the patient's airway history. Mask ventilation was difficult and there was gross hemoptysis. Direct laryngoscopies with Macintosh and Miller blades were unsuccessful. During attempted percutaneous cricothyrotomy, the patient died.

Discussion. The following points should be noted:

1. The enrollment of the patient into Medic Alert and the patient's understanding of his difficult airway enabled successful information exchange in an urgent setting (Figs. 2-3 and 2-4).

2. Although the critical information concerning this difficult airway was successfully communicated, there still existed a lack of appreciation as to its significance. Increased awareness by other medical specialties intimately involved in airway management must occur if required practice changes are to be made. In essence, this patient presented to the emergency department with an anticipated difficult airway and respiratory distress. Stated as such, with the clear understanding as to the degree of difficulty previously encountered, more serious consideration should have been given to securing his airway before transport. The anesthesiologist who was "stat paged" was thrust into a horrendous situation which could have been avoided.

CASE 2-4 *"I WANT TO SUE THE HOSPITAL AND MY ANESTHESIOLOGIST! THEY DIDN'T BELIEVE MY MEDIC ALERT BRACELET."*

Medic Alert operators received a phone call from an irate woman who related, "I have a Medic Alert bracelet that says 'Difficult Oral Intubation; Recommend Fiberoptics' and my anesthesiologist did not believe it! I went in for surgery; 3 hours later, I awakened as blood was being pumped from my stomach. I want to sue the hospital and my anesthesiologist. They didn't believe my Medic Alert bracelet."

Further investigation of the patient's complaint and direct communication with several of her former anesthesiologists revealed the following: The patient had undergone thyroid surgery with a history of uncomplicated general anesthesia (documentation unavailable regarding actual intubation of her trachea). The anesthesiologist had difficulty with intubation of her trachea and recommended enrollment into Medic Alert. The patient had undergone numerous surgeries in the same institution with successful airway management by fiberoptic bronchoscopy. On the last admission the anesthesiologist attempted, unsuccessfully, to manage her airway with rigid oral laryngoscopy. Numerous attempts with rigid laryngoscopes were unsuccessful, and fiberoptic bronchoscopy was limited by the presence of blood and secretions. The patient was awakened. She suffered nasal and oral soft tissue trauma, and the procedure was canceled.

Communication Issues. The last anesthesiologist relayed that, on the basis of the physical examination, the patient did not appear to have a difficult airway. Despite her Medic Alert bracelet, he was unable to solicit a history of her having undergone fiberoptic techniques. He was only able to access anesthesia records from before her enrollment into Medic Alert. He related that he informed her of his plan to induce anesthesia, establish mask ventilation, and attempt direct rigid laryngoscopy (with fiberoptic techniques available, if needed), and that she consented.

Following the cancellation, the patient related that the anesthesiologist appeared distressed and did not talk to her about the problems he encountered. A different anesthesiologist relayed the events to her. The procedure was rescheduled, and the patient's airway was successfully managed with fiberoptic techniques while the patient was awake.

Discussion. The following points are noted:

1. Members enrolling in Medic Alert are required to sign a statement printed in each Medic Alert brochure. Before the initiation of the Difficult Airway/Intubation Project, this statement simply verified patient information and assured confidentiality. As of January 1994, it has been noted that Medic Alert has never been sued by anyone for errors in medical information, errors in information transmission, or failure to protect patient confidentiality.[17] With initiation of The National Difficult Airway/Intubation Registry, Medic Alert expanded the statement to protect enrolling physicians and hospitals who were voluntarily releasing critical information about patients. Additionally, members agree to allow information collected to be used anonymously for education and scientific research.

2. In this case, specific recommendations regarding airway management appeared on the patient's emblem. The alert emblem is generically worded "Difficult Airway/Intubation." On the patient's wallet card, an initial noncommiting phrase, "Availability of Awake/Direct Visualization Techniques" was later replaced with details of primary difficulties encountered as identified by enrolling health care personnel.

3. Selective information from the enrollment data form is made available to physicians treating the patient.

CASE 2-5   *"WE ARE JUST GOING TO TAKE A LOOK, THEN REEVALUATE."*

An 83-year-old woman with a history of a substernal goiter underwent a diagnostic flexible bronchoscopy for further evaluation. Her medical history was significant for increasing respiratory difficulty. She was still fairly mobile and living independently. Radiographic studies showed marked tracheal deviation with compression from just below the glottis to just above the tracheal bifurcation, presumably from the retrosternal goiter. The consulting otolaryngologist scheduled the patient for a fiberoptic bronchoscopy to obtain detailed information on the dimensions of the airway and the distances that were still available for potential use. Pulmonary function tests and flow volume loops were obtained.

The patient underwent a fiberoptic bronchoscopy with local anesthesia and monitored anesthesia care. A videoscope for adults was placed orally after bilateral nasal obstruction was encountered. The instrument was passed through the vocal cords and, beginning approximately 1 to 2 cm below the cords, stenosis of the airway was noted, which prevented further passage of the instrument. The videoscope was replaced with a fiberoptic scope for pediatric patients. This was passed without difficulty through the stenotic trachea, revealing that the lower end of the stenosis ended approximately 2 cm above the carina. The carina and both main bronchi appeared to be perfectly normal. The mucosa throughout the stenosis was somewhat more vascular than usual but not particularly friable. The tracheal rings, although displaced, were well demonstrated. The instrument was removed, and the patient was taken to the recovery room in satisfactory condition.

Communication Issues. Photodocumentation from the videoscope was obtained, and hard copy was disseminated to the medical record, referring physician, and patient. Based on the diagnostic examination, recommendations were made for an additional surgical consultation, and a definitive procedure was planned. Specific technical information for definitive airway management was communicated to the anesthesiologist (Fig. 2-5). The patient underwent a total thyroidectomy without complications. The intraoperative airway management team included the otolaryngologist, an anesthesiologist, and a thoracic surgeon.

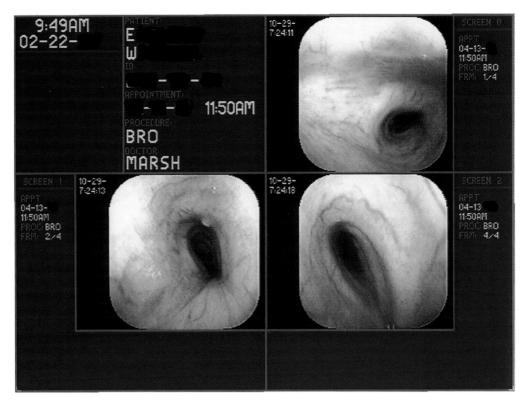

FIG. 2-5   Generation of videobronchoscopic images, showing severe tracheal compression from substernal goiter as seen by videobronchoscope.

Discussion. The following points should be noted:
1. The videobronchoscope was used to communicate information about distances, dimensions, significance, and dynamics. It facilitated a working diagnosis that fit with the radiographic image.
2. Use of the bronchoscope allows the anesthesiologist to share the information with the otolaryngologist about what is going on.
3. Photodocumentation facilitated an informed, educated patient decision regarding surgery.

CASE 2-6 *"SUBGLOTTIC STENOSIS 10 CM BELOW VOCAL CORDS."*

A 64-year-old woman with a recent infarct and postinfarction angina was transferred from an area hospital coronary care unit (CCU) and scheduled for coronary bypass surgery. Her medical history was significant for a CCU course complicated by congestive heart failure and flash pulmonary edema, requiring intubation of her trachea for 1 week, 2 months before this CCU admission. On the day of transfer she was observed to have stridor with increasing respiratory distress. She was treated for congestive heart failure, and consultation with an otolaryngologist was obtained. A bedside fiberoptic laryngoscopic examination was performed with the following recommendations: "Patient has subglottic stenosis 10 cm below her vocal cords. Recommend #5 endotracheal tube for general anesthesia."

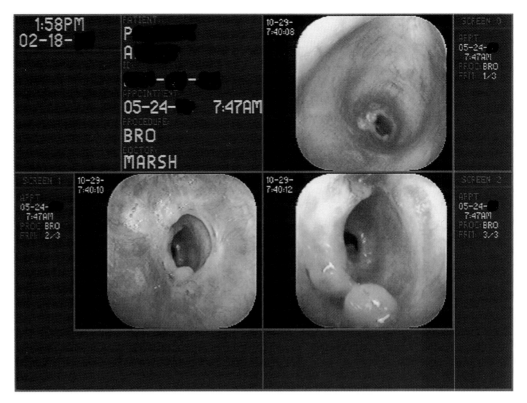

FIG. 2-6   Photodocumentation of severe subglottic tracheal stenosis using videobronchoscope.

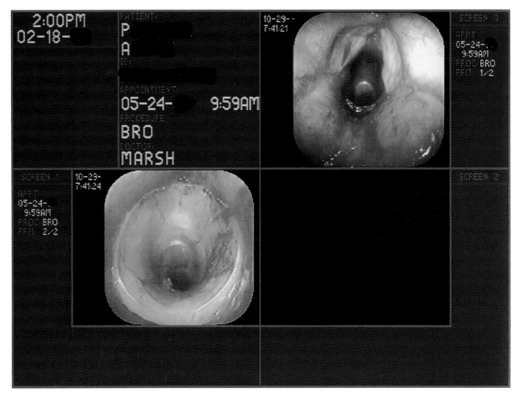

FIG. 2-7   Photodocumentation after placement of tracheal stent.

Communication Issues. The consultant anesthesiologist was concerned with the recommendations for airway management and asked for a second consultation with an otolaryngologist. The patient underwent a diagnostic fiberoptic bronchoscopy, which revealed a 4-mm diameter concentric stenosis of the trachea, which was located at a distance of 4 cm below the vocal cords. For a distance of approximately 1.5 cm distal to this, the posterior tracheal wall also had some granular tissue and was slightly constricted. A 4-mm fiberoptic bronchoscope was passed with difficulty through this stenotic segment. Based on that procedure the patient underwent tracheal stent placement. The coronary bypass surgery was rescheduled.

Discussion. The following points should be noted:

1. Photodocumentation as communicated to the referring physician and cardiac surgeon facilitated successful airway management for this patient's critical airway (Fig. 2-6).

2. For the endoscopist, photodocumentation is invaluable in clarifying issues as to what equipment could be used to most appropriately evaluate and document complex cases. With respect to equipment, an understanding of the various limitations, tradeoffs, and differences is crucial if results are to be optimized (for example, in this case, recommendations based on Machida scope findings resulted in confusing documentation). The commonly available fiberoptic laryngoscope has the following limitations:

   • It has a small diameter that does not allow for accurate assessment of airway lumen.
   • There is no channel for administration of anesthesia.
   • It was designed primarily to evaluate the subglottic region.

Because of these limitations, it is not prudent to use the fiberoptic laryngoscope to pass through a stenotic airway in a clinic or bedside setting. In this patient's case, recommendations based on the fiberoptic laryngoscopic examination resulted in imprecise documentation that only gave a clue as to the extent of the pathologic condition involved.

3. Communication regarding the tracheal stent to health care personnel unfamiliar with its use was easily facilitated with the hard copy (Fig. 2-7).

CASE 2-7 *"SOMETHING'S DOWN THERE. NO ONE CAN INTUBATE ME!"*

A 55-year-old woman was referred for airway management consultation for a left thyroid lobectomy. Her medical history was significant for failed intubation of her trachea 20 years ago when she underwent a hysterectomy with spinal anesthesia, 7 years ago before excision of a lipoma on her back (the procedure was canceled) and, most recently, 4 weeks before consultation for a left thyroidectomy (this procedure was also canceled). The referring otolaryngologist provided radiographic studies that revealed significant tracheal deviation without evidence of tracheal compression. The intraoperative events were relayed from written documentation and communication. Fiberoptic techniques were used. Subglottic resistance was encountered, and attempts to advance an endotracheal tube were unsuccessful. The procedure was canceled, and the patient was taken to the recovery room in satisfactory condition.

Communication Issues. During this consultation the patient expressed extreme anxiety regarding future attempts with airway management. She demanded that she be asleep for the procedure and that it be successful. She was assured that the surgery-anesthesia team would manage her to the best of their ability in an environment of optimal patient safety. She underwent a diagnostic fiberoptic bronchoscopy, followed by an oral fiberoptic intubation of her trachea while she was awake and had no complications. Photodocumentation was sent to the referring medical team.

Discussion. The following points should be noted:

1. In this case the videoscope confirmed the working diagnosis of significant tracheal deviation without compression. Hard copy readily communicated to the patient and referring physicians that no obstruction was "down there" (Fig. 2-8).

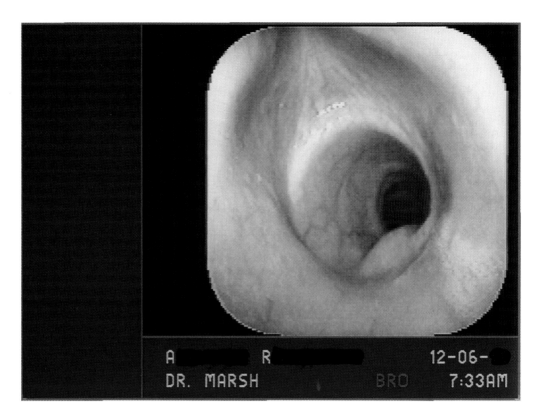

FIG. 2-8   Photodocumentation of videobronchoscopy showing no evidence of subglottic or tracheal compression.

2. Communication by means of a team approach for complex airway management was critical in the successful management of this patient.
3. Enrollment into Medic Alert will enable future health care providers to access the precise chronology of complex airway management events that this patient experienced.

CASE 2-8   *"WHAT DO I TELL MY DOCTORS ABOUT MY THYROPLASTY?"*

A 21-year-old man presented for medialization thyroplasty with Silastic implant. His medical history was significant for a Chiari malformation status postcervical syrinx excision and bilateral true vocal cord paralysis. Physical examination was significant for a soft, raspy voice. Examination of his airway revealed good oral excursion, good dentition, and partial visualization of his uvula (Mallampati Class 2). During the preanesthesia evaluation the patient informed his anesthesiologist that he must be awake during the surgery.

Communication Issues.   The anesthesiologist was unfamiliar with the surgery and its anesthetic requirements. Direct communication with the surgeon resulted in obtaining a more complete history regarding the patient's pathologic condition, photodocumentation of the patient's vocal cord condition, and explanation of anesthetic requirements during surgery. The procedure was completed with monitored anesthesia and minimal intravenous sedation with no complications.

At the postoperative visit the patient consented to enroll in Medic Alert Foundation.

Discussion. The following points should be noted:

1. Direct communication between members of the health care team resulted in a better understanding by the anesthesiologist of evolving surgical techniques for the management of vocal cord paralysis and secondary glottic insufficiency. Armed with that knowledge, specific recommendations regarding implications for future anesthetic management were communicated to the patient and included on his Medic Alert wallet card.

2. Enrollment into Medic Alert facilitates long-term follow-up care and evaluation of thyroplasty patients. Specific recommendations for future airway management are cited. Additionally, as these implants continue to undergo development, The National Difficult Airway/Intubation Registry database will facilitate scientific investigation.

Contributed by Dr. Paul Flint, Department of Otolaryngology—Head and Neck Surgery, The Johns Hopkins Medical Institutions.

CASE 2-9   *REALITIES OF CLINICAL PRACTICE*

A 44-year-old, 5'2"-, 90-kg woman was admitted for bilateral ethmoidectomies and revision septoplasty. Her medical history was significant for unanticipated difficult airway management, requiring urgent fiberoptic bronchoscopy and intubation of the trachea. Subsequent surgeries (secondary to a motor vehicle accident and cervical spine injury) were facilitated by fiberoptic bronchoscopy. On physical examination, the patient had limited neck extension, a small mouth, a jaw opening of 2 cm, and a limited oral view (Mallampati Class 4).

Six months earlier the intubation had been attempted with local anesthesia and intravenous sedation. The patient had become apneic early in the procedure, and mask ventilation was difficult to establish. Within minutes the patient resumed spontaneous ventilation. Shortly thereafter she showed signs and symptoms consistent with pulmonary edema. The procedure was aborted. Further diagnostic evaluation included an echocardiogram and thallium stress test, neither of which showed evidence of cardiac disease. The presumptive diagnosis was postobstructive pulmonary edema. The patient was billed for the canceled procedure and complained to hospital administration.

For this procedure the anesthesia team planned an elective oral fiberoptic intubation of the trachea while the patient was awake. The patient arrived in the operating room accompanied by the surgeon, who promptly explained to everyone present that the easiest and safest choice was local anesthesia with intravenous sedation. After polite, but extensive discussion, the anesthesia was administered as requested. The patient's operative course was rocky! She complained of headaches with the local anesthesia as well as nausea. The anesthesia team vigilantly struggled to control her symptoms by administering antiemetics. (Total intravenous sedation for a 4-hour procedure was 2 mg of midazolam; three different antiemetics were administered.) The surgeon commented, "You see. This is much easier than general anesthesia. It is less risky, and she gets to go home today."

Communication Issues. The anesthesia team again inquired as to the implications of the choice of anesthesia for surgery in an attempt to understand the surgeon. The surgeon finally admitted that the choice reflected his preference because the implications of the type of anesthetic used during the surgery were minimal. He asked for continued discussion regarding the anesthesiologist's concerns. What ensued was a pleasant, interactive, educational discussion of all of the information contained in this chapter. The patient's surgical procedure was completed without complications. Postoperatively, the patient was informed about and consented for enrollment into Medic Alert.

Discussion. The following points should be noted:

1. This case was chosen as the "grand finale" for this chapter. It is representative of those challenging clinical scenarios and dilemmas that anesthesiologists face in everyday clinical prac-

tice. The realities of clinical practice bring to the forefront issues such as these, which must be addressed if we are to effect change in the name of patient safety. Physicians must endeavor to effect responsible change that is supported by informed colleagues and educated patients—responsible change that acknowledges risk-benefit, economic, and medicolegal considerations.

CONCLUSION

This chapter presented nine cases with common themes and discussed specific strategies for communicating patient events. Information exchange is important for improving patient care. Intrinsic to the multispecialty nature of airway management, such exchange must be multidimensional to effectively communicate critical information.

If the single greatest incentive for precise documentation and effective dissemination is patient safety, the practitioner will also realize the added benefit of these incidental rewards: generation of innovative teaching materials for residents and colleagues, educational material for patients, creation of a clinically relevant airway database, and documentation that is legally acceptable and facilitates peer review.

Exciting advances in technologies and information systems combined with innovative use of existing resources facilitate rapid development of immediately accessible, multimedia, flexible information exchange. The future of successful airway management is limited only by our collective energies and creativity.

REFERENCES

1. *The Johns Hopkins Hospital Medical Staff Manual,* Baltimore, 1991, Johns Hopkins Hospital.
2. *1992 Annual Report,* Turlock, Calif, 1992, Medic Alert Foundation.
3. Mark LJ, Beattie C, Ferrell CL et al: The difficult airway: mechanisms for effective dissemination of critical information, *J Clin Anesth* 4:247-251, 1992.
4. Caplan RA: Anesthetic liability: what it is and what it isn't. In *1992 Review Course Lectures.* Presented at the IARS 66th Congress, San Francisco, March 13-17, 1992, International Anesthesia Research Society.
5. American Society of Anesthesiologists Committee on Professional Liability: Preliminary study of closed claims, *ASA Newsletter* 52:8-10, 1988.
6. Keats AS: Anesthesia mortality in perspective, *Anesth Analg* 71:113-119, 1990.
7. Eichhorn JH: Documenting improved anesthesia outcome, *J Clin Anesth* 3:351-353, 1991.
8. Orkin FK: Practice standards: the Midas touch or the emperor's new clothes? *Anesthesiology* 70:567-571, 1989.
9. Norton ML, Brown ACD: *Atlas of the difficult airway: a source book,* St Louis, 1991, Mosby.
10. Wilson ME, Spiegelhalter D, Robertson JA et al: Predicting difficult intubation, *Br J Anaesth* 61:211-216, 1988.
11. Mallampati SR, Gatt SP, Gugino LD et al: A clinical sign to predict difficult intubation: a prospective study, *Can Anaesth Soc J* 32:429-434, 1985.
12. Caplan RA, Posner K, Ward RJ et al: Adverse respiratory events in anesthesia: a closed claims analysis, *Anesthesiology* 72:828-833, 1993.
13. Task Force on Guidelines for Management of Difficult Airway Practice: Guidelines for management of the difficult airway, *Anesthesiology* 78:597-602, 1993.
14. Estafanous FG, Barash JG, Reves JG: *Cardiac anesthesia,* Philadelphia, 1994, JB Lippincott.
15. Mark LJ: *The consultant anesthesiologist: a new profile for the profession of the anesthesiologist,* Baltimore, 1991, The Foundation for Anesthesia Education and Research (unpublished grant).
16. Editorial: How to avoid small complaints about quality of care, *Maryland BPQA (Maryland Board of Physician Quality Assurance) Newsletter,* 1(4):1, 1993.
17. Wilbur RS: Personal communication, January, 1994.

CHAPTER 3

The Normal Practice of Endoscopy and Intubation

MARTIN L. NORTON

EXAMINATION

Of crucial importance is the need to do a thorough examination of areas not completely studied by the referring physician. Indeed, it is necessary to repeat parts of the history and physical examination. There is truth to the often-made comment, "I understand what I see for myself better than what I read on a chart."

This is particularly true when evaluating the airway because other medical specialists do not always give attention to some of the factors that the anesthesiologist must. For example, a patent nasal passage for intubation includes consideration of the outside and inside diameter of the tube to be inserted, particularly in the pediatric patient. Unfortunately, some anesthesiologists are reluctant to examine children who are in the awake state. They may have forgotten (or never learned) the ear, nose, and throat examination skills practiced by the family physician or otolaryngologist!

Examination must include a history, specifically related to the area of concern as well as other systems affected. It requires the *art* of visualization. It is interesting to note that indirect laryngoscopy originated with Manuel Garcia, a Professor of Signing at the Paris Conservatoire. In 1855 he read a paper before the Royal Society of Laryngology in England entitled *Observations on the Human Voice,*[1] based on his patient self-examination of his vocal cords with a dental mirror. Auscultation, palpation, and other exercises of the art of visualization constitutes the physical diagnosis.

Problems such as tonsillar enlargement, glossoptosis (the posterior and downward apposition of the base of the tongue to prevertebral tissues with resultant airway obstruction), or nasal passage obstruction are readily visualized with the simple and painless use of the otoscope and nasal or other speculae. In the infrequent case where it is necessary, the patient can be given appropriately small doses of midazolam, ketamine, or other medication, but always with the precautions of postexamination observation and the availability of airway support equipment. It is fallacious to call the latter *awake intubation.* This is a medicated intubation and, in some cases, borders on light general anesthesia.

The temporomandibular joint must be considered in the examination. Table 3-1 indicates the differential diagnoses of limited excursion of the mandible.

The physician must never wait until the moment of surgery to do an appropriate examination. Such strategy speaks ill of the profession by endangering the patient! One of the reasons for establishing the Difficult Airway Clinic (DAC) is to avoid the problems that ensue from last-minute examinations.

POSITIONING THE PATIENT

Dripps,[2] in his classic text, followed Jackson[3] in describing the axes of intubation as oral, pharyngeal, and tracheal. By opening the mouth properly and extending the cervical vertebrae at the atlantoaxial joint and flexing the lower cervical vertebral joints, these axes (especially the tracheal and the pharyngeal axes) can be brought together. This is the basis for placing the head in the "sniffing" or "pecking" position by means of a pad under the head for adults.

Table 3-1 Differential Diagnosis of Limited Excursion of the Mandible

Disorder	Diagnosis
Temporomandibular joint disorders	Congenital dysfunction
	Inflammation
	Trauma
	Neoplasia
Muscle disorders	Malignant hypothermia
	Myotonia
	Myopathy or myositis
Integumentary/fascia disorders	Neoplasia
	Infection
	Postirradiation
	Scleroderma
	Freeman-Sheldon syndrome
	Arthrogryposis
	Trismus
	Pseudocamptodactyly syndrome
Neurologic injury	Denervation

It can be noted that the area described (the atlantoaxial joint) is *not* the site of most movement (flexion or extension) of the neck. In fact this site lies between cervical vertebrae C4 and C7. Adding to the problem, endoscopists often put too large a pad under the head, thus limiting the available opening of the mouth. Similarly, what has become almost a reflex motion, that of snapping the head to extreme extension by pulling up the chin and pressing down and backward on the cranium, must be decried. As a consequence the airway narrows despite the greater room available to open the mouth. In addition, there is great risk of physician-induced trauma (euphoniously called *iatrogenic*) in older patients who are osteoporotic or who suffer from Paget's disease, rheumatoid arthritis with atlantoaxial instability, or other potential odontoid peg disorder.

Of particular importance is the relationship of the hyoid cartilage and its attached musculature. The importance of this "bone" is specifically related to the attachment of the middle constrictor and hyoglossus muscles at the greater cornua of the hyoid with the suspensory effect of the body of the hyoid and attached geniohyoid and with the genioglossus muscles shifting the base of the tongue anteriorly, thus opening the airway.

Anesthesia, sedatives, ethanol, and vagally mediated volume feedback from the lungs suppress motor output to the genioglossus in animals. Sleep deprivation has been shown to depress the phasic respiratory activity of this muscle in normal humans. In unanesthetized cats and sleeping human infants, neck position influences genioglossal activity and pharyngeal configuration. Neck flexion reflexly activates genioglossal discharge, which tends to maintain airway patency.

STANDARD TECHNIQUES

Standard techniques for establishing a patent airway with no instrumentation include jaw elevation. The object is to extend the head and elevate and project forward the base of the tongue. The latter is accomplished by means of the genioglossal muscles. Elevation of the laryngeal structures is facilitated by the hyoglossal muscles.

A problem arises when the knuckles press on the neck (Fig. 3-1) in the area of the angle of the mandibular ramus, thereby stimulating the glomus caroticum (carotid bulb) and producing a pressor response. **Creating the oropharyngeal airway by depressing the mandible, as is commonly done,**

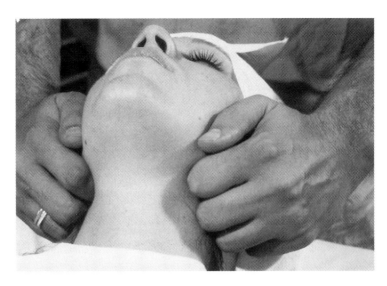

FIG. 3-1   Effects of knuckles pressing on neck in area of angle of mandibular ramus.

has the effect of locking in the condyloid process, which articulates with the articular disk of the temporomandibular joint. This actually limits mouth opening and prevents maximal extension of the tongue base.

A biomechanically efficient method is to open the mouth and then elevate and ventrally project both the mandible and the tongue base. In some cases this may require inserting the thumb into the mouth down to the tongue base, grasping both the base of the tongue and the mandible and lifting them anteriorly.

MONITORING CORRECT PLACEMENT OF THE ENDOTRACHEAL TUBE

The end point of endotracheal tube placement must be closely monitored. As discussed previously, the risk of esophageal insertion is real, and there are severe consequences to lack of timely recognition of this misplacement. Much of this monitoring is based on suspicion. The following should be observed during tube placement:

1. The top of the endotracheal tube cuff should be placed at or just below the level of the vocal folds.
2. With the use of translucent tubes, a fogging with expiration and clearing on inspiration is another index. However this may also appear from the gases within the upper gastrointestinal tract and thus is *not* a reliable sign.
3. Movements of the chest during assisted inspiration, especially the left thorax, should follow.
4. Comparative breath sounds should be determined by auscultation at the level of the fourth and fifth intercostal spaces at the mid-to-anterior axillary line. (NOTE: The practice of listening over the second or third intercostal spaces in the midclavicular line is fraught with the danger of deception from transmitted sounds from the trachea or even the esophagus.)
5. Listen for gurgling sounds in the stomach during assisted ventilation. (This step should be performed by auscultation of the epigastrium in conjunction with #2.)
6. Observe the end tidal CO_2 monitor for pattern of ventilation and level of CO_2 return, which does clearly indicate esophageal intubation but does not clearly isolate endobronchial intubation.
7. The level of red cell saturation should be monitored with the use of the pulse oximeter or other techniques of transcutaneous oxygen saturation monitoring. Unfortunately this may be a late sign but is certainly quicker and more accurate than #8.
8. Check the skin or mucosae for cyanosis (a very late sign).

9. Confirm the penultimate indicator by internal visual identification (flexible fiberoptic endoscopy) of the carina or bronchopulmonary segments.
10. Confirm tube positioning by radiologic means (x-ray).

Above all, constant vigilance and suspicion is the keystone when monitoring tube placement! It is important to keep in mind that **any changes of patient position on the table mandate rechecking of all parameters of endotracheal tube position!**

NASAL PASSAGE

One area of particular concern related to intubation is the rarity of direct examination using a nasal speculum. The common practice appears to be to determine nasal airway patency by asking the patient about ease of respiration while occluding one or the other of the nares or while passing a long cotton swab probe saturated with cocaine or a lidocaine-epinephrine solution. Passage of the long cotton swab probe only demonstrates that there is enough room for a 2- or 3-mm instrument and certainly yields no information as to obstructions when using a 6-mm internal diameter (ID) or 7.0-mm ID nasotracheal tube (in adults). It does give some guidance about the direction of the inferior turbinate passageway. However, this does not produce accurate measurements and certainly does not indicate the diameter of the passageway or its adequacy for passage of varying-sized endotracheal tubes. Even rhinomanometric values have not been reliable as a means of distinguishing between normal and abnormal passages based on rhinoscopic evaluation.[4]

In fact nasal resistance values have also been shown to be unreliable. Traditional medical practice has long taught the necessity of knowing the anatomy (Fig. 3-2), physiology (especially the functional suspension of the hyoid shown in Fig. 3-3), and pharmacology of the area of concern. Similarly, a proper diagnostic examination includes visualization, wherever possible, and the use of ancillary diagnostic methods to further illuminate an understanding of the passageway in the specific patient. The use of the otoscope with a long speculum has been found to be particularly advantageous in visualizing the nasal passageways, especially the regions of the nasal vestibule, turbinates, and the choanae. Nasal septal deviations, turbinate and conchael malformations, and simple polyps may be clearly visualized using this method.

Of particular concern is the palatal arch (hard palate). If a significantly high-arched palate is observed, the fact that the floor of the nose bulges into the nasal lumen as a result must be consid-

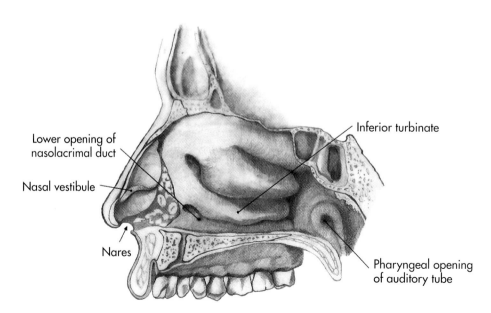

Lower opening of
nasolacrimal duct

Nasal vestibule

Nares

Inferior turbinate

Pharyngeal opening
of auditory tube

FIG. 3-2   Anatomy of nasal passage.

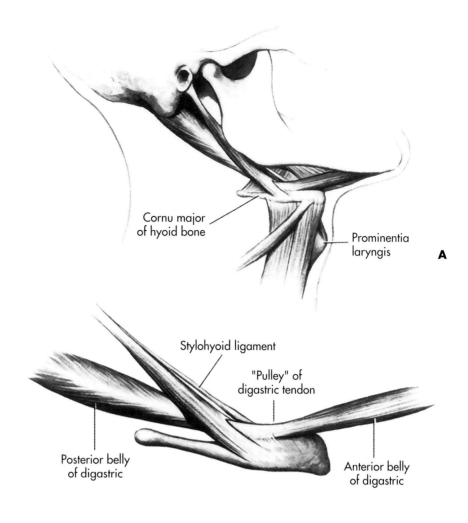

Cornu major
of hyoid bone

Prominentia
laryngis

A

Stylohyoid ligament

"Pulley" of
digastric tendon

Posterior belly
of digastric

Anterior belly
of digastric

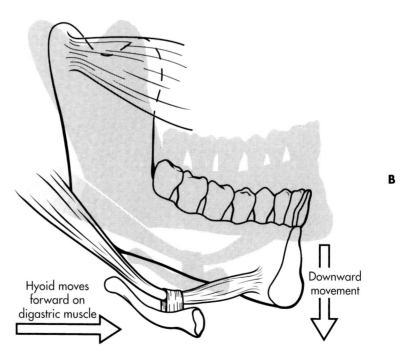

B

Hyoid moves
forward on
digastric muscle

Downward
movement

FIG. 3-3   Functional suspension of hyoid. **A,** Suspension; **B,** function.

ered. Possibly as a secondary phenomenon, the nasal septum is often buckled and deflected to one side or the other. The septal spurs impinge on the shelflike turbinates and complete the picture of nasal obstruction.

In children, and some adults, the factor of hypertrophied adenoid tissues and tonsils presents complicating concerns. The current deemphasis on tonsillectomy and adenoidectomy during childhood appears to have resulted in more obstructive tonsillar masses in adults, and these occasionally complicate nasotracheal intubations. The contribution of these masses to the presence of sleep apnea is yet to be fully elucidated.

An upper respiratory tract infection or allergy often manifested by nasal polyps also compromises the patency of the nasal airways.

After visualization, graded sizes of soft, well-lubricated nasopharyngeal tubes are used to reinforce visual observations and, indeed, to stretch up the diameter of the nasal passages. A small nasopharyngeal tube (about 6.0 mm in the adult) is used first, and then one that is one size larger than the nasotracheal tube that the physician wishes to insert is used.

This is particularly important in view of another consideration: the nasal passage is highly vascular. Therefore, the physician must be concerned about potential for severe hemorrhage from trauma and for definitive endotracheal tube softening in the nasal passage over a period. This leads to the risk of kinking or at least decreasing the internal diameter of the available imposed airway.

There appears to be less concern about tube sizes and their relationship to rheologic patterns than in previous years. The response heard is that any problem in this regard would be picked up by the end tidal CO_2 monitor.[5] This could be true, in part, if the end tidal pattern was closely analyzed. If major kinking occurs, the plateau portion of the end tidal capnograph would show the usual obstructive signs (i.e., the sudden drop to a low level). However, this is best seen in spontaneously breathing patients, which, unfortunately, the physicians are rarely dealing with at this point.

Additionally, the patient should be properly prepared. In most situations the patient is most comfortable in the sitting or semi-Fowler position. **For fiberoptic laryngoscopy and bronchoscopy, the upright sitting position is best because of the mechanical suspension of the larynx.** (The authors have been using a dental chair to great advantage because of its familiarity for patients and its ideal adjustability.)

A small dose of fentanyl or midazolam is of value in calming the patient. A mixture of 4% lidocaine mixed with 2% cocaine is then sprayed into the nasal passages as described previously.

As a precaution intravenous barbiturates and a source and system for providing controlled oxygen are available. A pulse oximeter is attached to each patient being examined, and, in patients for whom it is appropriate, an electrocardiogram (ECG) and blood pressure cuff (Dynamap) are attached as constant recording monitors.

Nasotracheal intubation airway management has become the procedure of choice in intensive care units (long-term intubations) and for plastic surgical and orosurgical procedures. Many colleagues in these specialties are particularly adamant about the need for nasoendotracheal intubation.

However, the procedure is not without its problems. Among these are the risk of reflex otic pain or internal ear infection (usually a serous otitis) related to the proximity of the pharyngeal orifice to the auditory canal, trauma to the posterior nasopharynx, or impingement of the endotracheal tube or endoscope on hypertrophied tonsillar or adenoidal tissue while the breathing tube is being advanced down past the soft palate and uvula. In addition, the tube is often further kinked by pressure of the inferior conchae of the turbinates. It is important to note that although dental surgery is easier (for the surgeon) in the patient who is intubated through the nose, there are few dental operations that cannot be performed with an orotracheal tube positioned behind the last molar and running along the buccal pouch and out of the mouth.

The convenience of nasotracheal intubation is counterbalanced by additional potential complications. Nasal bleeding, either from Kiesselbach's triangle anteriorly or trauma to the posterior nasal passage mucosa, suggests the wisdom of topical vasoconstrictor application and dilation of the inferior turbinate passage.

Postintubation earache following trauma to the Eustachian tube conus (tubus auditiva) and hypertrophic mucosae surrounding is not infrequent and is often missed by the endoscopist.

An unusual complication is extirpation of the inferior turbinate by rough intubation (Fig. 3-4), especially using a firm-walled endotracheal tube. A similar situation was reported by Muzzi, Losasso,

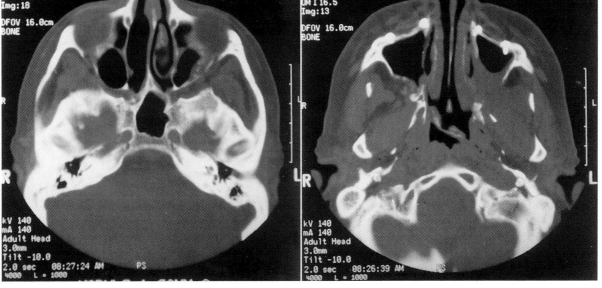

FIG. 3-4   Extirpation of the inferior turbinate by rough intubation. **A,** Extirpated specimen. **B** and **C,** Computed tomography scans.

and Cucchiara.[6] To avoid this the endotracheal tube should be softened in warm water. Sizing of the nasal passage by progressively sized, soft nasal trumpets described above is advised. Experience also suggests that the *maximum* size of endotracheal tubes required is 7.0-mm ID. **The convenience and comfort of the surgeon cannot take precedence over medical considerations of risk to the patient.**

There is an important difference between the adult and the infant in that the infant's large tongue is apposed to the palate during quiet respiration. Also, the infant's glottis is much higher, resting between C3 and C4 in the neonate and next to C6 in the adult. Furthermore, in the child the glottis is funnel shaped, and the narrowest portion internally lies at the cricoid cartilage, not the vocal folds. A presentation of the differences in the larynx between adults and children is found in Chapter 16.

Fiberoptic Intubation

Flexible fiberoptic laryngoscopy is the ideal approach to the difficult airway patient. It is believed that fiberoptic intubation is expedited with the least potential for trauma by *preplacement* of the endotracheal tube. In the transnasal approach the selected inferior turbinate area is topically anesthetized by spray technique or by use of nasal packing (Codman 1″ × 3″). This is followed by dilation by nasal trumpets, which is followed by insertion of a hot-water–softened endotracheal tube to, but not beyond, the posterior nasopharynx.

As a precaution the anesthetist must take care not to impact the tube against the prevertebral tissues. The lubricated fiberscope is then passed through the endotracheal tube down to the level of the carina, after which it is passed over the guided endoscope into the trachea.

When the oral route is chosen, the oropharynx is topically sprayed with anesthetic solution. Patients who have full upper dentures need not have the hard and soft palate anesthetized. However, patients who do not have prosthetic upper dentures and therefore are not accustomed to foreign body sensation should have thorough hard *and* soft palate topical anesthesia.

Occasionally, placement of the endoscope through the additus laryngis is extremely difficult. A Cook straight wire guide (SF, 145 cm, 0.89 mm flexible) (Cook Group Company, Bloomington, Indiana) is then used, using the section of biopsy pathway of the bronchoscope. When the flexible tip of the wire is seen through the endoscope or C-arm fluoroscope, it is aimed, using the bronchoscope angulation lever, and the wire is advanced into the trachea. It is necessary to have the distal end as close to the target *rima glottidis* as possible. After the guide wire has been passed, the fiberscope is advanced to the carina and endotracheal tube following to the appropriate depth. Then and only then should the wire and bronchoscope be withdrawn from the lumen of the endotracheal tube. NOTE: There is a somewhat different approach for the pediatric patient.

Following anesthetization the chosen lubricated intubation airway (Fig. 3-5) with well-lubricated endotracheal tube is preplaced (but *not* beyond the channel tip). Then, in the same fashion as for the nasal route, the fiberoptic instrument is advanced through the endotracheal tube.

Fiberoptic endoscopy must not be pursued as an afterthought or after the endoscopist has failed with other techniques. This approach requires a careful evaluation of the patient's anatomy, proper preparation of the passages, adequate anesthesia (whether topical or general), correct positioning of the patient, and an endoscopist with the requisite skill and experience. The *top* box on p. 44 lists those situations where fiberoptic endoscopy is recommended. Surgery for the patient who has had prior failed intubations should be postponed until the tissues have had time to recover from the incident trauma and to allow time for a thorough reevaluation of the airway per the procedures described for our DAC. Failure to do so risks complications, which include, but are not limited to, the extreme risk of unrecognized entrance into the superior mediastinum by laceration of the thin membrane at the level of the cricopharyngeal decussation.

It is believed that it takes at least 100 flexible fiberoptic intubations before the endoscopist can be called an expert in this field. Every residency program in anesthesiology should provide the opportunity for the house officer to attempt at least 25 fiberoptic intubations. It is suggested that at least 25 practice intubations on teaching models, followed by at least 25 intubations on patients be scheduled electively for nasotracheal intubation. This should then be followed by at least 10 orotracheal intubations. The patients included in this mix should include both awake (topical anesthesia) and lightly anesthetized (vocal folds functioning) subjects. Indications for awake fiberoptic evaluation are somewhat controversial. The *bottom* box on p. 44 gives a list of these indications.

These indications further imply the considered understanding of the anatomy and pathophysiology of the nasopharynx as well as the oropharynx. Once again physicians are reminded of the basics of medicine, anatomy, physiology, and pharmacology. A classic case wherein the fiberoptic instrument is of specific use is in the patient with glossoptosis. *Glossoptosis* is defined as basal tongue pressure on the cervical portion of the spinal column. Posterior positioning of the tongue causes pressure on the glottis. This closes the latter if the mouth is shut and limits it even with the open

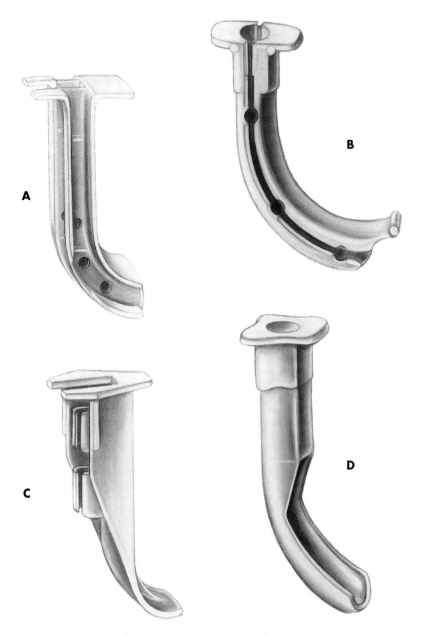

FIG. 3-5   **A,** Luomanen airway. **B,** Berman intubating airway. **C,** Ovassapian airway. **D,** Unidentified airway.

mouth position. The airways to the nasopharyngeal space are also closed. Consequently patients with severe glossoptosis are forced by anatomic mechanics to breathe and eat with open mouths.

Severe glossoptosis can often be recognized by the habitus of the patient. The head bends forward, the shoulders hang, the body seems bent and collapsed, the thighs appear excessively relaxed, and the facial expression is adenoidal. The teeth of the upper jaw are forward with reference to those of the retrograde lower jaw. The mouth responds to the condition of the weak receding chin by hanging open during breathing. The dull appearance of the patient combined with sloppy posture may suggest deficient mental development. However, this conclusion is not necessarily true. Children seem physically and psychologically stunted in growth because they constantly feel indisposed and are ventilating poorly without being seriously ill.

INTUBATIONS WHERE FIBEROPTIC ENDOSCOPY IS RECOMMENDED

Arthritis in airway or neck
Cicatricial burns or pemphigoid
Collagen vascular disease of neck or
    pharynx
Congenital abnormalities
Fixed neck
Foreign body
History of difficult intubation
Laryngeal tumors
Mallampati Classes 3 and 4
Mandibular hypoplasia

Morbid obesity
Myopathy or myositis
Neck masses
Old tracheostomy
Radiation therapy to upper airway
Radical neck dissection
Swallowing dysfunction
Temporomandibular joint disease
Unstable bridge work
Unstable neck fractures
Vocal fold paralysis

CONTROVERSIAL INDICATIONS FOR AWAKE FIBEROPTIC INTUBATION

Bronchopleural fistula
Dental disease
Epiglottitis
Evolving respiratory failure
Facial trauma
Full stomach
Mediastinal mass

Obstetric anesthesia
Pharyngeal mass
Sepsis or shock
Severe coronary disease
Status asthmaticus
Unstable neck

The differential diagnosis must also include macroglossia and its causes. Often, in this category of patients, there is a clear history of sleep apnea. However, this history must be sought out because this is one of the syndromes that is most often missed. The fact that these patients are often subjected to veloplasty, mandibular advancement procedures, or both makes this syndrome of particular interest to otolaryngologists, plastic surgeons, oral surgeons, and, of course, to anesthesiologists.

The insertion of a fiberoptic instrument through the oral route is reputedly more difficult than the nasal route. It has been found that this is not necessarily so. The key to success is the use of an appropriate oropharyngeal airway combined with proper topical anesthesia. The Berman Intubating Airway is (see Fig. 3-5, *B*) most useful, although the smaller sizes are, unfortunately, not currently available. (Others have found the use of the Ovassapian airway [see Fig. 3-5, *C*] of equal value.) This instrument has an added lip on its undersurface that protrudes into the vallecula epiglottis but that can also be inserted over the epiglottis. A slit along the entire side on the top allows for somewhat larger sizes of endotracheal tubes or can be used to open up the device for removal.

Finally, fiberoptic endoscopy is useful in a number of lower airway situations. Those are detailed in the box on p. 45.

LOWER AIRWAY PROBLEMS IN WHICH FIBEROPTIC EVALUATION IS STRONGLY RECOMMENDED

Anterior mediastinal masses	Recurrent atelectasis or plugging
Bronchial bleeding	Severe lung scarring—tracheal distortion
Bronchiectasis	Substernal thyroid-tracheal compression
Foreign body in airway	Superior vena cava syndrome
Intratracheal lesions	Suspected perioperative aspiration
Laryngoesophageal cleft	Tracheoesophageal fistula
Lung or airway resection	Tracheostomy or cricothyrotomy

TECHNIQUES FOR ESTABLISHING THE AIRWAY

What is the philosophy as to choice of airway management techniques? In the emergency situation, the physician should use the approach in which he or she is most expert and with which he or she feels most confident. In the elective case, or the situation where time permits, a visual technique is preferable. **As professionals, physicians are obligated not only to be sure of control, but also to see and review all tissues and pathways to rule out other pathologic conditions.** Other nonvisual methods (including light-wand or retrograde intubation) do not provide the same advantages as do flexible bronchoscopic direct visualization and assurance of proper airway control.

Regarding techniques of intubation, several approaches can be taken in the particularly difficult intubation situation. One technique is to pass a long arterial wire (often used in cardiac catheterization laboratory) through the suction channel of the intubating fiberoptic bronchoscope. The tip of the scope may then be positioned for full visualization of the larynx and the arterial wire passed under direct vision into the trachea. This is followed by passage of the fiberscope over the wire and then the endotracheal tube over the fiberscope, when indicated (see also Chapter 8). Another approach is to pass the fiberscope down to the additus laryngis transnasally and then to bring the endotracheal tube down the opposite nasal passage until it can be visualized at the rima glottidis through the optics of the fiberscope. Thus the tube would be further advanced under direct fiberoptic vision.

Perhaps the most important concept to be learned is that the best preparation of the patient includes a careful and sympathetic explanation of what an endoscopy entails, followed by a second, equally careful, step-by-step explanation during the procedure. Success probably depends more on rapport and resultant cooperation and, therefore, on the temperaments of the patient and the endoscopist than any other factor. *This takes time* and cannot be done in an environment of noise, confusion, and psychologic pressure!

Of great importance too is the positioning of the patient. The superb reference works by Fink[7] and Fink and Demarest[8] are commended to the reader. They certainly are the basis of consideration for efficient endoscopy and intubation. The reader will find the schematic to suggest the biomechanics of the unfolding of the larynx through use of its active and passive supports (Fig. 3-6) (refer also to Fink[7] [after Elze]). These studies present the rationale for considering the sitting position optimal for flexible fiberoptic endoscopy.

In making a decision on positioning the patient, the physician must consider the effect of the weight of the lungs and their fluid content (vasculature and cell fluid volume) when opening up the thoracic inlet as well as the unfolding of the larynx itself. Additionally, the proper manipulation of the mandible and patient cooperation in extending the tongue contribute to the efficiency of the procedure.

The sitting position is usually the most comfortable for the patient and most convenient for the operator, who should work facing (standing in front of) the patient. The pa-

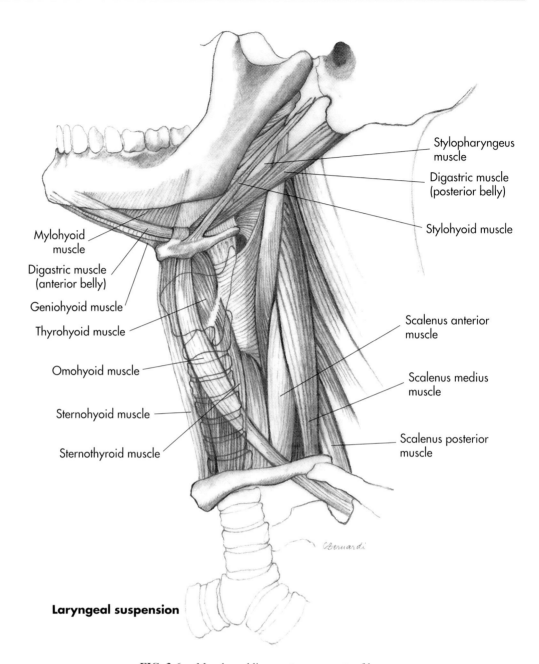

Stylopharyngeus
muscle

Digastric muscle
(posterior belly)

Stylohyoid muscle

Mylohyoid
muscle

Digastric muscle
(anterior belly)

Geniohyoid muscle

Thyrohyoid muscle

Scalenus anterior
muscle

Omohyoid muscle

Scalenus medius
muscle

Sternohyoid muscle

Scalenus posterior
muscle

Sternothyroid muscle

Laryngeal suspension

FIG. 3-6   Muscle and ligamentous supports of larynx.

tient's shoulders should be fully relaxed and the chin jutted forward. The tongue is protruded and held forward both while the topical anesthetic is applied and during the endoscopic procedure. If the patient is fully conscious, constant urging to breathe deeply slowly through the mouth can be of additional aid.

Endoscopy in the supine position is more familiar to the anesthesiologist and otolaryngologist when using rigid instrumentation. However, changes in support of the soft tissues of the upper respiratory tract lead to a "collapse" of the pharyngeal funnel. Head position becomes crucial with ventral movement of the C6-C7 vertebra presenting a further obstacle. Of course, use of ancillary aides such as the Berman, Williams, or Ovassapian intubating airway or preplacement of a nasotracheal tube to the point of maximal breath sounds can be of great value in overcoming these obstacles.

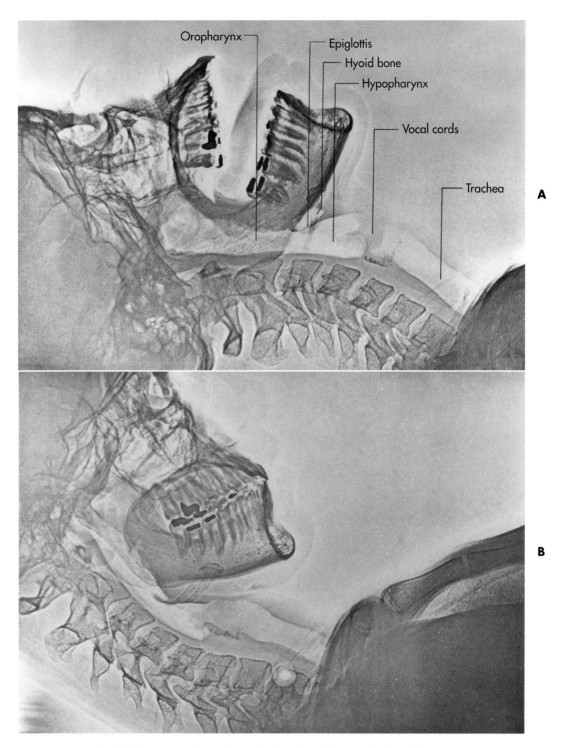

FIG. 3-7 Xeroradiographs of head and neck. **A,** Extension; **B,** flexion.

Cricoid pressure is an often recommended maneuver, originally described by Sellick[9] in 1961. It was developed to prevent regurgitant flow from the stomach into the airway. It involves backward pressure on the front of the cricoid cartilage, obstructing the upper esophagus and theoretically preventing regurgitation and aspiration before intubation. Some even believe that it prevents gastric distention during positive pressure ventilation by mask. However, the patient is often positioned with the head extended in the "pecking position" (Fig. 3-7).

The cricoid pressure technique was presented as an alternative to induction in the sitting position. However, anatomic distortion can occasionally result from pressure on the neck, rendering intubation more difficult, particularly in the obese or pregnant patient or in the patient who has a "short" neck. Posterior displacement of the larynx by pressure on the thyroid or cricoid cartilage is frequently used during difficult intubations when the larynx is not readily brought into adequate viewing. This also can distort the anatomy and may require contracricoid pressure[10] to the back of the neck (see also Chapter 4).

EXTUBATION

Of equal importance to endotracheal intubation are the considerations and techniques of extubation. The general rule holds that **a difficult intubation means a potentially difficult extubation.** Every time an endotracheal tube is removed (or a tracheostomy is decannulated), the physician must be prepared for a possible emergency reintubation. Examples of situations requiring emergency recannulation include, but are not limited to, tracheal collapse following total thyroidectomy of Riedel's struma, the recurarization syndrome, and sedative overdose of the postanesthesia patient.

One technique that is routinely used is to insert the long intubation guide (Norton, Teflon, or Eschmann woven) down to the level of the carina, to decannulate the endotracheal tube, and to leave the stylet in situ for at least 1 hour. Patients tolerate the retention of the stylet very well in comparison with the endotracheal tube and can even vocalize with it in place. Clinical observation of many patients over many years has demonstrated that airway obstruction (e.g., edema) following decannulation usually occurs within the first hour. If this does occur, it is simple to "railroad" the endotracheal tube over the long intubation guide into the trachea and thus bypass the obstruction until further treatment is provided. This approach has been and is being used routinely for both nasal and orotracheal intubation situations.

Table 3-2 Complications Associated with Intubation Techniques*

Technique	Complication or constraint
Jet (Venturi)	Pneumolarynx and trachea, pneumomediastinum, pneumothorax, infection
Retrograde	Trauma to vocal folds, infection, other laryngeal and tracheal trauma
Light wand	Tissue burn from heat of bulb
Fiberoptic (nasal)	Hemorrhage, nasal diameter (access by means of intubation airway)
Fiberoptic (oral)	Access through oral route only
Intubation guide (Norton, Teflon, or Eschmann woven)	Lateral wall disruption of second- or third-degree bronchial passages (pneumothorax)
Bullard laryngoscope	Access through oral route only, intubation guide
Tracheostomy	Tracheal infection, stenosis, loss of Valsalva mechanism, communication problems, cicatrix, hemorrhage
Nasal airway	Hemorrhage
Laryngeal mask	Leakage of liquids (e.g., regurgitant HCl), disruption of esophagopharyngeal introitus

*The above listing does not include reactions to topical anesthetics and adjuvants required for "shrinking" mucosa, reduction of sensation to passage of instruments, depression of gag reflex, and psychotropic effects.
HCl, Hydrochloride.

COMPLICATIONS

Even the most careful planning cannot anticipate every potential problem. Complications can and do occur. The first line of defense against them is to anticipate what may happen. Table 3-2 indicates the complications associated with various intubation techniques.

REFERENCES

1. Garcia M: Observations on the human voice. Paper presented to the Royal Society of Laryngology, London, 1855.
2. Dripps R, Eckenhoff J, Van Dam L: *Textbook of anesthesia,* Philadelphia, 1969, WB Saunders.
3. Jackson C, Jackson CL: *Diseases of the nose, throat, and ear,* Philadelphia, 1945, WB Saunders.
4. McCaffrey TV, Kern EB: Clinical evaluation of nasal obstruction: a study of 1000 patients, *Arch Otolaryngol,* 105:542, 1979.
5. Smallhout BA: *Quick guide to capnography and its use in differential diagnosis,* Hewlett-Packard Medical Products Group, Federal Republic of Germany: Hewlett-Packard GmbH, D-7030, 1983.
6. Muzzi DA, Losasso TJ, Cucchiara RF: Complication from a nasopharyngeal airway in a patient with a basilar skull fracture, *Anesthesiology* 74:366-368, 1991.
7. Fink BR: *The human larynx,* New York, 1975, Raven Press.
8. Fink BR, Demarest RJ: *Laryngeal biomechanics,* Cambridge and London, 1978, Harvard University Press.
9. Sellick BA: Cricoid pressure to control regurgitation of stomach contents during induction of anesthesia, *Lancet* 11:404, 1961.
10. Crawford JS: The "contra cricoid" cuboid aid to tracheal intubation, *Anaesthesia* 37:345, 1982.

CHAPTER 4

Airway Considerations in Emergency Medicine

CHARLES POLLACK

Emergency medicine is unique among the specialties that manage the airway because prehospital patient care is included within its scope. The prehospital setting is fraught with potential complications and confounding problems in emergent airway management, such as significant time pressure on frequently inexperienced providers, suboptimal conditions and equipment, unavailability of assistance, and a necessity to assume the worst (e.g., cervical spine injury in the multiple trauma patient) in a setting in which the worst cannot readily be disproved.

Nonetheless, studies have demonstrated for two decades that, in nontraumatic cardiopulmonary or pure respiratory arrest, prompt intubation, whether in the field or in the emergency department, is associated with a greater chance of survival.[1-3] For this reason, most organized prehospital care systems authorize and encourage intubation in the field, even when transport time to an emergency department is not prolonged. The motor skills required to intubate patients can be learned. The Advance Cardiac Life Support (ACLS) model of didactics followed by mannequin training is widely accepted; national paramedic certification standards also recommend observed intubations of anesthetized patients in the operating room. Experience, of course, is more difficult to attain. Even the best training loses its effectiveness if the trainee is not frequently retested, either in realistic simulations or in actual patient encounters. In addition, it is impossible to prepare paramedics for all of the untoward eventualities that may ensue. Therefore, it is important that emergency physicians who provide medical control for these paramedics stress repeatedly that successful resuscitations be carried out with bag-valve-mask ventilation and oral/nasal airway and that repeated attempts at intubation in the field are neither necessary nor appropriate when there is a better equipped emergency department with its more skilled personnel on the receiving end of the transport. Practicing anesthesiologists and anesthetists—and indeed many emergency physicians—would doubtlessly feel uncomfortable managing an acutely compromised airway in the prehospital setting. Many medications deemed "standard" in the emergency department or operating room setting are not carried in ambulance stock (see the box on p. 51); sedatives, for example, are ordinarily limited to diazepam or lorazepam and morphine sulfate. Neuromuscular blocking agents are generally unavailable. Monitoring capabilities are frequently limited to a cardiac monitor; few ground ambulances carry pulse oximeters because of their bulk and expense.

Intubation frequently must be performed either on the ground with the operator kneeling or lying supine above the patient's head or in the back of an ambulance traveling at high speeds over bumpy roads. In the ambulance there is insufficient space for an assistant to maintain cervical spinal stability while the operator intubates the patient.[4] (A hard cervical collar cannot be expected to provide sufficient stability during the intubating maneuver.) Rationally, it may seem difficult to believe that prehospital airway management has been repetitively found to be beneficial!

Although the prehospital scenario is handicapped in comparison with the emergency department, neither is the emergency department an ideal setting for managing the airway when compared with elective intubation in the operating room. Urgency is the watchword; unprepared patients are the rule. The old adage that trauma victims always eat a full plate of spaghetti and drink a pitcher of beer shortly before their accident is, distressingly, too frequently accurate!

**MEDICATIONS CARRIED ON PHOENIX, ARIZONA
FIRE DEPARTMENT AMBULANCES***

PARENTERAL PREPARATIONS

Adenosine
Aminophylline
Atropine
Bretylium
Calcium chloride
Dextrose ($D_{50}W$)
Diazepam
Diphenhydramine
Dopamine
Epinephrine 1:1000 solution
Epinephrine 1:10,000 solution
Glucagon
Furosemide
Lidocaine 100 mg/5 ml
Lidocaine 1 g/25 ml
Lidocaine 2 g/500cc D_5W premix
Magnesium sulfate

Methylprednisolone sodium succinate
Morphine sulfate
Naloxone
Neo-Synephrine
Oxytocin
Sodium bicarbonate
Thiamine
Verapamil

ORAL PREPARATIONS

Aspirin
Activated charcoal
Nifedipine
Nitroglycerine (sublingual)

OTHER PREPARATIONS

Albuterol for small volume nebulizer
Isoetharine for small volume nebulizer

*These medications are typical for urban prehospital systems in the United States.

Airway emergencies in the emergency department, which often present directly and have not been evaluated or stabilized by prehospital personnel, vary from combative overdose patients to those in status epilepticus or asthmaticus, to multiple trauma (or discrete airway trauma) victims, to a child with epiglottitis, to a patient in full cardiac arrest. The emergency physician must be comfortable with a variety of different approaches to handling airway emergencies because each patient presents a new challenge and might best be managed somewhat differently from the previous similar (or dissimilar) case. Emergency department personnel must have established protocols and comfortable working arrangements with their colleagues in the anesthesiology department, not only for the best possible management of expected difficult intubations, but also for those cases that are unexpectedly complicated.

Following is a review of seven "typical" scenarios in which prehospital and emergency personnel must be comfortable, along with general guidelines for managing each in their unique settings.

THE PATIENT WITH ACUTE RESPIRATORY FAILURE
Prehospital

The patient with impending or acute respiratory failure presents a difficult challenge to prehospital personnel. The initial decision faced is whether the patient should be intubated in the field or stabilized and "temporized," pending more aggressive support in the emergency department that might avert intubation. Nasal intubations are often preferentially used in the prehospital setting, particularly in the tachypneic, restless, hypoxemic patient. "Trigger tubes" (Endotrol endotracheal tubes) (Fig. 4-1) make this procedure more likely to be successful by providing the anatomic equivalent of a Sellick maneuver and allowing for entry into an "anterior" larynx.

Rapid sequence/crash induction. For many years "crash" induction has been the most common method of securing the airway and purportedly minimizing the chances of regurgitation and aspiration. Practitioners have suggested the head up, head down, or flat position. Preoxygenation

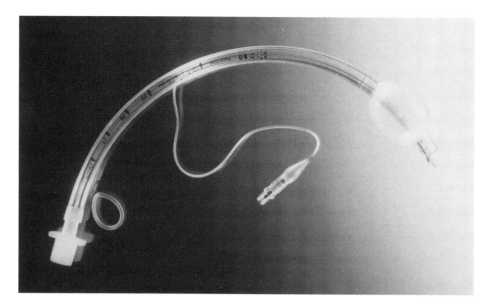

FIG. 4-1   Endotrol endotracheal tube.

effectively increases arterial oxygenation, but also adds to gastric distention, which predisposes to regurgitation and other vago-vagal effects. To minimize these, respiration should not be assisted until the airway is isolated and controlled.

The Sellick maneuver (cricoid pressure) is applied in an anteroposterior direction, occluding the esophagus. In fact this pressure may also distort the larynx, thereby making inductions more difficult. This has been discussed elsewhere.

Metoclopramide, a dopamine antagonist useful in aspiration prophylaxis because it promotes gastric emptying in addition to other agents, is often administered before induction of anesthesia.

Rapid induction techniques should *never* be considered unless the endoscopist is sure there is no impediment to intubation. Further, rapid intubation techniques should be severely limited to specific indications—not to routine inductions—because of the risks of unanticipated difficult airway problems.

The risks of managing the patient with a difficult airway after administering muscle relaxants or bringing the patient to deep anesthetic levels cannot be underestimated.

The unavailability of medications for rapid sequence induction in the field (such as sodium thiopental, ketamine, or neuromuscular blockers) makes the oral route less appealing unless the patient is in full arrest. Particularly, if the anticipated transport time is brief, the preferred management may be a nasal trumpet assisted with bag-valve-mask ventilation.

Emergency Department

Once in the emergency department, patients in impending respiratory failure are managed initially with the goal of avoiding intubation if the underlying process is a readily reversible one. Pharmaceutic intervention, such as specific therapy for bronchospasm in the form of aerosolized beta-adrenergic agonists, or therapy for pulmonary edema, such as diuretics or nitrates, and physical adjuncts, such as bilateral continuous positive airway pressure support with a nasal mask (nasal bi-PAP)[5,6] may sufficiently improve the patient to the point that intubation and mechanical ventilation may no longer be necessary. Emergency Department use of modalities such as bi-PAP reflects a growing trend toward therapies previously limited to other critical and intensive care areas. Although long-term studies have yet to be completed, anecdotal evidence indicates that severity of illness and lengths of stay are being affected by such strategies.

When intubation and ventilation are indicated in the emergency management of patients with respiratory failure, nasal intubations are generally preferred because frequently these patients are expected to require mechanical ventilation for extended periods. If the patient is not apneic and oxygenation, as measured by pulse oximetry, is satisfactory, the nostril can be prepared with a spray of Neo-Synephrine and subsequent insertion of a large nasal trumpet (one-half to one size larger than the anticipated nasotracheal tube) for dilation. A standard or Endotrol tube (Endotrol endotracheal tubes are marketed by Mallinckrodt Critical Care, Glens Fall, New York) can then be inserted. Occasionally, intubation over a fiberoptic scope is used for respiratory failure in the emergency department, but only in those patients sufficiently stable to undergo a procedure with which most emergency physicians have limited experience. If oral intubation is preferred by the physician or indicated clinically (e.g., in apneic patients, combative patients, or those with nasal obstruction), rapid sequence induction is usually performed with sodium thiopental, midazolam, or lorazepam and then succinylcholine or atracurium.

The use of succinylcholine in the Emergency Department occurs almost by tradition. Although an ever-burgeoning array of options are available for neuromuscular blockade, *emergency department physicians, who do not manage airway emergencies every day but who must be prepared to manage a variety of airway insults at all times,* tend to rely on a medication that has a rapid onset of action, few (if any) absolute contraindications, and a short duration of action in case intubation attempts are unsuccessful. Therefore, it is common for succinylcholine to be used in the rapid sequence induction of patients in the emergency department, regardless of the etiology of their airway compromise. Sedatives and other adjunctive medications, for example, lidocaine in head trauma, are the ones that are modified from case to case.

THE PATIENT IN CARDIOPULMONARY ARREST
Prehospital

Once the patient is in full arrest, nasal intubation is no longer available as an option. The most expeditious orotracheal intubation is indicated because data support the efficacy of definitive prehospital airway management.[1-3] If intubation is unsuccessful, the paramedics' next best option is prompt transport to the nearest emergency department, while supporting the patient with bag-valve-mask ventilation over an oral airway or with an airway adjunct.

In the past, esophageal obturator airways were used for the latter; esophageal obturator airways are inserted blindly and intentionally into the esophagus. They provide a means for assisted positive pressure ventilation in the setting in which the prehospital provider is either unable or unqualified to endotracheally intubate the patient. An improved version of the esophageal obturator airway is the Combitube (Sheridan Catheter Corp., Argyle, New York), which is also inserted blindly but is then functional even if the tube is inadvertently inserted into the trachea[7-9]; the esophageal obturator airway is not.

The Combitube (Fig. 4-2) is a double-barrel tube with designated esophageal and distal balloons. It can be attached to an Ambu bag without a face mask and seal, which is another advantage over the esophageal obturator airway. If positive pressure ventilation (PPV) through the esophagus-designated lumen yields gastric insufflation, the tube is assumed to be in the trachea and the Combitube acts as an endotracheal tube. If PPV yields lung expansion, the Combitube acts as an endotracheal tube. If the tube is inadvertently placed in the esophagus, ventilation occurs through side holes and a gastric tube can be passed through the trachea-designated lumen.

Emergency Department

The patient in medical arrest in the emergency department is intubated orally in the quickest manner possible. Occasionally a lighted stylet[10] or fiberoptic scope[10-12] is used as an adjunct. In contrast to the prehospital setting, it is unacceptable to temporize with bag-valve-mask ventilation in the emergency department; if oral intubation is unsuccessful, an emergent surgical airway is indicated.

THE MULTIPLE TRAUMA PATIENT
Prehospital

The primary consideration in the multiple trauma victim with a compromised airway is expeditious airway management with stabilization of the cervical spine. Many studies[4,13-15] have compared the various methods of intubation with respect to cervical spine stability; in the prehospital setting the

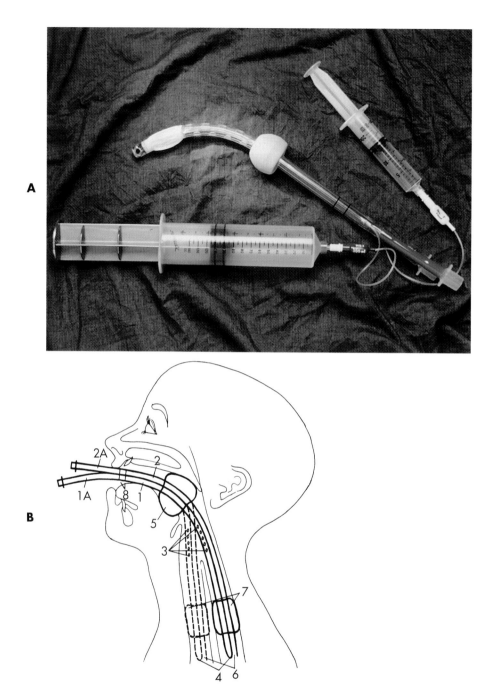

FIG. 4-2 **A,** Combitube dual-lumen airway. **B,** This tube is preferable to the esophageal obturator airway for prehospital use and for potential use in emergency departments. It is shown in cross section in esophageal *(solid lines)* and tracheal *(dotted lines)* positions. *1,* Esophageal lumen; *1A,* longer, blue connector leading to lumen 1; *2,* tracheal lumen; *2A,* shorter, clear connector leading to lumen 2; *3,* perforations of lumen; *4,* distal blocked end of lumen 1; *5,* pharyngeal balloon (holds 140 cc of air); *6,* distal open end of lumen 2; *7,* distal cuff for sealing esophagus or trachea (holds 20 cc of air); *8,* printed rings indicating depth of insertion. (From Frass M, Rödler S, Frenzer R et al: *J Trauma* 29:1476, 1989.)

orotracheal route is probably preferred. Many trauma victims have associated facial and head injuries that may complicate or contraindicate blind nasal intubation, and cricothyrotomy in the field (which is not permitted in many regions) is frequently associated with a poor outcome, although often because of overall injury severity, not necessarily because of the procedure.[16,17] When permitted, cricothyrotomy should be attempted in the field only when orotracheal intubation is repeatedly unsuccessful or is impossible, that is, when one is unable to visualize cords, massive upper airway bleeding occurs, or distorting injury exists; and when other temporizing modalities, such as bag-valve-mask, laryngeal mask, or transtracheal jet ventilation are unavailable or are unsuccessful.

Emergency Department

Although it may seem obvious, it is worthwhile to mention that when the airway is exposed, as might be the case for the unfortunate patient with a shotgun blast to the neck (Fig. 4-3), it should be directly intubated.

Fig. 4-4 illustrates classic examples of the admonition never to judge airways by first impressions. Fig. 4-4, *A* shows a patient with a tree branch through his neck. He was holding on to the branch to prevent it from moving. Fig. 4-4, *B* shows the wound site after removal of the branch. By some trick of fate, neither the airway nor major vessels were traumatized. This situation also high-

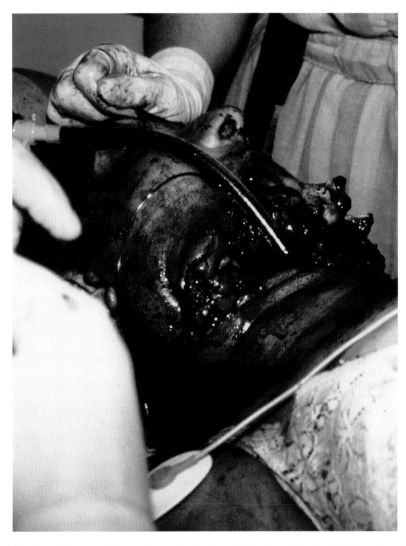

FIG. 4-3   Victim of shotgun blast to the neck, intubated directly with visualization of trachea through wound.

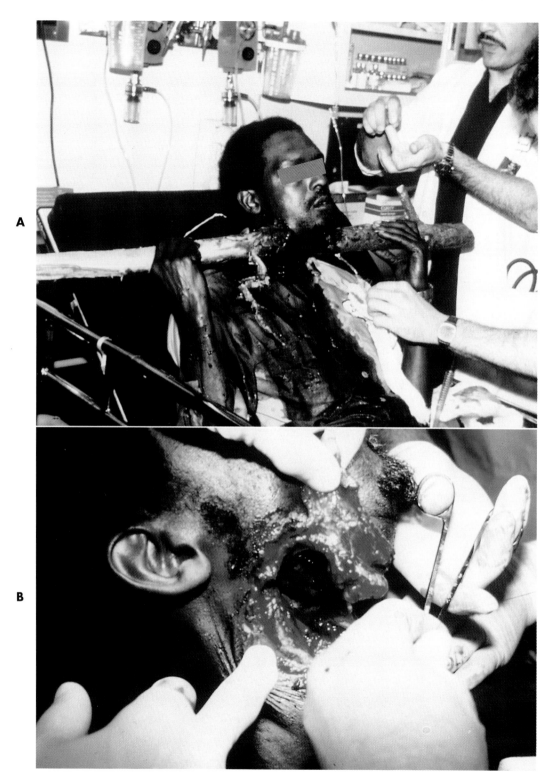

FIG. 4-4   A, Victim of tree-trunk penetration through neck. **B,** After removal of tree trunk, it was discovered that neither the airway nor major vessels were traumatized. (Courtesy Dr. Charles Pollack.)

lights the truism that foreign bodies should not be removed until the patient is in a controlled environment with assured airway and major vessel control.

In the emergency department the additional options of controlled paralysis before orotracheal intubation, intubation over a fiberoptic scope, and transtracheal jet ventilation are available. Every blunt trauma patient in the emergency department is presumed to have a cervical spine injury. Even with normal radiographs the patient with altered mental status caused by intoxication or injury must be treated as if an unstable injury is present because ligamentous disruptions may occur with minimal damage to static bony integrity. Cervical spine concerns in intubation are best addressed by balancing speed with expertise, that is, with a number of options available (blind nasal intubation, oral intubations with in-line stabilization with or without neuromuscular blockade, or cricothyrotomy). **The best option for a given patient is careful accomplishment of the method with which the operator is most facile!**

Blind nasal intubation is an option when the patient is breathing and cervical spinal (c-spine) control is adequate. Although it appears to be safe in the c-spine–injured patient, drawbacks include the potential for aspiration in a restrained patient, the unpredictable level of difficulty encountered, unexpected movement or gagging by the patient in response to laryngeal stimulation, and concurrent midface instability. Oral intubation in the blunt multitrauma patient is difficult primarily because of the need to protect the cervical spine. The intubating maneuver itself can cause c-spine shifts even when immobilization is adequate; cricoid pressure may also cause untoward movement. Axial traction on the neck may be inadvertently applied by an assistant who is straining to avoid blocking the view of the intubator. Only immobilization is needed. If neuromuscular blockade is induced, unsuccessful intubation becomes an even more apprehensive situation in the trauma patient when bag-valve-mask ventilation is precluded by facial trauma or oropharyngeal bleeding. Furthermore, paralysis and sedation compromise monitoring of the patient's neurologic status. Cricothyrotomy requires technical skill and some experience; it also has its own accepted set of complications. In skilled hands, however, cricothyrotomy provides a rapid, definitive airway that should not compromise c-spine integrity unless cricoid pressure is too excessively applied. In less experienced hands, one of the several commercially available cricotome kits, for example, NuTrake (International Medical Devices, Inc., Northridge, California) or the Melder catheter (Cook Critical Care, Bloomington, Indiana), may be helpful.

Transtracheal jet ventilation. Similarly, transtracheal jet ventilation may be an effective temporizing measure to support the ventilation of the trauma patient who cannot be intubated. The only universal contraindications to the technique are inadequate equipment and complete airway obstruction. Transtracheal jet ventilation is a positive-pressure ventilation technique that is probably significantly underused. There are animal studies and multiple anecdotal clinical reports to support its use, but, as of this writing, no prospective human trials have been published. The technique for establishing transtracheal jet ventilation is described as follows: Transtracheal jet ventilation is a method that requires expectant planning, specialized equipment, and familiarity with the anatomy and techniques involved. Improvisation with nonstandard equipment or untrained personnel should not be attempted in any clinical situation that demands such advanced airway management. The indications for transtracheal jet ventilation are the same as those listed in the chapter for other surgical airway modalities, namely, inability to intubate the airway from above because of direct trauma, adjacent trauma (e.g., profuse oropharyngeal bleeding), or nonvisualization of landmarks from other causes.

The only absolute contraindications to transtracheal jet ventilation are inadequate equipment and complete expiratory airway obstruction at or above the level of the vocal cords. The necessary equipment includes the following:

1. A source of oxygen of 50 psi, *in circuit preferably with a variable pressure regulator1*; (Hospital wall sources have this capability if no flow regulator is interposed.)
2. A transtracheal cannula of at least 14-gauge size, preferably with side holes[2];
3. A method of interrupting the flow of oxygen through the cannula to allow for exhalation through spontaneous relaxation of the chest wall. Commercial trigger valve kits with pressure-reducing valves are available for this purpose. The patient must be approached to as-

certain that, first, there is no complete expiratory obstruction (so that barotrauma does not result from inadequate lung emptying) and, second, the cricothyroid membrane can be physically identified just below the thyroid cartilage prominence. The catheter-over-needle assembly is then placed on a 10-cc syringe that may, at the operator's discretion, be filled with 1 to 3 cc of 2% plain lidocaine.

The catheter is then introduced at a 45-degree angle through the skin overlying the cricothyroid membrane. (Some authorities recommend making a nick in the skin with a #11 scalpel blade to each entry.) The right-handed operator should constantly exert negative pressure on the syringe plunger with the right thumb and with the left thumb and forefinger steadying the airway (see Chapter 5). When the trachea is entered, air is readily aspirated. If the syringe contains lidocaine, this may now be injected into the trachea, expelling any tissue plugs and suppressing the subsequent cough reflex. *It should be noted, however, that the lidocaine may provoke a cough in the unprepared patient, prompting unexpected movement of the patient's neck.* In the potentially c-spine–injured trauma patient, this is a most untoward complication.

Once free flow of air has been established, the catheter should be advanced over the needle into the neck until the hub reaches the skin. The catheter should be secured; then the tubing is connected to it. Positive-pressure ventilation is gently begun in short bursts while the patient is monitored for evidence of satisfactory lung inflation and the absence of appearance of subcutaneous emphysema.

After placement is deemed acceptable, the ventilatory rate should be 12 to 20 insufflations/min in adults and up to 30 insufflations/min in children. Manual insufflations should be held for around 1 second each, with a pressure (if a variable pressure regulator is in place) only sufficient to allow adequate chest rise. Arterial blood gases should be monitored frequently during transtracheal jet ventilation. Successful ventilation can generally be maintained for 30 minutes or more while a more definitive airway is established.

The following are complications of transtracheal jet ventilation that can occur:

Arterial perforation	Hematoma
Bleeding	Hemoptysis
Erosion of tracheal mucosa	Mediastinal emphysema
Esophageal puncture	Pneumothorax
Exhalation difficulty	Subcutaneous emphysema

Finally, in the semielective intubation of a stable patient with a known c-spine injury, fiberoptic-aided intubation should be considered. This technique allows for minimal disturbance of the neck trauma to the airway. Adequate topical anesthesia should be applied before inserting the fiberscope because an untoward cough could jeopardize c-spine stability.

In a recent review, Walls[18] concluded that there is no literature to support advocating any one individual approach over another in managing the traumatized airway. Therefore the operator is the critical variable; the emergency physician must be skilled in a variety of standard and surgical airway maneuvers and must exercise sound judgment in determining which approach to apply in a given clinical situation.

The other major concern in emergency department airway management is the patient with a head injury. Frequently patients present with a deteriorating airway and obvious or indirect evidence of elevated intracranial pressure. These patients are best managed with a rapid sequence induction using pharmacologic agents that blunt the adverse hemodynamic and intracranial pressure effects of intubation. Current recommendations for these patients are pretreatment with a defasciculating dose of vecuronium, then lidocaine (1.5 mg/kg IV) and fentanyl (3 µg/kg IV); this is followed by sedation with thiopental (3 to 5 mg/kg IV, 0.5 to 1 mg/kg IV if the patient is hypotensive) and paralysis with succinylcholine.[19] Atracurium (0.4 mg/kg IV) is a safer paralytic agent with respect to induced increases in intracranial pressure, but when using it, the physician must accept its slower duration of action in comparison with succinylcholine.

THE SEIZING PATIENT
Prehospital and Emergency Department

The primary objective in airway control during ictal events is to support oxygenation until clonic contractions of the jaw and mouth subside. This includes placing bite blocks for protection of the tongue, positioning maneuvers such as jaw thrust to keep the tongue from occluding the airway, suctioning of secretions, and providing supplemental oxygen. Thiamine and glucose should be considered for treating underlying metabolic derangements. Benzodiazepines should be administered promptly to treat the seizure activity if it does not resolve spontaneously. Should the seizure activity persist to the point of cyanosis or other objective evidence of desaturation, these drugs also serve as sedation if used before emergent paralysis and oral intubation. Patients who are paralyzed should promptly be given a loading dose of intravenous phenytoin or, occasionally, phenobarbital because neuromuscular blockade prevents ongoing monitoring for recurrent ictal activity.

During the postictal period, when patients who are having seizures arrive in the emergency department, the primary concerns are hypoventilation, lingual airway obstruction, and vomiting with aspiration. These complications can frequently be addressed without endotracheal intubation if the patient did not require a definitive airway during the seizure.

THE COMBATIVE PATIENT

Prehospital

The agitated, combative patient is all too frequently encountered in the prehospital setting, where resources for both chemical and physical restraint are frequently limited and the safety of medical personnel is often uncertain. The combative patient should always be presumed to be hypoxemic and should be managed as such until proven otherwise. Although in certain scenarios hypoglycemia, intoxication, or head trauma may readily appear to provide an explanation for erratic behavior, airway management and provision of supplemental oxygen remains the first priority. **When restraint is required in the prehospital setting to assess and manage the airway, physical means are generally preferred over pharmaceutic agents. Physical control, when possible, allows for definitive intervention aimed at potentially correctable causes of agitation that, once addressed, should alleviate the need for chemical restraint.** This policy also avoids possible interactions between administered sedatives and intoxicants that are already affecting the patient. Still, if the safety of the patient or prehospital personnel is at risk, sedation is clearly indicated to allow safe and prompt transportation of the patient to the emergency department.

Most prehospital systems do not stock their ambulances with neuroleptics, which are the first-line drugs for chemical restraint in the emergency department. However, benzodiazepines such as diazepam and lorazepam are available in the field because of their use in seizures. Therefore the combative patient who requires chemical restraint in the prehospital setting should be given a benzodiazepine. The goal of sedation is to secure the patient for safe transport and to allow for intervention that might stabilize him or her while in the field. The airway must be managed expectantly because of the possibility of respiratory depression with these drugs, particularly if alcohol or narcotics have been ingested by the patient. Patients who are combative with an unstable airway should be pretreated with benzodiazepines to facilitate endotracheal intubation.

Emergency Department

As in the prehospital setting, physical restraint is generally preferred over chemical sedation in managing the combative patient. Hypoxia, hypoglycemia, intoxication, and head injury are, again, the initial etiologies to be considered and immediately addressed. When chemical restraint is necessary to carry out these evaluations and stabilizing measures, haloperidol may be the drug of choice.

Haloperidol has been demonstrated to be safe and effective in a broad clinical experience.[20-22] With proper patient monitoring, an appropriate starting dose is 5 mg IV or IM, if necessary. The routes are roughly equivalent in terms of effect, but not speed of onset. Subsequent doses are given every 5 to 10 minutes until the desired level of sedation is achieved. A good guideline for subsequent doses is to double the preceding dose, for example, the second dose of haloperidol is 10 mg IV and the third, 20 mg IV.[21,23,24] However, this introduces the possibility of ventilatory compromise that haloperidol alone does not cause.

It should be noted that haloperidol is *not* recommended for patients who are thought to be acutely intoxicated with cocaine because neuroleptics lower the seizure threshold and may thereby contribute to airway compromise. In this specific case, benzodiazepines alone are indicated for behavior control. Neuromuscular blockade with succinylcholine remains the modality of last resort.

Other medications useful in airway management in the combative patient, either as part of a rapid sequence induction or for brief sedation, include short-acting barbiturates such as methohexital (Brevital) and rapidly metabolized narcotics such as fentanyl (Sublimaze).[23]

THE POISONED PATIENT
Prehospital

Overdoses comprise a significant proportion of ambulance calls and emergency department visits. Fortunately, it is rare that toxicity from prescription, over-the-counter, or illicit drugs and intoxicants results in true airway compromise. Aggressive airway intervention in the poisoned patient should always await treatment with glucose (or a prompt bedside blood glucose assay) and nalozone. Vomiting with aspiration is a primary concern in this setting and must be anticipated before any airway intervention is attempted. Gastric decontamination in the field after known toxic ingestion is fraught with complications and, barring a prolonged transport time, should probably be limited to alert patients voluntarily drinking activated charcoal. The key to successful prehospital management of the poisoned patient is prompt and accurate recognition of deterioration or the potential for deterioration as early as possible.

Emergency Department

Overdose patients in the emergency department fall into one of several categories: alert with a protected airway, lethargic with a compromised airway, combative, seizing, or comatose. Glucose, thiamine, naloxone, and any specific antidote for the toxin should be considered in all cases. Management of the alert patient is dependent on the need for gastric emptying. The indications for lavage have narrowed considerably over the past several years[24,25] but remain beyond the scope of this text. If, however, gastric emptying is deemed necessary in an alert patient, the need for airway protection with sedation and blind nasal intubation or rapid sequence induction and intubation depends on the potential of the ingestant or intoxicant to produce sudden deterioration in mental status or seizures (see the box on p. 61). If lavage is deemed unnecessary, activated charcoal may be given orally or via a nasogastric tube as the sole method of detoxification with only expectant airway management.

Lethargic patients with respiratory distress, a poor gag reflex, or bradypnea should be intubated, particularly if there is a long-acting toxin on board that is likely to result in a persistently decreased level of consciousness. Combative patients should be managed as outlined previously to protect themselves and emergency department personnel from injury. Combative behavior should never automatically be ascribed to intoxication; hypoxia, head injury, and infectious encephalopathy must always be considered! Seizing toxic patients are properly managed as outlined previously for other ictal states, with intubation indicated only for obvious hypoxemia or prolonged seizure activity. Benzodiazepines are first-line therapy; failure of seizures to respond to these drugs should prompt suspicion of significant head injury, severe hypoxia, or isoniazid ingestion (for which the antidote is pyridoxine). Comatose poisoned patients are managed as arrest patients (after failure of naloxone)[26] if the airway is not protected, if there is significant hypoxemia, or if gastric emptying is required. If the patient is ventilating well but is unresponsive to external stimuli (as in a deep alcoholic inebriation), the patient may be managed expectantly with close observation. In the rare case of caustic ingestion with a compromised airway, fiberoptic intubation is useful for visualizing tissue damage and thereby minimizing the trauma associated with passing an endotracheal tube along the injured tissues.

THE PEDIATRIC PATIENT
Prehospital and Emergency Department

The primary airway problems encountered in emergency pediatrics center around (1) differences in anatomy between infants, children, and adults and (2) the anxiety that generally attends pediatric resuscitations. The latter concern is to be expected. Only repeated exposure and practice—unusual in all but high-acuity dedicated pediatric emergency departments—address it directly.

Anatomic differences are important in four primary areas: the availability of the proper equipment, adequate cord visualization during intubation, the significance of acute epiglottitis, and the typical sites of upper airway obstruction. There are several memory aids to determine the appropri-

TOXINS LIKELY TO PRODUCE COMA OR SEIZURES

Coma	Seizures
Narcotics	Anticholinergic agents
Sedative hypnotics	Organophosphates
Benzodiazepines	Physostigmine
Barbiturates	Antihistamines
Cyanide	Antidepressants
Hydrogen sulfide	Antipsychotics
Carbon monoxide	Beta-adrenergic blockers
Nicotinic acid	Camphor
Phencyclidine (PCP)	Chlorambucil
Glutethimide	Cocaine, lidocaine
Alcohols	Cycloserine
Methanol	Cyclosporin A
Ethylene glycol	Ergonovine
Ethanol	Folic acid
Isopropanol	Hypoglycemic agents
Anticonvulsants	Isoniazid
Phenytoin	Methylxanthines (theophylline)
Valproic acid	Metronidazole
Others	Nalidixic acid
Monoamine oxidase inhibitors	Narcotics
Tricyclic antidepressants	Phencyclidine (PCP)
Antihistamines	Sympathomimetics
Bromides	Amphetamines
Tranquilizers	Ephedrine
	Terbutaline
	Phenytoin

From Tesar GE, Murray GB, Cassem NH: *J Clin Psychopharmacol* 5:344, 1985.

ate size for an endotracheal tube and laryngoscope blade when intubating an infant or child. Some involve arithmetic (for example, age in years + 16 ÷ 4), and others involve body parts (for example, the size of the fifth finger or the nare). These are available in standard textbooks such as *Pediatric Advanced Life Support.* It is incumbent on the emergency department and medical control physicians who supervise paramedics to assure that a sufficient array of equipment is available to address these measurements once they are made. A useful tool is the Broselow Resuscitation Tape (Armstrong Medical Industries, San Diego, California), a body-length–based algorithm that folds into the physician's pocket and gives ready guidelines for tube sizes, medication doses,[27] and other information useful in pediatric resuscitations.[28]

The pediatric larynx is relatively more anterior and superior to the oropharynx than in adults and may be partially obscured by adenoidal, tonsillar, or epiglottic hypertrophy. The tendency to hyperextend the neck in an attempt to bring the airway structures into the viewing line of the laryngoscope is counterproductive in children in whom laryngeal cartilaginous support is lacking. The larynx is usually too anterior for this maneuver to afford significant benefit, and the trachea will collapse against the cervical vertebral bodies, further compromising ventilation during the procedure. It is more helpful to place the infant's head in the sniffing position and then gently, so as to avoid damage to the esophageal introitus, pass the laryngoscope blade as far into the airway as possible. Careful, methodic withdrawal of the laryngoscope then allows the larynx to "fall into view" for the operator.

The management of epiglottitis (supraglottitis) has prompted establishment of protocols in essentially every acute care hospital. The primary concerns in the prehospital and emergency department care of these children are to avoid stressing them as much as possible, as long as they are oxygenating well (pulse oximetry is essential in this scenario); to arrange promptly for definitive airway management in the operating room where adequate facilities, medications, and personnel are available for orotracheal intubations, fiberoptic-aided intubation, or tracheostomy; and to realize, before moving the patient in the operating room, that reasonable oxygenation can generally be maintained through positive pressure ventilation with a bag-valve-mask with a tight face seal. The key to successful management of these patients is to avoid delay in establishing a definitive airway. Preestablished cooperative protocols between emergency medicine, anesthesiology, and otolaryngology are the best way to do this.

Finally, the point of minimum diameter in the pediatric airway is subglottic, as opposed to the level of the true cords in adults. This indicates that cricothyrotomy as a surgical airway is contraindicated in children under the age of 6 to 8 years with upper airway obstructions because it places an airway likely proximal to the point of obstruction. Children also are poor candidates for cricothyrotomy because of the lack of cartilaginous airway support in this area with subsequent poor healing. Tracheostomy, therefore, is the surgical airway of choice in the pediatric age group. This is a procedure with which few emergency physicians and even fewer paramedics will ever gain sufficient familiarity; furthermore, it is technically more difficult than cricothyrotomy. Commercially available kits use either the Seldinger techniques or serial dilations (an example is Rapi-Trach, Premier Medical Products, Norristown, Pennsylvania), procedures with which emergency physicians are more comfortable for tracheostomy, and these may warrant investigation in individual institutions.

CONCLUSION

Airway management by the emergency physician is complicated by (1) his or her responsible role as medical control for prehospital personnel, (2) the variety of emergent insults to airway integrity for which he or she must be prepared, (3) the concern and responsibility for the detection and stabilization of associated injuries in the trauma victim, and (4) the frequent absence of preparation prompted by the unexpected arrival of a critically ill or injured patient. Of these, the first, second, and fourth complications are addressed by compulsive training, retraining, and clinical testing of the emergency physician and his or her subordinates. The third concern is best confronted by a methodic, algorithmic approach to the multiple trauma patient by the emergency physician in cooperation with surgery, anesthesiology, and ancillary colleagues, just as airway emergencies in the critically ill patient are managed in consultation with internists, intensivists, and anesthesiologists. Interdisciplinary collaboration is essential to the efficacious care of the emergency department patient with a compromised airway.

REFERENCES

1. Siegel JH, Farrell EJ, Miller M et al: Cardiorespiratory interactions as determinants of survival and the need for respiratory support in human shock states, *J Trauma* 23:976-981, 1973.
2. Copass MK, Oreskovich MR, Bladergroen MR et al: Prehospital cardiopulmonary resuscitation of the critically injured patient, *Am J Surg* 148:20-26, 1984.
3. Pepe PE, Copas MK, Joyce TH: Prehospital endotracheal intubation: rationale for training emergency medical personnel, *Ann Emerg Med* 14:1085-1092, 1985.
4. Knopp RK: The safety of orotracheal intubation in patients with suspected cervical spine injury, *Ann Emerg Med* 19:603-604, 1990.
5. Benhamou D, Girault C, Faure C et al: Nasal mask ventilation in acute respiratory failure: experience in elderly patients, *Chest* 102:912-917, 1992.
6. Meduri GU, Abou-Shala N, Fox RC et al: Noninvasive face mask mechanical ventilation in patients with acute hypercapnic respiratory failure, *Chest* 100:445-454, 1992.

7. Atherton GL, Johnson JC: Ability of paramedics to use the Combitube in prehospital cardiac arrest, *Ann Emerg Med* 22:1263-1268, 1993.

8. Frass M, Rödler S, Frenzer R et al: Esophageal tracheal Combitube, endotracheal airway, and mask: comparison of ventilatory pressure curves, *J Trauma* 29:1476-1479, 1989.

9. Verdille VP, Chiang JL, Bedger R et al: Nasotracheal Combitube in prehospital cardiac arrest, *Ann Emerg Med* 22:1263-1268, 1993.

10. Delaney KA, Hessler R: Emergency flexible fiberoptic nasotracheal intubation: a report of 60 cases, *Ann Emerg Med* 17:919-926, 1988.

11. Purcell T: Fiberscopic assisted intubation. In Daily RH, Simon B, Young GP et al (eds): *The airway: emergency management,* St Louis, 1992, Mosby.

12. Afialo M, Guttman A, Stern E et al: Fiberoptic intubation in the emergency department: a case series, *J Emerg Med* 11:387-391, 1993.

13. Rhee KJ, Green W, Holcroft JW et al: Oral intubation in the multiply-injured patient: the risk of exacerbating spinal cord damage, *Ann Emerg Med* 19:45-48, 1990.

14. Holley J, Jorden RC: Airway management in patients with unstable cervical spine fractures, *Ann Emerg Med* 18:151-153, 1989.

15. Joyce SM: Cervical spine immobilization during orotracheal intubation in trauma victims, *Ann Emerg Med* 17:145, 1988.

16. Spaite DW, Joseph M: Prehospital cricothyrotomy: an investigation of the indications, technique, complications, and patient outcome, *Ann Emerg Med* 19:101-107, 1990.

17. Miklus RM, Elliot C, Snow N: Surgical cricothyrotomy in the field: experience of a helicopter transport team, *J Trauma* 29:506-508, 1989.

18. Walls RM: Airway management in the blunt trauma patient: how important is the cervical spine? *Can J Surg* 35:27-30, 1992.

19. Walls RM: Rapid-sequence induction in head trauma, *Ann Emerg Med* 22:1008-1013, 1993.

20. Adams F: Emergency intravenous sedation of the delirious, medically ill patient, *J Clin Psychiatry* 49(Suppl):22-26, 1988.

21. Silverstein S, Frommer DA, Marx JA et al: Parenteral haloperidol in combative patients: a prospective study (abstract), *Ann Emerg Med* 15:636, 1986.

22. Clinton JE, Sterner S, Steimachers Z et al: Haloperidol for sedation of disruptive emergency patients, *Ann Emerg Med* 16:319-322, 1987.

23. Tesar GE, Murray GB, Cassem NH: Use of high dose intravenous haloperidol in the treatment of agitated cardiac patients, *J Clin Psychopharmacol* 5:344-347, 1985.

24. Rosen P: Vitamin H and how to use it, *J Emerg Med* 10:753-755, 1992.

25. Magnusson R: Overdoses. In Dailey RH, Simon B, Young GP et al (eds): *The airway: emergency management,* St Louis, 1992, Mosby.

26. Rumack BH: *POISONDEX Information System,* Denver, 1990, Micromedex.

27. Lubitz A, Seidel JS, Chameides L et al: A rapid method of estimating weight and resuscitation drug dosages from length in the pediatric age group, *Ann Emerg Med* 17:576-581, 1988.

28. Kulig K, Bar-Or D, Cantrill S et al: Management of acutely poisoned patients without gastric emptying, *Ann Emerg Med* 14:562-567, 1985.

CHAPTER **5**

General Anesthetic Management

ALLAN C. D. BROWN

One of the most frightening experiences for the practicing anesthesiologist is to find unexpectedly that, having induced anesthesia, he or she is unable to maintain the patient's oxygenation. Fortunately, the truly difficult airway that requires heroic methods to control occurs infrequently, although unanticipated difficulties with intubation have been variously reported in 3% to 5% of all patients requiring general anesthesia.[1] As other elements of anesthesia practice become more sophisticated, from the precision of anesthetic pharmacology to the refinement of anesthetic gas machines and monitors, the relative importance of airway management is increasing as a major contributor to anesthetic morbidity and mortality.[2] Because death or serious morbidity can and does result from these technical misfortunes, the anesthesiologist is obliged to become familiar with the several management techniques that may be applied to avert disaster.

MANIFESTATION OF THE COMPROMISED AIRWAY

It is useful to divide patients with airway problems into three general groups according to the manner in which they present to the anesthesiologist: (1) patients in extremis (near death), (2) patients in distress, and (3) patients with occult impending obstruction.

Patients in extremis have severe airway obstruction associated with hypoxia, hypercarbia, delirium, or unconsciousness. This is an emergency, and cardiac arrest supervenes unless the airway is reestablished quickly. The overwhelming consideration is time, and the prime objective is to reestablish patient oxygenation immediately. The treatment for hypoxia is to reestablish or maximize oxygenation. Because a patient in extremis may already be unconscious with total airway obstruction or in extreme distress with some residual airway, rapid assessment is required to determine initial management. If the airway is totally obstructed, an attempt to reoxygenate by mask with an oral airway is required as a first step. Rapid laryngoscopy can then be used to ascertain whether an oral endotracheal tube may be passed. If these maneuvers should prove, in any way, difficult (i.e., cannot be achieved with one attempt), all further efforts should be abandoned and an airway should be secured from below the larynx. This may be effected with emergency tracheotomy, cricothyrotomy, or transcricothyroid or transtracheal jet ventilation and should be undertaken where the patient is first seen. Only when adequate oxygenation has been reestablished should the patient be moved to the operating room for formal intubation or tracheotomy.

If the airway is not totally obstructed when first encountered, the patient is usually agitated and may be sufficiently hypoxic to be confused and uncooperative. In this circumstance the prime consideration is to maximize effective oxygen intake with minimum airway interference with the intent of avoiding turning partial obstruction into total obstruction. Thus 100% oxygen is administered by mask, and, if hypoxia is relieved, the patient is transferred to the operating room before any further intervention.

The reader is cautioned not to take these two separate scenarios in a dogmatic context. A partial obstruction may turn into total obstruction with minor stimulus and little warning. The purpose of the description is to concentrate attention on the fact that the prime consideration is to reestablish patient oxygenation. If a patient is moving any air into the lungs past an incomplete obstruction, he or she may respond well to 100% inspired oxygen by mask, but the airway still can become totally obstructed during transport. Thus the means for laryngoscopy, intubation, and sublaryngeal airway control must accompany the patient to the operating room. The patient who does not respond well to raising the inspired oxygen concentration alone may be improved by having an oral airway placed. Note that this action can also precipitate total obstruction in an irritable airway, requiring the more invasive immediate intervention described earlier. Many such patients require nothing more than laryngoscopy to raise a relaxed tongue bulk or a swollen epiglottis to remove the obstruction and permit oxygenation. Intubation of the airway itself may pose no difficulty when the prime problem is an incidental pathologic condition superimposed on an essentially normal airway. However, this fact cannot be known in advance of laryngoscopy, and, because time is short, alternative means for gaining control must be available. **The one pitfall that should be avoided in those patients who are confused and uncooperative is the use of sedative and anesthetic drugs, which can abolish any airway remaining to the patient.**

Patients in distress represent the largest group of patients who require anesthesia with a compromised airway. Such patients may exhibit stridor, labored breathing, tracheal tug, intercostal retraction, and agitation, but they are alert and cooperative. The distressed patient is usually becoming fatigued by the time the anesthesiologist arrives but is still able to compensate for airway difficulties sufficiently to maintain adequate oxygenation. With such patients the anesthesiologist and the surgeon are permitted the luxury of time to plan for careful airway management. Patients with respiratory distress through established or progressive partial obstruction of the airway are usually agitated and conscious of dyspnea. They tend to adopt a sitting or erect posture and endeavor to "straighten" their airway to reduce resistance to breathing. The neck is flexed and the head extended, sometimes with protrusion of the tongue. The fists are clenched and arms rigid and forced into the bed, thereby fixing the pectoral girdle, which enables the full force of the accessory muscles of inspiration and expiration to be brought into action. Such an appearance of struggling for air must be recognized as characteristic and calls for prompt but not immediate action to relieve the situation.

Patients with occult impending obstruction on cursory physical examination give few clues to suggest the management problems that follow the induction of anesthesia. They volunteer little information in their histories to suggest airway difficulties, and the first intimation that the unwary anesthesiologist may have of an occult airway problem is when the patient is medicated or manipulated. This situation occurs in patients with some supraglottic tumors and base of tongue neoplasms or with congenital deformities, usually arising from the second branchial arch for which the patient normally compensates with muscular effort. The major challenge in this group of patients is to detect that a problem exists before anesthesia is induced. This enables a full evaluation to be undertaken in a facility such as a difficult airway clinic and the formulation of an anesthetic plan that has some assurance of success. The detection of the initial problem frequently relies on eliciting a careful detailed history, with specific leading questions as required. Of particular interest are previous anesthetic intubation difficulties, a history of heavy snoring, or obstructive sleep apnea. Sleep apnea may be represented only as a story of unexplained early wakening, but when the patient's spouse or bedmate is questioned, a more accurate history of "choking" followed by the patient's awakening is obtained. A history of congenital abnormalities of hearing or of the heart should also alert the anesthesiologist to the possibility of involvement of structures arising from the second branchial arch.

For convenience, the problems posed as falling into these three distinct groups for the following reasons are discussed: (1) the short time available for successful management of the patient in extremis, (2) the urgent but carefully considered management of the patient in distress, and (3) the diagnostic acumen and experience required to detect a patient with occult problems that require careful anesthetic management. However, this division is artificial, and, in reality, the groups tend to merge into a continuum, in which management depends on the degree of hypoxia, hypercarbia, and distress, which, in turn, dictates the rapidity of intervention.

Within this continuum two distinct problems may exist: (1) the truly difficult airway in which abnormal anatomy and a superimposed pathologic condition render the maintenance of a mask airway or the technical feat of intubation difficult and (2) the relatively more normal airway with only pathologic changes leading to obstruction, which, once bypassed, do not pose intubation or mask problems. In the absence of hypoxia there is sufficient time to unravel these problems in the individual patient and to develop a cogent anesthetic plan in conjunction with the operating surgeon.

GENERAL PRINCIPLES OF MANAGEMENT OF THE COMPROMISED AIRWAY

When the absence of hypoxia permits the time required for patient evaluation, an anesthetic plan may be made, offering some reasonable hope for success in every patient with a compromised airway. The options for anesthetic management depend greatly on the preferences and skills of the anesthesiologist. **Whatever options are decided, two precautions should be observed in every patient:**

1. **The patient's spontaneous respiration should not be abolished until the airway is secured.**
2. **The surgeon should be scrubbed and standing by in the operating room, ready to do an immediate tracheotomy, if required.**

The prime objective in management is to bypass the obstruction and to gain control of the airway, either from above the larynx with an endotracheal tube or from below with a tube passed through either a tracheotomy or a cricothyrotomy incision. Passing an endotracheal tube through the larynx from above is always more desirable because the long-term morbidity associated with this approach is less than that associated with a tracheal incision.[3] However, the anesthesiologist must consider whether the patient's obstructive process can be expected to resolve within the time limit that an endotracheal tube may be left in place. The surgeon should be consulted. If the technical difficulties posed by the patient's condition are great and a tracheotomy would be needed later in any case, the patient's interest may be best served with a tracheotomy under local infiltration anesthesia in the first instance. However, whenever possible, the airway should be controlled with a cuffed endotracheal tube before a tracheotomy is performed to protect the airway against operative bleeding or technical difficulties in placing the tracheostomy tube.

If the airway cannot be controlled from above, a tracheotomy must be performed under local infiltration without the benefit of a cuffed endotracheal tube and its protection against aspiration of blood and secretions, thus precluding any sedation until after the airway is controlled.

Premedication

The patient should be brought to the operating room without any narcotic or sedative premedication. **Even small doses of sedatives can turn a partial obstruction into a complete obstruction with alarming rapidity.** Should this occur on the ward, unseen and remote from those with the means to intervene effectively, the result can be fatal. The use of an antisialagogue such as atropine, glycopyrrolate, or scopolamine is optional when general anesthesia is planned. On the one hand, in patients with pathologic conditions that lead to difficulty in handling secretions, a preoperative antisialagogue may improve their agitation and general condition; on the other hand, the drying effect of antisialagogues can increase airway irritability and make the gentle positioning of instruments more difficult. When an awake intubation with topical anesthesia is intended, an antisialagogue is usually required to enhance the effectiveness of topical "paint-up" and to facilitate fiberoptic visualization.

The patient's usual medication for chronic medical conditions should not be forgotten. In patients with distress, swallowing may have been difficult for some time and routine oral medications may have been ignored, requiring appropriate evaluation and parenteral administration before operation.

Transport to Operating Room

The patient in severe distress should be transported to the operating room on a stretcher accompanied by a source of oxygen with a mask and a means of giving positive pressure assistance for ventilation, such as an Ambu bag (Mercury Medical, Tampa, Fla.). In addition, a means of controlling the airway from below the larynx must accompany the patient, for example, an emergency tracheostomy tray, a cricothyrotomy kit, or a jet ventilation cart. The purpose of the trolley is to permit the switch from spontaneous to controlled ventilation in the supine position. **The patient should not be forced to lie down if the dyspnea is better tolerated in the sitting position.** In a patient who is in less distress, it is appropriate to permit transport in a hospital wheelchair. In either situation it is important that the anesthesiologist and the surgeon fetch the patient in person, accompanied by at least one assistant, thereby providing two pairs of trained hands and a "runner" in the event of an emergency.

Preparation and Monitoring

Once the patient has arrived in the operating room, three options for positioning for anesthetic induction are available, depending on the clinical circumstances:

1. The sitting position with the operating table appropriately conformed for the patient's comfort is the most common position for the patient in distress. It facilitates respiratory excursion and permits the patient to maintain the fixity of the pectoral girdle. It is the ideal position for the application of a topical anesthetic and for most intubation maneuvers in the awake patient. However, should direct rigid laryngoscopy be required, the anesthesiologist must still work from behind the patient's head and usually requires something stable on which to stand, such as an operating room lift, to achieve the correct working height relative to the patient's head.

2. The right tonsil position is used much less commonly for those patients who have active bleeding or free pus in the airway. The tonsil position, with or without a minimum of head-down tilt on the operating table, facilitates the passive drainage of liquids away from the larynx out of the mouth and dependent nostril. This position is used in conjunction with inhalation induction of general anesthesia. The type of problems managed in this way include a posttonsillectomy secondary hemorrhage, bleeding from biopsy sites in or around the larynx, and ruptured retropharyngeal abscess. The position is particularly useful in managing induction in the patient with active hematemesis.

3. The supine position is suitable only for patients with airway difficulties in the absence of significant respiratory distress. Thus it tends to be limited to those patients with occult problems for which a viable anesthetic plan has already been formulated, with alternative approaches, should obstruction occur during induction of anesthesia. If vomiting or loss of the airway occurs before intubation is achieved in this position, disaster may be averted by turning the patient into the tonsil position, which aids drainage maneuvers and tends to throw the patient's tongue forward, thus making a mask airway easier to maintain. In an emergency situation, turning a patient from one position to another requires the help of several trained assistants.

Two particular groups of patients are worth noting in passing: the morbidly obese patient and the woman in labor. The morbidly obese patient may derive airway difficulties from obesity itself or from several more usual causes of abnormal basic anatomy or disease. However, the sheer bulk of the patient makes it difficult to manage the induction of general anesthesia in anything other than the supine position. A moderate reverse Trendelenburg position on the table may facilitate respiratory excursion, although at some risk of hypotension and aspiration, should vomiting occur. The parturient requires that particular precautions be taken against hypotension, which makes the sitting position for induction of general anesthesia less desirable. The tonsil position is usually too uncomfortable for most of these patients, and the usual left lateral wedge tilt in the supine position must be remembered to guard against supine hypotension at term.

Once the patient has been placed in the appropriate position for the procedure intended, monitors are applied. The extent of invasive monitoring is dictated by the patient's overall medical condition. However, the minimum standards of noninvasive monitoring recently promulgated by the American Society of Anesthesiologists[4] should be adhered to with all patients, including end-tidal CO_2, pulse oximetry, indirect blood pressure, temperature, and electrocardiogram. A well-secured intravenous line is started as a conduit for drugs, but the patient's arms should not be strapped to armboards or to the table but should be restrained by assistants in the event of excitement during induction. This ensures that the patient's position can be changed quickly, as needed, and that the intravenous line and monitor attachments remain functional during induction.

ANESTHETIC OPTIONS
The Question of Intubation

Once the patient with known or potential airway difficulty has been evaluated, an anesthesia plan can be formulated. Because a difficult airway usually translates into a difficult intubation to the anesthesiologist, the first question to be asked is whether intubation may be avoided, thereby nullifying the difficulty.

As a matter of convenience, it is too often forgotten that endotracheal intubation, like all other invasive medical procedures, has the following formal indications:

- Ventilatory support
- Airway protection
- Airway patency
- Access for surgery
- Tracheal toilet
- Special techniques
- Reduction of dead space

The indication for intubation in the particular patient should be established. Many patients who have airways that are difficult to intubate may be managed perfectly well with a mask for general anesthesia, provided the operative procedure is suitable. Even better, general anesthesia may be avoided altogether with local infiltration or conduction blockade.

However, the reverse of this argument must also be considered. **Just because an operation can be managed with a local anesthetic technique does not relieve the anesthesiologist of the responsibility of planning for general anesthesia with endotracheal intubation.** Intubation may be required in a hurry during a local anesthetic procedure for several reasons. Even light sedation may lead to obstruction of a marginal airway in an awake patient. A spinal anesthetic may migrate too high. A technical complication (e.g., pneumothorax in association with a supraclavicular block) may demand emergency intubation. The patient's airway problem may worsen acutely during the operation, or he or she may not be able to tolerate the positioning for the time required to complete the operation.

Awake intubation. As a basic rule, no anesthetic drugs of any sort should be given to the patient until a formal plan to secure the airway has been developed and the necessary equipment and personnel have been assembled. If the anesthesiologist decides that intubation is a reasonable course, a decision must be made between awake intubation and passing the tube while the patient is under general anesthesia. Some physicians maintain that awake intubation is safer because the patient's protective reflexes are maintained, but experience suggests that this argument has been exaggerated. The technique of awake intubation is not pleasant for the patient, and, even with the utmost care and concern, the patient's cooperation cannot be guaranteed. If the physician takes the time to meticulously prepare the patient with topical anesthesia to the oral structures, the base of the tongue, and the larynx, there certainly is a better chance for atraumatic intubation, but this obviates the original argument of maintaining protective reflexes. The addition of sedative drugs may compound the problem further and indeed on occasion lead to loss of the airway. Spraying the larynx with a local anesthetic agent can itself produce laryngospasm in an irritable airway. It is true that with some patients, usually in the older age groups, complete faith in the physician may permit a trouble-free intubation, but this is not so in many cases.

It is suggested that awake intubation be reserved for those patients in whom there is no firm indication for tracheotomy under local anesthetic but about whom the anesthesiologist has doubts in regard to safe airway management with the patient under general anesthesia. The "balance" of this decision between topical and general anesthesia changes with increasing levels of skill, experience, and confidence on the part of the endoscopist. However, the basic conflict between patient comfort with sufficient muscle relaxation to achieve intubation with sedation or general anesthesia versus the risk of losing the airway or not reducing patient muscle tone sufficiently to achieve intubation remains.

The larynx and its adjacent structures are part of a muscular organ of great strength. This muscle strength is required to fulfill the function of the "glottal stop" mechanism that allows the fixation of the thorax to bring the full potential power of the muscles of the pectoral girdle to bear. These closure muscles are under both voluntary and reflex control and, if not suitably obtunded, may prevent successful intubation of the trachea. The following clinical maxims may help the practitioner decide where the balance lies for a particular patient:

1. The problem highest in the airway usually dictates the choice of intubation technique.
2. Always beware of edema in the airway.
3. If fiberoptic technique is considered a good option, *use it first!*

4. Fiberoptic techniques can be used while the patient is either awake or asleep, but the narrow pharyngeal airway is almost always widest open in the sitting position.

5. The patient who cannot maintain his or her own airway when awake and supine is not suited for general anesthesia induction except in limited circumstances (e.g., bilateral fractures of the mandibular ramus).

6. The patient with copious secretions, blood, or pus in the pharynx is rarely suitable for fiberoptic techniques.

7. The greater the degree of "audible" dyspnea and visible distress, the more likely the patient's airway is to be lost with either sedation or the induction of general anesthesia.

8. The patient's previous endoscopist who failed is rarely incompetent. Do not repeat failed techniques.

9. Failure occurs in less than an hour—do not persevere beyond reason! Back out and think again whenever possible. The methods available for preparing a patient for awake intubation and the details of fiberoptic technique are dealt with elsewhere in this atlas.

Intubation under general anesthesia. If the physician accepts the premise that the careful passage of an endotracheal tube through the glottis under direct vision in a fully relaxed and asleep patient is the least likely means to cause any lasting damage to the patient's psyche or anatomy, general anesthesia must be considered the method of choice for gaining control of the airway. The purpose of the preoperative assessment is to determine whether there are sufficiently weighty reasons involving patient safety or whether the experience of the anesthesiologist might dictate the less desirable approaches of either performing a tracheotomy under local infiltration or passing an endotracheal tube in the airway of a conscious patient who may not cooperate.

Factors likely to influence the anesthesiologist to recommend a tracheotomy under local anesthesia include a friable tumor above the larynx that is likely to bleed and thus to obscure vision or a large retropharyngeal or peritonsillar abscess, particularly if it is "pointing," which could rupture on contact with either the laryngoscope or the tube and contaminate the airway with pus. Any history of previous complete failure to intubate requires that serious consideration be given to awake techniques and tracheotomy.

INDUCTION OF ANESTHESIA BY INHALATION

If the physician decides to induce general anesthesia by inhalation, the patient is brought to the operating room with no premedication other than antacids or an H_2 blocking drug and is made comfortable on the operating table, in the sitting position, if necessary. The patient's neck is prepared for tracheotomy, and he or she is then preoxygenated by mask for at least 5 minutes. Preoxygenation does not improve the moment-to-moment oxygen supply to the tissues to any great extent, but it does create an oxygen reserve in the patient's functional residual capacity (FRC) that may be of importance if induction is subsequently troublesome. Denitrogenation also facilitates and expedites inhalation induction.

When everything is prepared, the anesthesiologist should check that the surgeon is scrubbed and ready before beginning induction. Intravenous induction agents are avoided, and relaxants should not be used; either can result in loss of muscle tone that can lead to complete obstruction before it is known whether the patient can be ventilated artificially. A reliable estimate of dose response cannot be made with even small doses of thiobarbiturates, particularly in the patient who is already fatigued. The patient should be instructed quietly, in simple language, as to what to expect. He or she should be told about the characteristic smell of inhalation agents and be reassured that the experience is not unpleasant.

The patient should not be requested to breathe deeply because in the presence of anxiety it can lead to hypocapnia and periods of apnea that interfere with the induction process. Deep breathing also leads to increased peak inspiratory flow rates, perceived by the patient as an increase in the obstruction to breathing, leading to further agitation. The patient should be talked down quietly and with confidence and should not be asked any questions after induction has begun. Particularly stormy inductions have been observed in patients struggling against the depressant effects of anesthesia in an attempt to answer a question from the anesthesiologist, which, as far as the patient knows, may be critical to his or her care and safety. However, the anesthesiologist should be talking to the patient constantly until the patient has lost consciousness, remembering that hearing is the last special sense to be obtunded.

During induction the anesthesiologist must ensure that nothing is done to stimulate the patient during the first or second stage of anesthesia. This includes the nurse making any last-minute adjustments or the surgeon palpating or trying to prepare the neck for tracheotomy. Similarly, the anesthesiologist must be gentle in his or her manipulations to minimize stimulation. The support given to the patient's jaw must be gentle, and the pressure used to maintain a good seal with the mask must be the least possible. Along with these precautions, it is preferable not to make any cuff blood pressure measurements during the early stages of induction but to rely on an impression of blood pressure from the continuous gentle palpation of the temporal or facial pulse. Silence should be maintained by other personnel in the operating room until induction is complete. Patients will usually tolerate an initial inhaled concentration of 1% of any of the three commonly used halogenated agents (fluothane, enflurane, or isoflurane) in oxygen while conscious. The vaporizer with the chosen agent is turned on after preoxygenation. The patient is allowed to breathe this mixture for 10 to 15 breaths, then nitrous oxide is introduced to the extent that permits the maintenance of a satisfactory inspired oxygen concentration in that patient.

The patient moves more rapidly through the second stage of anesthesia because of the second-gas effect. The percentage of inspired vapor is increased 1% at a time, allowing 5 to 10 breaths between each increment so that the anesthesiologist may detect any developing irritable response to the new concentration. The total carrier gas flow is maintained at a high level (8 to 10 L/min), particularly if a circle absorber is being used, so that the set concentration is presented to the patient as soon as possible. The factors limiting the rapidity with which the inspired concentration may be increased are airway irritability and the maintenance of adequate blood pressure. During this whole process the anesthesiologist should be watching for developing difficulty in maintaining the patient's airway. He or she must develop that nicety of judgment required to decide at which point signs of increasing obstruction or a tiring patient dictate the abandonment of induction, while still permitting the agents to be vented spontaneously. Should total obstruction occur without warning, an oral airway should be inserted. If the airway is inserted too early, this manipulation may itself result in laryngeal spasm. If an oral airway is already in place or does not lead to immediate improvement, rapid but gentle laryngoscopy should be attempted. Frequently, lifting a swollen epiglottis is all that is required to reestablish the airway, and intubation may be possible even if the patient is not fully relaxed. The physician should insert a nasal airway only as a last resort because nasal bleeding may add more difficulties to be overcome.

If the obstruction is not caused by the epiglottis or the base of the tongue, the problem may be at the glottis itself. Even if the anatomy is grossly abnormal or distorted, some residual entrance to the trachea can usually be detected. This may amount to nothing more than a dimple in the edematous folds of the false cords. In such circumstances, if an antisialagogue has not been used, the anesthesiologist can "follow the bubbles" in the spontaneously breathing patient. Once the entrance has been found, with the laryngoscope still in place, a soft flexible stylet may be inserted as an endotracheal tube guide, or a small rigid pediatric bronchoscope may be passed to control the airway. If anesthesia is too light or if, even with gentle probing, the entrance to the trachea cannot be found, the surgeon should be called on to perform an immediate tracheotomy before hypoxia develops.

Should the induction process prove stormy, the anesthesia assistants should be instructed to restrain the patient's movements rather than prevent them. If the patient tries to sit up, the anesthesiologist should not resist. Rather, he or she should maintain a gas seal and try to continue induction without disturbing the patient's pattern of respiration any further. The anesthesiologist should follow the patient's movements, restraining only those that are likely to cause injury to the patient. A high-volume suction capability must be available, together with a hard suction tip (Yankauer) to deal with any vomiting during the excitement stage. The objective of the whole exercise is to achieve a smooth transition from consciousness to stage 3 anesthesia, at which time laryngoscopy and intubation may be undertaken safely. Spontaneous respiration must be maintained so that the process can be reversed in the face of insurmountable difficulty. This is why intravenous drugs are not given. Obsessive attention to the details of technique is required.

As the stages of anesthesia are traversed, the patient can be lowered to the supine position, if he or she was previously sitting. Any interference with the airway is delayed as long as possible. The initial rate of induction should be sufficiently rapid to minimize the chance of excitement, but as induction proceeds and the relaxation of muscle tone becomes apparent, the rate should be slowed to assess any loss of airway in time to retreat. Once the anesthesiologist is satisfied that the patient is in the third stage of anesthesia, vital signs should be checked and the carrier gas mixture should be adjusted to increase the oxygen reserve in the FRC before intubation maneuvers. Any loss of the nitrous oxide anesthetic effect because of the increase in oxygen percentage must be compensated for by increasing the inspired vapor concentration if a stable level of anesthesia is to be maintained. A variation of this procedure is required if a patient is bleeding in the oropharynx or the airway (e.g., posttonsillectomy hemorrhage). If the patient is a child, the problem is complicated further by the small airway. Children with secondary hemorrhage usually swallow the blood and may develop signs of shock before the situation is recognized. If irritability is observed in a postoperative patient after hypoxia has been excluded as a cause, secondary hemorrhage should always be considered before pain medication is prescribed.

The anesthesiologist is presented with several concurrent problems in the case of a patient who has just had an anesthetic with persisting drug effects and who has hypovolemia with a stomach full of blood and active bleeding above the larynx. A large-bore needle for intravenous infusion should be inserted immediately. If shock is evident, transfusion is indicated, even though a rise in blood pressure may make the pharyngeal bleeding worse. The situation will not improve until the bleeding points are secured, therefore the patient should be returned to the operating room in the tonsil position (i.e., semiprone) without delay (Fig. 5-1).

Once in the operating room, the patient should be placed on the operating table in the same tonsil position, on the right side (if the anesthesiologist holds the laryngoscope in the left hand) with no support under the head, to facilitate gravity drainage of blood away from the larynx. Assistants are instructed to stand on either side of the table to hold the patient in position. The same preparations for induction are made.

An endotracheal tube of appropriate size (a full size smaller) is selected to deal with any narrowing of the glottis following the previous intubation. When possible, a transparent plastic mask is selected. The same induction procedure is followed, but the oxygen concentration in the carrier gas mixture is maintained at 50% or higher. Blood accumulating under the mask is allowed to drain intermittently by raising the lower edge. When an adequate depth of anesthesia is achieved for laryngoscopy, the table is raised to the appropriate height for the individual anesthesiologist, and the assistants are asked to roll the patient gently into the full right-lateral position and to hold him or her there. With no supports under the head, the bleeding points are below the larynx and a few degrees of head-down tilt prevents the passive draining of any blood down the trachea. The laryngoscope is introduced, but instead of being lifted in the usual sagittal plane, the direction of lift is now 45 degrees upward and outward from the sagittal plane, exposing the larynx for intubation over any blood pooling inside the right cheek. When intubation is complete, the table is lowered and the patient is turned into the supine position, secured, and presented to the surgeon.

INTUBATION TECHNIQUES

The following section illustrates how techniques may be assigned utility and priority within an anesthetic plan for difficult intubation based largely on experience with the patients and problems presented in this atlas.

Difficult airways are either anticipated or unanticipated. If a difficult airway is anticipated, this atlas describes a systematic method of evaluation of the airway problems involved and the management options available to maintain the patient's spontaneous respiration and oxygenation while a methodic sequence of techniques is applied to control the airway. If difficulty is unanticipated, the patient has usually received an intravenous induction agent followed by a muscle relaxant before the problem is recognized, and now the overriding concern is the supply of oxygen left in the patient's functional residual capacity, which dictates the time available to recoup the situation.

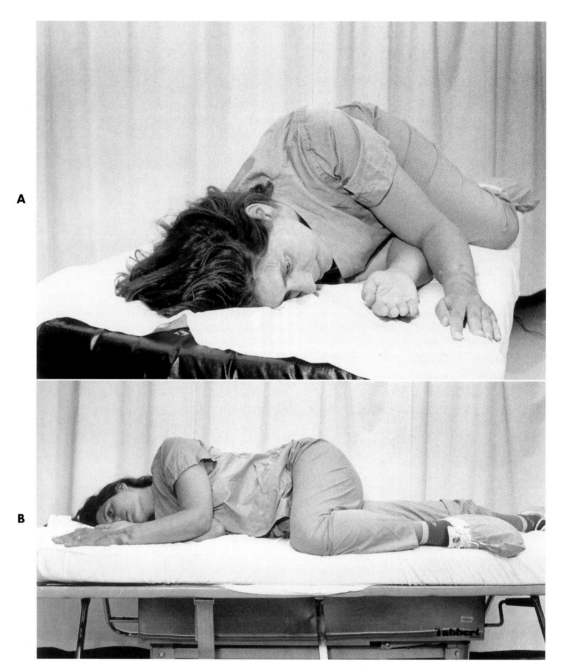

FIG. 5-1   Right tonsil position permits anesthetist, holding laryngoscope in left hand, to visualize larynx in normal way. **A,** Patient lies on right side with body leaning forward at 45 degrees. **B,** Position of left leg and arms stabilizes pelvic and pectoral girdles. No pillow under head permits width of shoulder to incline pharynx downward to facilitate drainage away from larynx.

However, in both presentations, the same four groups or combinations of problems are noted:

1. Access: Can the endotracheal tube be introduced into the pharynx?
2. Visualization: Can the larynx be visualized by normal anesthetic laryngoscopy?
3. Target: Can the glottis be seen within the laryngeal "funnel," and is it narrowed or obstructed?
4. Escape: If an endotracheal tube cannot be passed from above, does the anatomy of the neck permit rapid oxygenation from below the larynx? In all patients in whom neck anatomy suggests a difficult escape route, even in situations in which airway difficulties are not anticipated, anesthesia management should be more circumspect.

In the following description, certain techniques have been selected as examples with particular utility in overcoming one of the groups of problems posed in either access, visualization, or intubating a difficult airway. The emphasis in the examples is on simplicity, ease, and rapidity of use. The use of fiberoptic instruments as intubation guides is not discussed in any detail. Other published sources cover this aspect of management well.[5-7]

In addition, the time available and bleeding following early attempts at intubation frequently preclude the use of fiberoptic instruments in patients with unanticipated difficult airways. The need for every anesthesiologist to be able to perform a selection of simple intubating techniques is emphasized.

Careful repositioning of the patient's head into the true "sniffing" positing and the selection of an endotracheal tube 1 mm smaller than the anticipated size is frequently all that is required to turn a failed intubation into a success on the second attempt. Fig. 5-2 shows the order of choice of simple techniques that one group of experienced anesthesiologists has found useful in difficult situations. However, where simple maneuvers fail, other techniques must be used.

Although each of the following may be used in more than one situation, each is described as being particularly suited to a given set of problems under the classification previously described.

Problems of Access

Access to the oropharynx may be sought through the mouth or nose. The nasal route may be obstructed by polyps, bony spurs, septal deflections, or tumors requiring oral intubation. The oral route itself may be restricted by limited mouth opening because of temporomandibular joint disease or trismus, enlarged tongue, or tumors in the oral cavity. Thus even though there may be room for a laryngoscope, it may be impossible to manipulate an endotracheal tube as well. If the nasal route is dictated because of the patient's condition, blind nasal intubation may be the technique of choice using the classic blind technique or nasal lightwand or nasal fiberoptic visualization, depending on the circumstances.

The major risks associated with the nasal route are infection, bleeding, and trauma to the posterior pharyngeal wall. With base-of-skull fractures, a remote possibility exists of the tube entering the cranium (see Chapter 3). The inherent risks are minimized by preparing the nose with vasoconstrictors and using a properly designed nasal tube that has a longer bevel than is usual with oral tubes but that does not have a Murphy's port, which can act as a curette during nasal passage. This nasal tube should be made of a material that is soft but that does not lose its shape at body temperature, thereby allowing accurate manipulation. These properties are best embodied in the red rubber Magill nasal tubes, although plastic copies are now available. If access through the nose is not feasible and oral access is also restricted, the retrograde catheter technique (Fig. 5-3) offers much. However, this technique takes time and requires the patient to be breathing spontaneously, either awake or asleep. If the patient is awake, the hypopharynx is left unanesthetized initially and the patient is encouraged to spit the slack catheter fed into the pharynx from below the larynx out through the mouth. Once the catheter is retrieved, topical anesthesia may be applied to the hypopharynx and the tube may be guided into the larynx blindly or the catheter may be passed up the suction channel of a fiberscope and the tube placed under direct vision.

Problems of Visualization

Normal visualization of the larynx depends primarily on the ability of the laryngoscopist to reduce the angle between the planes of the oral and pharyngeal cavities in the sniffing position with the se-

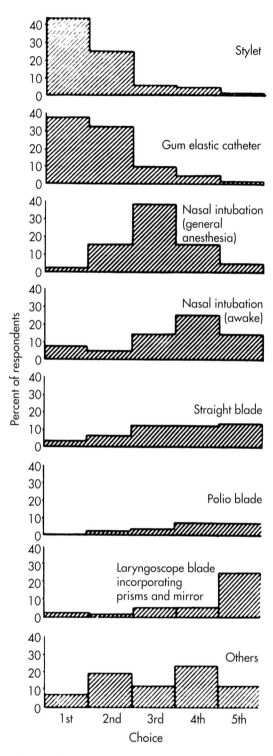

FIG. 5-2 Survey results with regard to initial choice of technique for management of difficult airway. Simple methods were chosen initially and are shown in order of preference. One third of respondents used these methods alone and had not experienced more complex methods. (Courtesy James Q, Latto IP: Unpublished data presented to the Welsh Society of Anaesthetists, 1982).

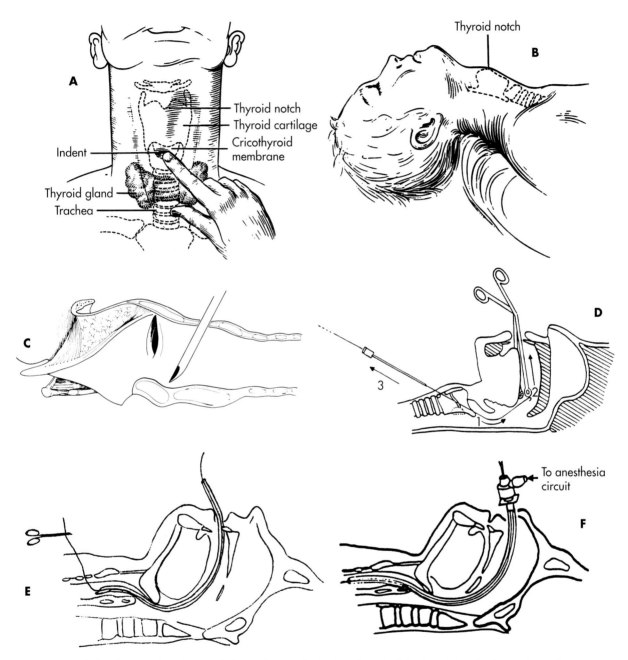

FIG. 5-3   Retrograde catheter technique using standard epidural set. **A,** Palpation of thyrohyoid membrane for retrograde intubation. **B,** Position for retrograde intubation. **C,** Introduction of catheter through pharynx. **D,** Catheter wire retrieved through mouth. **E,** Retrograde catheter in position. **F,** Connection to anesthesia circuit.

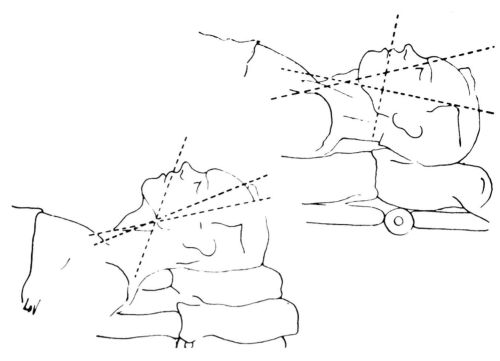

FIG. 5-4   Sniffing position.

lected laryngoscope blade (Fig. 5-4). This requires compression or deflection of the tongue mass within the arch of the mandible and the larynx being in its normal position.

If the arch of the mandible is small or the tongue is large or less than normally compressible because of infiltration or scarring, normal laryngoscopic techniques may not bring the glottis into view. Similarly, if the larynx is high and immobile, tucked under the base of the tongue, normal laryngoscopy is ineffective. However, it is often remarkable how the simple "BURP"[8] maneuver may improve the situation. Knill[9] reports a high success rate by displacing the laryngeal cartilage with *B*ackwards, *U*pwards, and *R*ightwards *P*ressure (i.e., toward the laryngoscope blade) in dealing with laryngoscopic views.[9]

If simple maneuvers are not sufficient in such a situation, two approaches may achieve success. A gum-elastic intubation guide (Eschmann) or a hollow tube-changer may be introduced under direct vision, then passed (blindly, if necessary) anterior to whatever part of the posterior larynx can be seen in the midline. Once in place the guide is sufficiently stiff to pull at least part of the larynx back into view in most cases. The guide then permits a range of endotracheal tubes to be introduced as required.

Another technique that is useful in such a situation is the light wand (Fig. 5-5), which may also prove successful when fiberoptic intubation attempts have failed. The disadvantage of the technique is that most larger diameter tubes must be trimmed to a suitable length for the light wand. This may not be acceptable for some surgical procedures. However, new designs of wands will soon be available to overcome this problem. With increasing neck obesity or skin pigmentation, the chances of success diminish. Both techniques may also be used when oral intubation is a necessity but access through the mouth is restricted.

Problems with Target

The ability to pass an endotracheal tube through the glottis may be limited by the physical size of the glottic chink or the airway below. The position of the glottis may not be immediately evident because of swelling of supraglottic laryngeal structures or because of rotation and deformities of the larynx

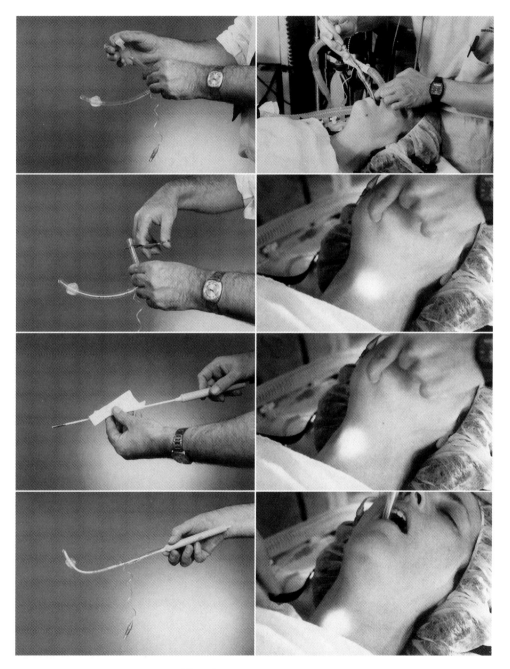

FIG. 5-5 Light-wand technique.

itself. A profuse crop of laryngeal papillomas may effectively camouflage the entrance to the airway. The problem in such situations is to first find the entrance to the airway then determine the size of tube that will fit through the opening. These problems require the ability to probe for the glottic opening without traumatizing the larynx. This is better done with a small-diameter soft stylet rather than the endotracheal tube itself. Again, the gum-elastic guide (modeled on the Tiemens urinary bougie) is ideal for this purpose, but other equally effective tube guides are also available.

The guide is introduced with the endotracheal tube, but, unlike an ordinary stylet, 2 to 3 inches of it are allowed to protrude beyond the tube tip to be used as the probe and then the guide over which the tube is slid into place. It is of great help in this situation if the patient is breathing spontaneously, without an antisialagogue, because the laryngoscopist can "follow the bubbles" with the guide tip. Should the initial tube be too big for a fixed glottic or subglottic restriction, the original tube may be withdrawn from the larynx over the guide and smaller tubes may be passed over or beside it. If the problems are complex, involving a mixture of laryngeal rotation and other factors, continued oxygenation and ventilation of the patient under general anesthesia may be ensured by transcricothyroid jet ventilation (Fig. 5-6) while supralaryngeal probing takes place. When using jet ventilation, special care must be exercised to prevent barotrauma. The possibility of a fixed restriction in the expiratory pathway should be excluded, if possible. If any doubt exists, jet ventilation should be commenced at low inflation pressures (<14 psi), at a low rate, and at high inspiratory/expiratory ratio while chest deflation and the escape of gas through the larynx are confirmed. Once the adequacy of gas escape is established, the patient should be relaxed to prevent him or her from raising the intrathoracic pressure by straining against ventilation. While still in the recovery room, all patients

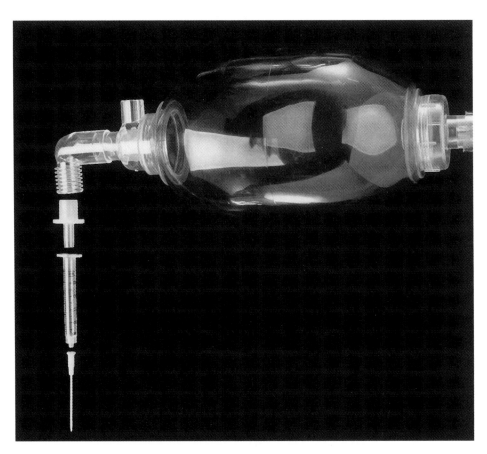

FIG. 5-6   Transcrycothyroid jet ventilation equipment.

who have undergone jet ventilation should have a postoperative chest radiograph taken to check for barotrauma. If there is any suggestion of restricted gas egress with the difficult airway, jet ventilation techniques should be avoided.

Escape Routes

The potential for failure of anesthetic management must be considered in every patient with a difficult airway, and a clear plan of action to retrieve the situation must be made in advance. This means not only formulating a plan, but also assuring that all personnel involved in the operating room understand what is expected of them and the signal to implement it. The most desirable escape plan is to maintain the patient's spontaneous respiration during anesthetic manipulations, and, if the decision is made that the anesthetic intubation attempts have failed, a reasonable trial should be made to allow the patient to recover from whatever medications have been given. The physician may then proceed to a calm, elective tracheostomy with the patient locally anesthetized. However, should the ideal prove elusive, several methods of achieving oxygenation of the patient from both below and above the larynx are available in an emergency. The recent addition of two devices to the anesthesiologists' armamentarium offer the ability to retrieve a lost airway rapidly without resorting to a sublaryngeal airway.

The laryngeal mask (Fig. 5-7) and the esophageal-tracheal Combitube can both usually be inserted into the hypopharynx when intubation attempts have failed and mask ventilation is lost so that oxygenation can be reestablished.[10] Neither device reliably protects against aspiration of stomach contents, but this is of lesser concern in the face of hypoxemia. Both devices have their proponents for easiest placement, but the laryngeal mask has some additional advantages in that its smaller sizes may be used in children and its largest size (#4) will permit the passage of a 6.0-mm cuffed endotracheal tube through its lumen into the trachea to give better protection against aspiration. Facility with both devices can be gained with prior use on suitably selected elective cases. If intermediate measures fail, jet ventilation can be effective as a lifesaving measure in an emergency and the catheter-injector can be placed anywhere in the trachea, if required. If the expiratory pathway is obstructed or barotrauma has occurred, a second catheter placed beside the first may improve the situation and may allow enough time for an emergency tracheotomy to be completed. Jet ventilation depends on special equipment that may not always be available in an emergency, thus some have de-

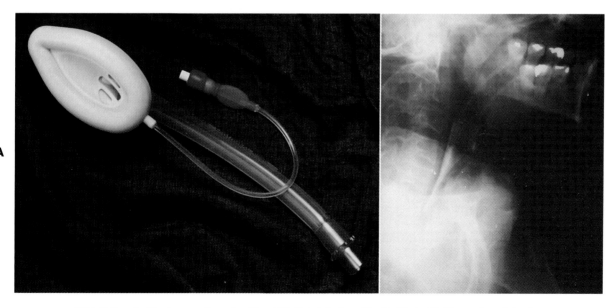

A   **B**

FIG. 5-7   A, The laryngeal mask with cuff inflated designed by Dr. Brain. **B,** X-ray of mask in situ.

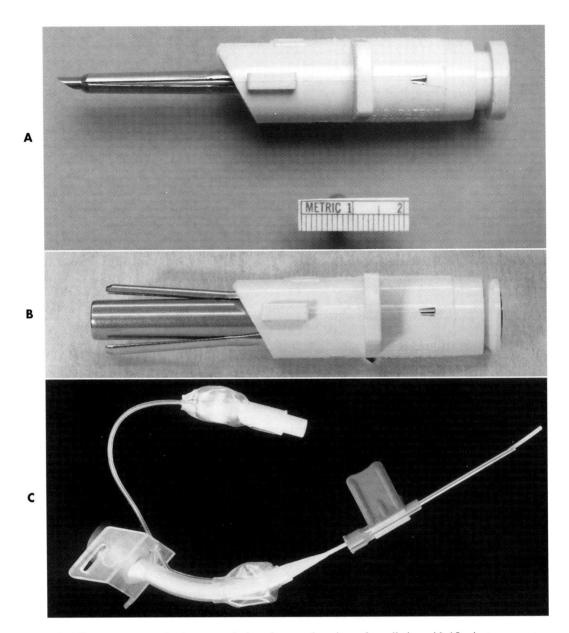

FIG. 5-8 Emergency cricothyrotomy devices that permit reciprocal ventilation with 15-minute connectors. Nutrake configured for **A,** insertion, and **B,** ventilation. **C,** Pertrach device. Tube on dilator shown with split needle to introduce filiform section into trachea. After insertion of filiform part of dilator through needle into trachea, needle is split apart and removed.

scribed the use of various ad hoc combinations of widely available equipment to achieve low-pressure oxygenation through an injector. This buys time but is far less effective than jet ventilation.

The final alternative is the sublaryngeal airway.[11] Several devices are now available in presterilized packaging for performing an emergency cricothyrotomy large enough to allow not only oxygenation but also sufficient reciprocal ventilation to control CO_2 levels and protect the airway either by suction or the introduction of a cuffed tube (Fig. 5-8).[12] All such emergency maneuvers rely on the operator's ability to identify the exterior anatomic landmarks of the airway in the neck. Patients with gross fat deposits in the neck, fixed flexion deformities, or extreme swelling from any cause are not good candidates for such procedures. Therefore the original anesthetic management plan should take this lack of a reasonable escape route into account.

Extubation of the Difficult Airway

Although the difficult airway and its management have achieved increasing prominence in the anesthetic literature over the last decade, it is only recently that attention has been focused on the postoperative management of the problem.[13] **Patients whose difficult airways were successfully and safely overcome for intubation have suffered both death and permanent injury as a result of ill-considered management at the time of extubation. This should be borne in mind by the attending anesthesiologist when the patient with a difficult airway arrives in the recovery room. A plan for extubation should be formulated in advance, with the interventions that may be required if the endotracheal tube is removed and, in spite of all precautions, the airway is still lost.** The following preparations, suitably modified for each patient's circumstances, are suggested as a guide for postoperative management.

The intubated patient with a difficult airway should be checked in the operating room while still in third-stage anesthesia to see if the glottis can be visualized with normal laryngoscopy with the endotracheal tube in place. This is to ensure that the patient has not been unnecessarily "labeled" as a patient with a difficult airway. However, it must be remembered that, in some patients, the endotracheal tube can pull the larynx into view, and when removed, the larynx returns to a hidden position. Knowledge of the successful maneuvers used and ease of intubation helps clarify this situation. During examination of the glottis, care should also be taken to identify any developing edema of the larynx and pharyngeal walls. If edema is present, extubation management should be more cautious and dexamethasone treatment should be considered. The patient should be taken to the recovery room, stabilized, and allowed to awaken fully. The patient should have stable vital signs and adequate spontaneous ventilation and should be awake, alert, oriented, cooperative, and sitting, if physically possible, before any attempt at extubate is considered. If these prerequisites are not met, extubation should be delayed.

Once the patient is ready for extubation the means for establishing an emergency airway should be assembled at the bedside. When everything is prepared, an oral endotracheal tube may be removed as follows:

1. An antisialagogue is given intravenously.
2. The pharynx is suctioned to remove secretions and to check for pus or active bleeding.
3. The stomach is emptied through a nasogastric tube, if required.
4. A final check is made for developing edema.
5. The patient is preoxygenated with 100% O_2.
6. An appropriate dose of lidocaine is instilled down the endotracheal tube.
7. While coughing subsides during a 2- to 3-minute wait, a suitable tube guide (e.g., the Eschmann gum-elastic bougie or a ventilating stylet) is selected with a new endotracheal tube of the same size and one that is 1 mm smaller. These are lubricated and tested.
8. When everything is prepared, the cuff on the patient's endotracheal tube is deflated and the tube lumen is stopped with the attendant's thumb. The patient's ability to breathe around the tube is tested. If the patient cannot breathe in this way, extubation attempts are abandoned for the moment and the cuff is reinflated. If the patient is able to breathe with the lumen stopped, preoxygenation with 100% O_2 is repeated.
9. The selected tube guide is then passed 1 to 2 cm beyond the end of the patient's endotracheal tube, and the tube is withdrawn over it until the tip is clear of the larynx, leaving the tube guide in the trachea.
10. If the patient appears to be breathing satisfactorily, the tube is then withdrawn from the mouth and an oxygen mask with 100% O_2 is applied. The tube guide is left in situ, having been led up through the mask and secured firmly.
11. The patient is then observed for up to 1 hour for developing signs of obstruction. If all is well at the end of the observation period, the tube guide is withdrawn and the patient is discharged to the ward clearly labeled as a difficult intubation, in case late obstruction occurs.

Should signs of obstruction start to develop earlier rather than later, one of the new endotracheal tubes should be "railroaded" back into the trachea over the tube guide. If the same size tube will not pass, the smaller one almost always will. In the unusual event of the airway being lost, the same emergency techniques are available as discussed earlier. If a nasal endotracheal tube is in place, a slight variation is required.

A longer, thinner, more flexible, preferably Teflon tube guide is selected and advanced through the tube into the trachea. The nasal endotracheal tube is then withdrawn into the pharynx and is left in that position during the observation period. This acts as a partial nasal airway because it is partly obstructed by the tube guide. The patient usually breathes partly through the mouth as well as the nasal airway. Should any difficulty be encountered, the same tube is then "railroaded" back into the trachea.

If the patient is unable to breathe around the endotracheal tube when the lumen is first stopped, it is necessary to consult with the surgeon on future management options. The surgeon may prefer, in the light of the surgical procedure done, to take the patient back to the operating room to do a formal tracheotomy over the existing, secure endotracheal tube. Or, together, the surgeon and anesthesiologist may decide to leave the patient intubated overnight and try extubating the following day. If the latter is decided upon, the patient should be prepared as though for elective surgery and returned to the operating room area for the actual extubation. An antisialagogue should be given as premedication, and H_2-blockers and oral antacids should be considered. If there is any question of the patient swallowing blood overnight, strenuous efforts should be made to empty the stomach before extubation. Edema is the usual cause of airway obstruction on extubation. This may be caused by fluid overload, surgical interference with lymphatic drainage from the area, or the trauma of laryngoscopic and intubation maneuvers. If one of the first two causes is suspected, it is better to wait for the edema to subside before considering extubation. However, if airway trauma is thought to be the cause of marginal edema, inhaled racemic epinephrine immediately after extubation may make the difference between a successful or failed extubation.

CONCLUSION

Several published reports suggest that difficulty with intubation is more common than generally supposed. The contribution of the difficult airway to anesthetic morbidity and mortality is significant and probably of increasing importance as other causes are overcome by improved monitoring and pharmacologic techniques. It has been estimated that at least 90% of difficult intubations should be anticipated,[8] but this can be achieved only by careful, routine examination of the airways in all patients requiring anesthesia. If a problem is detected, successful management can be expected only if a full preoperative evaluation is undertaken to establish the nature of the problem and the level in the airway involved.

Most problems can be conveniently compartmentalized into problems of access, visualization, or target, and combinations thereof. Most intubation techniques are particularly suited to overcoming one of these problem types but may be useful in more than one. Simple techniques are commonly successful in most patients with difficult airways, and the equipment required for simple techniques is more generally available in an emergency. Therefore the anesthesiologist should make every effort to ensure facility with several simple techniques suited to overcoming the problems posed by each of the three groups described, as well as with fiberoptic skills. Thus an argument is made for mastering a group of techniques applicable in terms of access, visualization, or target, remembering that the problem highest in the airway is the usual determinant of the primary technique that can be used. This approach is recommended to formulate an elective anesthetic management plan and to simplify the management decisions under the pressure involved with the unanticipated difficult airway, rather than trying to memorize one of the more complex decision trees that have been published in the literature. In all patients requiring anesthesia, the anesthesiologist should cultivate the habit of examining the neck to identify the feasibility of a sublaryngeal emergency airway. Patient safety is best ensured by maintaining spontaneous respiration until the airway is secured and by exercising sufficient caution, combined with experience, to know when the management plan has failed, always remembering that a falling oxygen saturation level on the pulse oximeter is a late manifestation of impending disaster.

REFERENCES

1. Aro L, Takki S, Aromaa V: Technique for difficult intubation, *Br J Anaesth* 43:1081, 1974.
2. Caplan RA, Posner KL, Ward RS et al: Adverse respiratory events in anesthesia: a closed claims analysis, *Anesthesiology* 72:828, 1990.
3. Stauffer JL, Olson DE, Petty TL: Complications and consequences of endotracheal intubation and tracheostomy: a prospective study of 150 critically ill patients, *Am J Med* 70:65, 1981.
4. American Society of Anesthesiologists: *Standards for basic intraoperative monitoring: ASA Directory,* Chicago, 1990, American Society of Anesthesiologists.
5. Shaw JD, Lancer JM: *A color atlas of fiberoptic endoscopy of the upper respiratory tract,* Chicago, 1987, Year Book Medical.
6. Patil V, Stehling L, Zander H: *Fiberoptic endoscopy in anesthesia,* Chicago, 1983, Year Book Medical.
7. Ovassapian A: *Fiberoptic airway endoscopy in anesthesia and critical care,* New York, 1990, Raven Press.
8. Sia RL, Edens ET: How to avoid problems when using the fiberoptic bronchoscope for difficult intubations, *Anaesthesia* 36:74, 1981.
9. Knill RL: Difficult laryngoscopy made easy with a "BURP," *Can J Anaesth* 40:3:279-282, 1993.
10. Cormach RS, Lehane J: Difficult tracheal intubation in obstetrics, *Anaesthesia* 39:1105-1111, 1984.
11. Wies S: A new emergency cricothyroidotomy instrument, *J Trauma* 23:155, 1983.
12. Toye FJ, Weinstein JD: Clinical experience with percutaneous tracheostomy and cricothyroidotomy in 100 patients, *J Trauma* 26:1034, 1984.
13. American Society of Anesthesiologists: Practice guidelines for management of the difficult airway: a report by the ASA task force on management of the difficult airway, *Anesthesiology* 78:597-602, 1993.

CHAPTER 6

Topical and Regional Anesthesia of the Upper Airway

VILDAN MULLIN

Anesthesia for the upper airway has been performed for various reasons,[1-3] including tracheobronchial toilet in the conscious patient, transesophageal echocardiography, and glossopharyngeal nerve block for carotid sinus syndrome and endotracheal tube insertion. More refined techniques have developed after the invention and widespread application of the fiberoptic endoscope as a diagnostic tool in the evaluation of upper respiratory diseases and for difficult intubation in conscious patients.

If the problems presented are complex and both oral and nasal routes are accessible, it is essential to prepare both routes for instrumentation. The focus of this chapter is on anesthesia for awake intubation and instrumentation, regardless of the route being used.

PREPARATION
Communication

Nothing is more gratifying than having happy and grateful patients at the end of a procedure. This requires, at the onset of a procedure, an unhurried interview with the patient, a professional, caring attitude, and a comprehensible practical explanation of all procedures to be performed. Instrumentation of the upper airway is a potent stimulus to gagging in some patients. **It is just as important in regional anesthesia as it is in general anesthesia for the patient to not have had any food, liquid, or other intake by mouth 6 to 8 hours before the procedure.**

Resuscitation Equipment

The anesthetist must be aware of the possible complications and thus take all necessary precautions before inducing anesthesia or undertaking endoscopic procedures. The procedure room should be supplied with basic resuscitation equipment, which includes an Ambu bag, mask, oxygen source, cricothyrotomy set, and, if possible, additional personnel. Intravenous access must be established, and basic blood pressure, electrocardiogram, and pulse oximeter monitors should be applied.

Instrumentation Tray

A well-organized and uncomplicated anesthetic procedure requires proper selection of instruments. Fig. 6-1 illustrates the standard instrumentation tray used in the Difficult Airway Clinic.

LOCAL ANESTHETICS

Commonly used local anesthetic drugs are listed in Table 6-1. A 1% to 4% concentration of lidocaine and 2% to 4% concentration of cocaine is most commonly used. They are applied alone or as a mixture, according to needs. High concentrations are used for mucosal surfaces and the lowest concentrations for nerve blocks. Lidocaine, when applied topically, has an onset of 1 to 5 minutes and a duration of 60 minutes.

Toxic reactions from local anesthetics may occur regardless of the route of administration and most frequently after intravascular application. Most toxic reactions from local anesthetics are as-

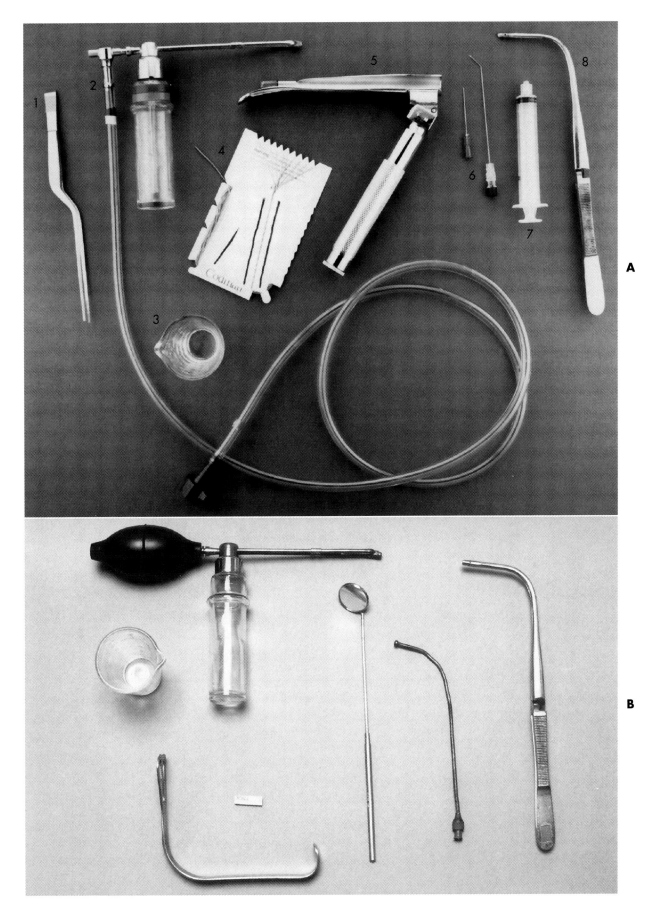

FIG. 6-1 Standard instrumentation tray used in the Difficult Airway Clinic. **A,** DeVilbis spray (oxygen-activated). **B,** Hand-activated DeVilbis.

Table 6-1 Local Anesthetic Drugs for Airway Management

Drugs	Topical			Injection		
	Respiratory tract	Total dose without epinephrine (mg)	Duration (min)	Nerve block	Duration (min)	Maximum dose without epinephrine (mg)
ESTER GROUP						
Cocaine HCl	2% to 4% (4 to 5 ml)	200	30 to 60	Not used		
Procaine	Ineffective			1% to 2% (50 to 100 ml)	30 to 60	1000
Benzocaine	Lozenges	100	30 to 60	Not used		
AMIDE GROUP						
Lidocaine	2% to 4% (5 to 10 ml)	200	30 to 60	1% to 2% (25 to 50 ml)	60 to 180	500
Bupivacaine	Not used			0.25% to 0.75% (65 to 200 ml)		

sociated with high plasma drug levels from rapid absorption.[4] In practice, slow application usually causes slow build-up without toxic reactions.

Vasoconstrictors

Instrumentation of the nose may cause epistaxis. Once epistaxis occurs, visualization, especially through the fiberoptic scope, becomes impaired and thus use of vasoconstrictors with local anesthetics is essential. In our practice, 2% cocaine mixed with 2% or 4% lidocaine is used.

Phenylephrine, another topical vasoconstrictor, can be mixed with local anesthetics at 0.25% or 0.5% concentration. If the physician chooses to use a pure vasoconstrictor without local anesthetics, 0.05% oxymetazoline is an alternative.

Anticholinergic and Antisialagogue Agents

It is important to dry the airways before instrumentation for fiberoptic bronchoscopy and laryngoscopy because secretions may obstruct the view and make visualization impossible. It is also important to dry the airways before applying topical anesthesia because it allows the drug to make contact with the airway mucosa and to avoid dilution with secretions. Because most sensory innervation to the upper airways is derived from the vagus nerve, adequate vagolytic premedication prevents the problem of profound vagal response. Tables 6-2 and 6-3 show the three drugs generally available for this purpose and their effects. Glycopyrrolate is preferred.

Sedation

The need for sedation depends on the patient's emotional and physical condition and the anesthetist's clinical judgment. Patients who require sedation may receive 1 to 3 mg of midazolam intravenously combined with 25 to 75 µg of fentanyl intravenously, titrated to effect. The advantages of sedation are that the patient usually feels more comfortable, is more cooperative, and experiences less emotional and physical trauma. **The oversedated patient may be unable to follow commands and runs the additional risk of aspiration, respiratory depression, and oxygen desaturation.** Amnesia, although usually a desirable effect of midazolam, on occasion can create uncomfortable side effects for the patient.

Table 6-2   Effects of Anticholinergic Drugs Used for Premedication

Drugs	Sedation and amnesia	Vagolytic action	Antisialagogue effect
Atropine	0	3+	1+
Glycopyrrolate	0	2+	3+
Scopolamine	3+	1+	2+

Table 6-3   Complications of Local Anesthetics

Secondary to local anesthetic toxicity	Secondary to nerve blocks	Secondary to vasoconstrictors
During spraying or application with swabs	Intravascular injection (CNS and cardiovascular effect)	Epinephrine ($\uparrow$BP, tachycardia)
Primarily involves the CNS and cardiovascular systems	Unintentional blocking	Neo-Synephrine ($\uparrow$BP) other nerves
	Hematoma formation	Cocaine ($\uparrow$BP, $\uparrow$HR, CNS) stimulation
	Hypotension and bradycardia secondary to vagal block	
	Aspiration (if patient has full stomach)[9]	

CNS, Central nervous system; *BP*, blood pressure; *HR*, heart rate.

POSITIONING

A comfortable patient usually means a cooperative patient, thus he or she should receive reassurance before any attempt is made to anesthetize the airway. In the clinical setting the author usually chooses the sitting position with the legs resting on a reclining leg support and the knees slightly bent. The dental chair used has power and mobility in all directions.

UPPER AIRWAY ANESTHESIA

The upper airway has three main anatomic zones, innervated by the trigeminal, glossopharyngeal, and vagus nerves (Fig. 6-2). A working knowledge of anatomy is one of the most important factors for success. Many techniques are available to anesthetize the upper airways, and each should be tailored according to the patient's need, the type of procedure, and the route of intubation.

Regardless of the route used, the patient is asked to gargle with 5 ml 4% viscous lidocaine solution for 1 minute, keeping the solution in the mouth for that length of time. This helps anesthetize not only the hypopharynx but also the tongue sufficiently to do basic manipulations such as inserting a blade and extruding the tongue with a gauze pad.

Methods

Step-by-step topical spray technique. The technique of anesthesia used most frequently in the Difficult Airway Clinic is topical spraying using 2% lidocaine with 2% cocaine in a 5:1 ratio as the agent of choice. This mixture is placed in a DeVilbis sprayer powered by 100% oxygen at a 6 to 8 L/min flow rate. **The patient is placed in the full sitting position and instructed to inhale and exhale deeply and slowly during spraying.** It should be noted that inhalation of nebulized local anesthetics allows satisfactory topical sensory anesthesia without specific nerve blocks. The process is initiated using transnasal spraying, regardless of which route of intubation is intended. The key is

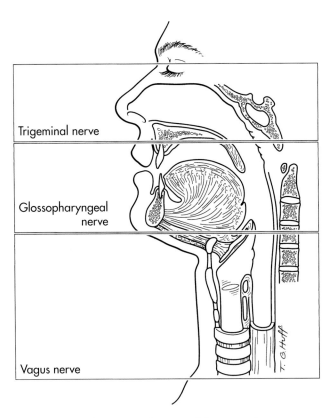

Trigeminal nerve

Glossopharyngeal
nerve

Vagus nerve

FIG. 6-2   Anatomic zones of the upper airway.

to anesthetize the posterior nasopharynx and posterior aspect of the uvula. The variable tip of the
DeVilbis sprayer is placed superficially in the external orifice of the nasal passage (Fig. 6-3). The oral
passage is then sprayed, beginning with the anterior surface of the uvula, base of tongue, soft palate,
and oropharynx. If oral intubation is planned in a patient without dentures, the hard palate is anesthetized as well. This is not usually required in patients who use full upper dentures and who, therefore, are used to a foreign body in the airway. If the patient coughs initially, the physician can be sure
that the spray is reaching the desired anatomic structures.

This technique should take at least 30 minutes and *must not be rushed.* The added time permits
a further opportunity for building rapport and ensures adequacy of anesthesia of the anatomic structures down to the carina. Indeed, the key to awake intubation is patience, rapport, and adequate topical anesthesia.

Spray with topical anesthesia.   Topical anesthesia is induced as previously mentioned and
continued with bilateral nasal anesthesia. Cotton swabs soaked with a 4% cocaine and 4% lidocaine
mixture are inserted into the nasal cavity and gently advanced posteriorly to demonstrate the existing nasal passage. This is followed by a 3″ × 1″ Codman pack (Johnson & Johnson Co., Randolph,
Mass.) with a string tie, inserted using a Harrison or a Cohen nasal packing forceps. Note that the
nasal passage is not dilated if this route of intubation is chosen. This is followed by progressive sizes
of nasal trumpets up to and including one size larger than the intended endotracheal tube, which is
placed before fiberoptic endoscopy through the lumen. The author cautions that no tubes should ever
be forced in and that the trumpets, endotracheal tube, and intubating airways should be liberally lubricated with lidocaine jelly (4%). In adults the maximum nasotracheal tube recommended is 7.0
mm internal diameter (ID). Bilateral nasal anesthesia is preferable even if a nasal tube is to be inserted only on one side. This ensures bilateral blockage of the sphenopalatine fibers that produce
partial posterior pharyngeal anesthesia. The pledgets should be allowed to stay in place for 5 minutes.

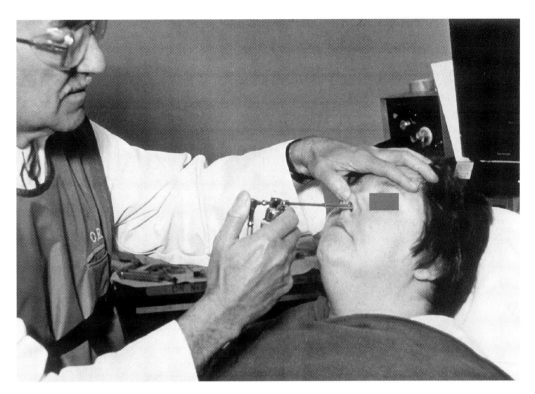

FIG. 6-3   DeVilbis varidirectional anesthetic spray powered by oxygen cylinder pressure.

Topical anesthesia for the superior laryngeal nerve (sensory anesthesia from the epiglottis to the vocal cords) can also be performed with Jackson (Krause) forceps (Pilling Instruction Co., Philadelphia, Pa.). A surgical sponge is rolled into the shape of a ball, soaked with local anesthetic (4% lidocaine), and grasped with Jackson forceps that are designed to conform to the curve of the tongue. The patient is asked to open his or her mouth as wide as possible, and the tongue is held with a gauze sponge and extruded. The forceps is introduced over the side of the tongue and the sponge placed into the piriform fossa (Fig. 6-4). With the handle held horizontally, the patient is asked to hold the forceps in place for 2 to 3 minutes. The procedure is repeated on the contralateral side. This technique is only possible, of course, if the patient can open his or her mouth.

With the above techniques the patient will readily tolerate the intubation airway (Berman, Ovassapian, or Williams) and anesthesia of structures down to the carina.

Topical anesthesia and nerve blocks. Many patients may be comfortable with only the spraying technique being used. Some patients with active airway reflexes may require topical anesthesia and nerve blocks in addition to spraying. For patients with active gag reflexes, bilateral glossopharyngeal nerve block can play a major role in abolishing this reflex, because it produces an anesthetic effect of the posterior third of the tongue, tonsillar region, and oropharynx.

The major disadvantage of this block is that it produces extremely rapid paralysis of the pharyngeal muscles, relaxation of the base of the tongue, and sudden respiratory obstruction.[4] For this reason, topical anesthesia followed by a superior laryngeal block before glossopharyngeal block is recommended.

COMMON NERVE BLOCKS USED IN UPPER AIRWAYS
Superior Laryngeal Nerve Block

Superior laryngeal nerve block will block sensory innervation to the base of the tongue, epiglottis, piriform fossa, and valleculae. Bilateral block provides laryngeal anesthesia from the epiglottis to the

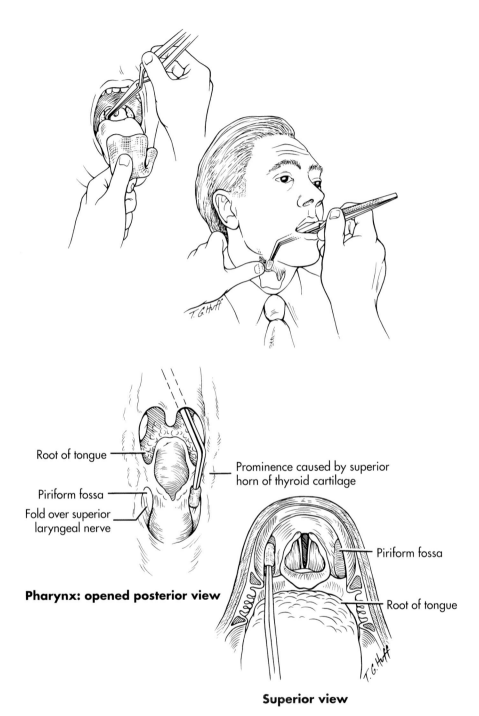

Pharynx: opened posterior view

Root of tongue

Piriform fossa

Fold over superior
laryngeal nerve

Prominence caused by superior
horn of thyroid cartilage

Piriform fossa

Root of tongue

Superior view

FIG. 6-4   Jackson forceps with anesthetic-soaked gauze pad in self-retaining jaws are advanced over the
tongue into each piriform fossa.

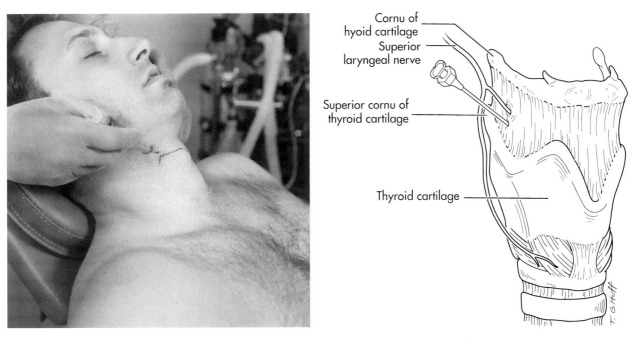

FIG. 6-5   Superior laryngeal nerve block, percutaneous approach.

vocal folds, and, most important, it anesthetizes the posterior surface of the epiglottis, something that is usually difficult to anesthetize with the spray technique.

Two approaches to anesthetize the superior laryngeal nerve include: the intraoral approach, which was previously described (see Fig. 6-4) and the percutaneous approach (Fig. 6-5). The patient should be in a semisupine position. Palpation of the hyoid bone in most patients can be extremely difficult.[5,6] Because of this problem, the author prefers to use the superior (greater) cornua of the thyroid cartilage as a landmark. The boundaries of the thyroid cartilage are palpated, and the cartilage itself is pushed from the contralateral side to make it more prominent. A 25-gauge needle attached to a 3-cc syringe filled with 2 cc of 1% lidocaine is inserted perpendicularly to the superior horn of the thyroid cartilage. If the needle rests on the cartilage, it may be met by resistance and should be redirected in an anterior and superior direction. This places the needle between the thyroid cartilage and the hyoid bone, approximately 1 cm anterior to the superior cornua of the thyroid cartilage, the area of the superior laryngeal nerve. After sliding over the superior horn of the thyroid cartilage, the needle should be advanced until penetration of the thyrohyoid membrane is felt. After careful aspiration for blood and air, 2 cc of 1% lidocaine is injected. If air is aspirated, the needle should be withdrawn until this ceases to occur. The procedure should be repeated on the contralateral side. Completion of a successful block should take place within 5 minutes.

Glossopharyngeal Nerve Block

Intraoral approach.   The patient should be in a supine or semisupine position with his or her mouth open as wide as possible. A Mac #3 blade or Miller #2 blade is used to depress the tongue and expose the posterior tonsillar pillar (palatopharyngeal fold) (Fig. 6-6, *A*).[4,7] Either an angled 22-gauge, 3.5-inch spinal needle with a 1-cm distal protrusion or a tonsillar needle is inserted behind the posterior tonsillar pillar at its midpoint into the lateral pharyngeal mucosa to a maximum depth of 1 cm to avoid intravascular injection into the internal carotid artery. After careful aspiration, 3 cc of 0.5% or 1% lidocaine is injected. The procedure is repeated on the contralateral side.

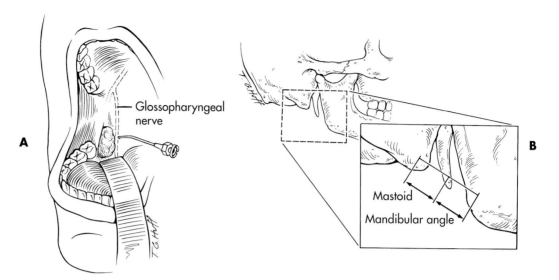

FIG. 6-6   Glossopharyngeal nerve block. **A,** Intraoral approach. **B,** Extraoral (peristyloid) approach.

Extraoral approach. The intraoral approach is recommended over the peristyloid approach for the following reasons. In the peristyloid approach, the glossopharyngeal nerve is in close proximity to the internal jugular vein, internal carotid artery, vagus nerve, and sympathetic chain. Injection in this area may produce unwanted intravascular injection or blockade of the neighboring structures. Technically, it is much more difficult to achieve glossopharyngeal block using the peristyloid approach.

The patient should be supine or semisupine with his or her head in a neutral position. The tip of the mastoid process and the angle of the mandible are marked, and a line is drawn between the two points. The midpoint on this line is marked, and a skin wheal raised. A 22-gauge, 3.5-inch spinal needle with a rubber marker is inserted perpendicularly to the skin until it contacts the styloid process (Fig. 6-6, *B*). The depth should be no more than 3 cm. At this point a rubber marker is adjusted approximately 0.5 cm above the skin, and the needle is withdrawn more than half way. The needle is redirected posteriorly to the styloid process until the marker reaches the skin. After careful aspiration a total of 3 to 4 cc of 0.5% lidocaine is injected. The procedure can be repeated on the contralateral side if needed.

Transtracheal Injection of the Recurrent Laryngeal Nerve

Transtracheal injection is done for branches of the recurrent laryngeal nerve. Percutaneous cricothyroid block of the lower larynx and trachea may be required in addition to block of the internal branch of superior laryngeal nerve if intubation in the awake patient is to be attempted. Both sensory and motor innervation of the intrinsic muscles of the larynx arise from the recurrent laryngeal nerves. Because the laryngeal nerves lie submucosally in the trachea, they are amenable to topical blockade. The patient should be in a supine or semisupine position.

A skin wheal is raised in the midline over the cricothyroid membrane that connects the inferior edge of the thyroid cartilage above and the superior edge of the cricoid cartilage below. A short 22-gauge needle on a syringe containing 4 ml of 2% lidocaine or 2 ml of 4% lidocaine is introduced vertically through the skin wheal into the trachea (Fig. 6-7). During this part of the procedure the anesthetist should maintain continuous negative pressure on the syringe. As the trachea is pierced, air is aspirated. On occasion the patient may also cough. At this point the anesthetist should inject the lo-

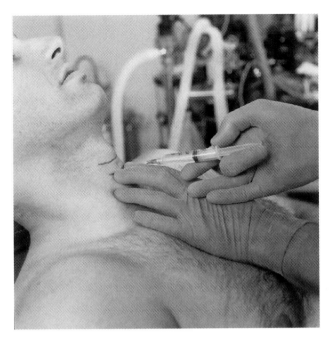

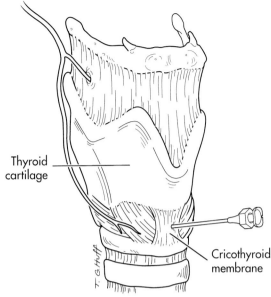

Thyroid cartilage

Cricothyroid membrane

FIG. 6-7   Recurrent laryngeal nerve block, transtracheal injection.

cal anesthetic rapidly and withdraw the needle. If the patient coughs, it usually ensures a good spread of the local anesthetic. Without transtracheal injection, sensory anesthesia of the vocal folds may be incomplete in most cases.

COMPLICATIONS

The mucosa of the upper airway is well perfused, which results in rapid uptake of the local anesthetics applied or injected in this area.[8] Local anesthetics mixed with vasoconstrictors may retard the speed of absorption. **The physician must never forget to calculate precise doses. The total dosage and resulting plasma levels play a major role in the development of toxicity.**[9] Allergic and anaphylactoid reactions from local anesthetics are extremely rare.

Treatment of Complications

Treatment of complications requires the following considerations:
1. Central nervous system stimulation leading to convulsions requires establishing an airway, ventilation with O_2 and a small dose of short-acting barbiturate such as thiopental (1 to 1.5 mg/kg) or methohexital (0.5 mg/kg) intravenously.
2. Hypotension and bradycardia should be treated with atropine (0.4 to 0.8 mg) or ephedrine in 5 to 10 mg IV doses titrated to effect.
3. Rare allergic and anaphylactoid reactions may require rapid control of the airway, O_2 administration, and intravenous medications, which should include Benadryl (25 to 50 mg IV) or dexamethasone (8 to 12 mg IV) or both. For extreme cases, epinephrine (0.1 to 1 mg IV) may be needed.
4. Acute and expanding hematoma will require immediate surgical intervention.
    Adequate oxygenation, as well as the ability to breathe unobstructedly during regional anesthesia procedures, decreases or prevents related complications, except those related to pharmacologic actions of the agent used.

REFERENCES

1. Zuch D: A technique for tracheo-bronchial toilet in the conscious patient, *Anaesthesia* 6(4):226, 1951.
2. Risk C, Richard F, D'Ambra M et al: New application for superior laryngeal nerve block: transesophageal echocardiography, *Anesthesiology* 72:746-747, 1990.
3. Kodama K: Glossopharyngeal nerve block for carotid sinus syndrome, *Anesth Analg* 75:1036-1037, 1992.
4. Reed A, Han D: Preparation of the patient for awake fiberoptic intubation, *Anesth Clin North Am* 9:69-81, 1991.
5. Cooper M, Watson R: An improved regional anesthetic technique for peroral endoscopy, *Anesthesiology* 43:372-375, 1975.
6. Shultz E, Chin F, Williams J: Superior laryngeal nerve block, *Radiology* 97:94, 1970.
7. Barton S, Williams D: Glossopharyngeal nerve block, *Otolaryngology* 93:186-188, 1971.
8. Gotta A, Sullivan C: Anaesthesia of the upper airway using topical anaesthetic and superior laryngeal nerve block, *Anaesthesia* 53:1055, 1981.
9. Campbell D, Adriani J: Absorption of local anesthetics, *JAMA* 168(7):873-877, 1958.

PART II

MANAGEMENT OF THE DIFFICULT AIRWAY

CHAPTER 7

Instrumentation and Equipment

MARTIN L. NORTON

"Diseases desperate grown
By desperate appliance are reliev'd
or not at all."

WILLIAM SHAKESPEARE

Hamlet, Act IV, Scene iii, Line 9

An old saying suggests that the shoemaker must not blame the equipment for faulty work. An analogy for the physician could be extended to his or her care of equipment. Equipment has a design and a need for understanding of its construction and handling in relation to anatomic configuration. **The problem airway occasionally becomes much more difficult from the use of improper instrumentation techniques.**

RIGID LARYNGOSCOPE BLADES

A classic example of iatrogenic airway problems relates to rigid laryngoscope blades. Often anesthesiologists pass the endotracheal tube through the channel of the laryngoscope. Although this technique sometimes may be useful in difficult situations, the channel was originally designed to serve as a visual pathway, and using the technique usually obstructs vision. This can lead to inadvertent esophageal intubation or trauma from insertion of the tube.

Similarly, all rigid laryngoscope blades were designed to be inserted along the right side of the pharynx, with the flange of the blade used to displace the bulk of the tongue to the left, providing a larger pharyngeal area through which to pass the endotracheal tube.

Chevalier Jackson taught insertion of the straight blade along the right pharyngeal area, directing it into the pharynx over the pathway delineated by the molar dentition and tonsillar area, bypassing the right root of the tongue, and lifting up the epiglottis from the lateral side by making a small C-shaped motion with the tip of the blade.[1] This simple maneuver allows the physician not only to bypass the bulk of the tongue, but also to elevate the epiglottis, even if the latter is floppy, long, or bulky (e.g., from epiglottic cyst, hemangioma, or other lesion).

In patients with full dentition, the jaw should not be depressed when it is opened and the laryngoscope blade should not be inserted into the mouth. The optimum opening of the mouth should be with a motion that approximates the gliding motion of the temporomandibular joint (TMJ). Thus a thumb-over-index finger approach is advised, with the index finger on the upper dentition as far to the right as possible and the thumb placed on the lower dentition.

In essence, the resultant motion should be the same as that for the elevation of the mandible and tongue—down, out, and finally elevated on to the laryngoscope blade. The mandible is lifted onto the blade rather than the blade being placed under the tongue. Thus in allowing this motion, the TMJ is "dislocated" anteriorly. (Because the usual intubation is done with muscle relaxants, this dislocation is readily achieved.) The larynx and its component parts are then brought superiorly and in close approximation to the lighted tip of the laryngoscope blade.

We often hear about the *anterior larynx* when discussing difficult intubation problems with clinicians. This term is incongruous in light of the fact that the most prominent cartilage of the larynx is directly under the skin. In fact, what is meant is that the tracheal cartilage is positioned higher than usual and may be enfolded within the arch of the hyoid cartilage, thus narrowing the additus laryngis.

STRAIGHT VS. CURVED BLADE LARYNGOSCOPES

Advocates of straight vs. curved blade rigid laryngoscopes (Fig. 7-1) warrant an analysis of their origin, application, advantages, and disadvantages. Certainly there is a place and a need for both types. The choice of instrumentation in the airway is as important as any other facet of the diagnostic-therapeutic plan.

In the early era of anesthetic and laryngologic endoscopy the most common type of blade was exemplified by the Wisconsin (Foregger) blade (Foregger Corp., Allentown, Pa). Subsequently the Macintosh blade came into vogue.[2]

The technique for insertion of the straight blade is as follows: The laryngoscope should be held in the left hand with the thumb and first finger of the right hand separating the lips and teeth and preventing the lips from being caught between the blade and the teeth. The blade is then inserted on the right side of the mouth, advancing it alongside the molars until the root of the tongue is reached (near the tonsillar pillars). The straight blade must *never* be inserted in the midline. Following insertion on the right side of the mouth, the tip of the blade is deflected toward the midline under the right root of the tongue, serving to visualize the epiglottis. The tip of the blade is inserted under the epiglottis (dorsal surface) and advanced a few millimeters. The proximal end of the blade is moved toward the midline only far enough to allow passage of the endotracheal tube or bronchoscope.

Rarely it may be necessary to reverse this to a left-handed approach. This would be applicable for bulky tumors of the right side of the tongue and right tonsillar fauces, particularly if friable. An upward and outward lift of the instrument in a 45-degree angle from the face should provide exposure of the rima glottidis. Overinsertion of the blade results in elevation of the larynx as a whole rather than exposure of the glottic opening. Occasionally the blade exposes the esophagus, which is recognizable by its transverse oval opening and lack of arytenoid cartilages.

The tip of the laryngoscope should never be advanced without visualization and identification of the orifice and tissues being approached. The three rules of endoscopy are (1) identify, (2) identify, and (3) identify. One risk relates to the cricopharyngeus decussation at the level of C6 and C7 vertebrae (posterior wall of the esophagopharynx), where there is only a thin layer of fibrofascial tissue that can readily be perforated and lead to a potentially life-threatening mediastinitis, particularly if the trauma is unrecognized.

The technique with the curved blade approach is the same—through the right pharyngeal pouch—except that exposure of the glottic opening should not be obtained through elevation of the laryngoscope blade placed under the laryngeal surface of the epiglottis. The tip of the blade remains in contact with the tongue and rests in the area between the epiglottis and the base of the tongue (vallecula). Elevation causes retraction of the epiglottis toward the blade and exposure by the pull on the glossoepiglottic ligament. If the tip of the blade is inserted too deeply, retraction cannot occur and exposure becomes difficult.

The theoretic neurologic advantages of a curved blade are derived from the fact that the sensory innervation of the laryngeal surface of the epiglottis arises from the superior laryngeal branch of the vagus nerve (X). Stimulation of this surface by the blade may lead to reflex vocal fold spasm and coughing. Conversely, innervation of the pharyngeal surface is derived from the glossopharyngeal nerve (IX). Stimulation of this surface is less likely to cause laryngeal spasm. This does not account for the minor branch interdigitations of the ninth and tenth nerves in the dorsal ganglion of the vagus, the nucleus salivatarius, and in the glossopharyngeal ganglion. Further, any stretching of the mucosae of the dorsal surface of the epiglottis is similarly reflected in the mucosal tissue of the ventral surface, thereby still producing activation of both nerve endings to some degree. In fact, when healthy subjects were fully anesthetized before their airways were intubated, no variation in cardiovascular response could be demonstrated.[3] However, the curved blade does allow more room for the

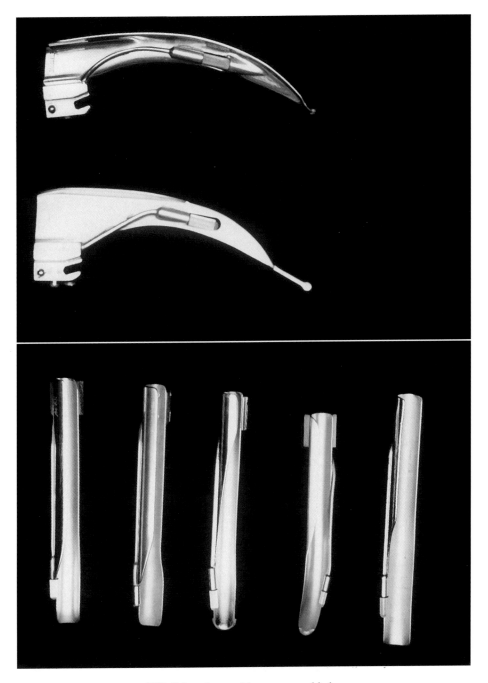

FIG. 7-1   Assorted laryngoscopy blades.

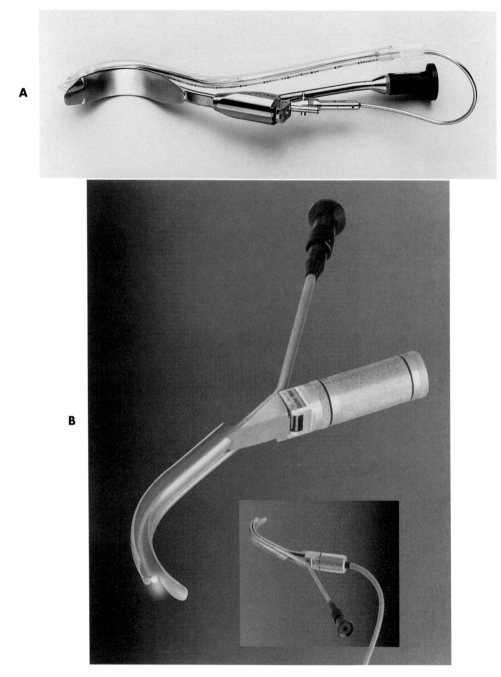

FIG. 7-2   **A,** Bullard laryngoscope. **B,** Upsher laryngoscope.

SPECIFIC INDICATIONS FOR RIGID BRONCHOSCOPY

1. The oropharynx shows major disruption with endoluminal suction of blood and mucus. A tracheostomy may be impossible to accomplish because of massive edema or cervical swelling from hematoma. Direct endotracheal intubation can be established using the bronchoscope with an endotracheal tube preplaced over the rigid tube. An alternate approach includes the use of the Bullard laryngoscope (Fig. 7-2, *A*) and the Upsher laryngoscope (Fig. 7-2, *B*).

2. Tracheal luminal disruption, with or without cartilaginous disruption, requires early reestablishment of luminal integrity. Direct vision insertion of the rigid tube accomplishes this objective and, if a ventilating bronchoscope is placed and left in the lumen, can meet the additional need of providing a route for supporting ventilation. Thus an emergency situation is converted to an elective one for further airway procedures.

3. A patient in labor has recently eaten, then regurgitated and aspirated. Endoluminal foreign body removal from the aerodigestive tract can be accomplished *only* by means of the rigid tubular endoscope (bronchoscope or esophagoscope). The key here is *not* to attempt to pull the foreign body through the bronchoscope.

   Proper procedure involves inserting the endoscope down to a point of direct visualization of the foreign body. The foreign body is then grasped by endoscopic grasping forceps. Following that, it is impacted against the distal orifice of the endoscope and *both* instruments are gradually removed from the airway. The endoscope should be reinserted to be sure that the entire foreign body has been removed and to search for resultant tissue trauma.

passage of the tube than the average straight blade in patients with large bulky tongues (macroglossia), prominent lower dentition, and some lower jaw malformations (Fig. 7-2).

Occasionally exposure of the glottis is not as good as that obtained with the straight blade, as in cases of *floppy epiglottis,* and it is evident that an intubating stylet or guide must be used in a much higher proportion of cases. Despite this, in short, thick-necked individuals and those with more superiorly situated larynxes the curved blade may prove to be the instrument of choice.

STYLETS AND GUIDES

Long intubation guides are occasionally used when direct rigid laryngoscopy does not permit visualization of more than the arytenoids or perhaps demonstrates only an air bubble. Other indications also dictate the use of indirect or fiberoptic laryngoscopy (see the box above). Sometimes they are inserted blindly (by digital manipulation) along the laryngeal surface of the epiglottis.

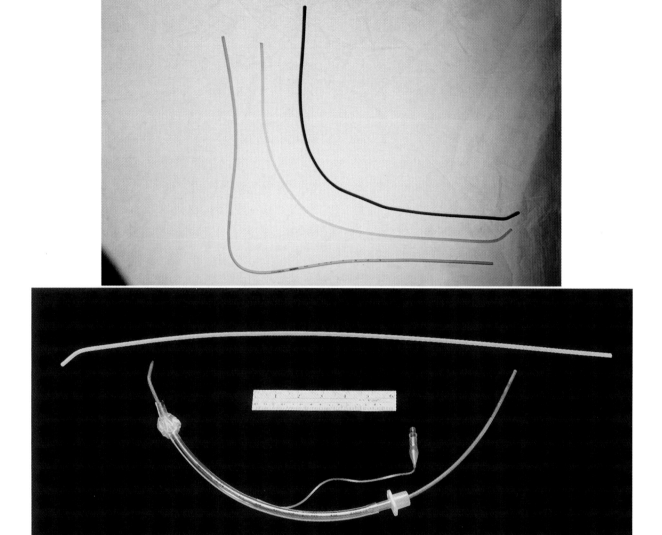

FIG. 7-3   Intubation guides.

A plethora of stylets is available for insertion of endotracheal tubes. Most of these keep the tube in a predetermined, flexed position. However, most useful are the long, semiflexible, intubation guides, i.e., Eschmann woven brown, the Norton (Teflon), and the JEM77400 (Instrumentation Industries, Inc., Bethel Park, Pa) white or clear hollow tubes (Fig. 7-3).

Hollow guides provide a lumen, purportedly for the patient to breathe through during the manipulative phase of intubation. However, the length and cross-sectional diameter of the lumen create a great deal of resistance, resulting in excessive ventilatory efforts for the patient. Thus its value is questionable. Additionally, the tube tends to kink, thus obstructing the lumen.

These guides may be used for changing tubes as well as providing guidance for blind or direct vision in situations where immediate insertion of the endotracheal tube is limited by size of the evident airway or visual obstructions. Our experience also has indicated that quality control of the guides may not be sufficient to guarantee that the distal end is smooth. There have been several indications of mucosal tears, probably secondary to rough distal ends. Also, unless the guides are relatively stiff, they may whip out of the airway during the threading of the endotracheal tube. In this sense only the long guides act more as stylets by molding the threaded endotracheal tube in the direction of the airway. Note that the tubes should be threaded over the introducer with a rotary motion.

These guides have been used in adult extubation situations where there are demonstrated or potential difficulties for reintubations, such as found in high-intensity care units. Here, after the usual suction and other precautions, the intubation guide is inserted through the extant endotracheal tube. The tube is then removed over the guide. The guide is left in situ for approximately 1 to 1½ hours after removing the endotracheal tube. If the patient shows a need for reintubation during this time, it is a simple matter to thread the replacement tube over the long guide. Patients tolerate the guide readily and can even talk around it. Note that the diameter of the guide is only a few millimeters and therefore, in relation to the average adult endotracheal tube, presents a negligible obstruction to closure of the vocal folds.

These long guides should be used with caution, however. There is a remote risk of forcing the long guide into a bronchopulmonary orifice and segment, causing disruption of the wall of the peripheral bronchus and resultant pneumothorax. This could occur if the proximal end of the guide catches on the edge of the endotracheal tube Rovenstine adapter or if too small an endotracheal tube is threaded over the guide. The guide should never be inserted against resistance. It is imperative to remove the endotracheal tube adapter to allow an unimpeded threading and passage without force. Consideration of the possibility of complications must always be a part of stylet and guide-assisted maneuvers.

Many types of rigid laryngoscope blades are described in the literature; most of them are rarely used today. With the advent of fiberoptic laryngoscopes, rigid blades are progressively being relegated to museum status. Herein are described some of the examples for the sake of completeness. The Snow blade with the Eversole blade are specifically recommended and are limited to insertion of rigid bronchoscopes. All aspects of these blades have not been fully described. Further study will reveal differences even in the standard Macintosh blades, such as the height of the flange, which is crucial in situations in which the patient has prominent upper dentition ("buck teeth").

LIGHT WAND

Another concept in guidance for intubation is the Trachlight (Laerdal Medical Corporation, Long Beach, Calif.) light wand. The Trachlight (Fig. 7-4) is comprised of a rigid internal stylet, a flexible wand with a bright light bulb at the tip, and a handle. To accommodate a cut tube or a full-length tube, the wand can be adjusted by squeezing the wand connector and sliding it along the grooves of the handle. The tip of the Trachlight should be placed close to but not protruding beyond the tip of the endotracheal tube. Following lubrication the wand can be inserted into the endotracheal tube. The connector of the endotracheal tube can be attached to the Trachlight by pressing it into the clamp and closing the clamp lever. The wand and tube should be bent to a 90-degree angle in the shape of a field hockey stick. The wand and tube become pliable following the retraction of the rigid inner stylet. The head of the patient should be placed in a neutral or slightly extended position. The intubator's nondominant hand should grasp the patient's mandible to allow jaw lift, which pulls the tongue and epiglottis upward. To identify the glottic opening, the wand and tube should move in a rock and roll motion in the midline direction. A well-defined, circumscribed glow can be seen readily to the left of the larynx if the tip of the endotracheal tube is placed at the right piriform fossa. When the Trachlight enters the glottic opening, a well-defined, circumscribed glow can be readily seen midline, slightly below the thyroid prominence. Retracting the rigid stylet from the wand facilitates the entry of the pliable wand and tube into the trachea. Because the sternal notch has been shown previously to be at the midpoint between the vocal cords and carina following the entry into the trachea, the wand and tube should be advanced until the light glow just disappears at the sternal notch as shown. Fig. 7-5 illustrates a step-by-step use of the light wand.

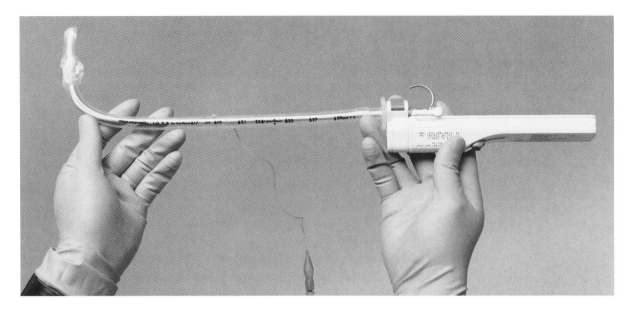

FIG. 7-4 Trachlight light wand.

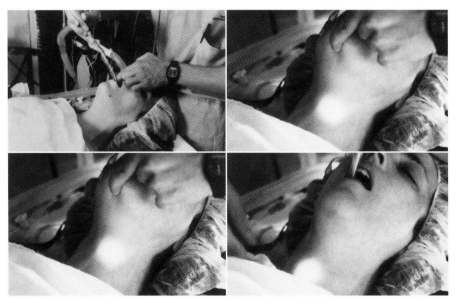

FIG. 7-5 Insertion of light wand.

RIGID BRONCHOSCOPE

Visualization of the larynx under reflected light was first accomplished in about 1858. Von Mikulicz used rigid tubes with reflected light for esophagoscopy. Killian[4] (the "father" of bronchoscopy) removed a foreign body from the bronchus in 1897. Einhorn devised a light carrier extending to the distal end of the bronchoscope. Chevalier Jackson,[5] the dean of American bronchoesophagology, combined Einhorn's light with Killian's rigid tube and brought endoscopy to a highly developed field of specialization. The rigid bronchoscope has found less application since the development of the flexible fiberoptic endoscope.[6]

The specific indications for use of the rigid bronchoscope include the following:

1. Bronchoscopic introduction of an endotracheal tube by direct vision
2. Transection or partial disruption of the integrity of the laryngotrachea, as in clothesline or handle-bar (i.e., motorcycle or bicycle) injuries
3. Removal of airway foreign bodies

Bronchoscopic technique as taught by Jackson used two approaches to insertion of a rigid tube. Currently, many surgeons insert the instrument directly through the mouth and into the laryngotracheal lumen after having roughly estimated the appropriate distance from the ear to the additus laryngis. Although the mechanics of insertion can be met by this approach, the entire area from the teeth and oropharynx down through the rima glottidis and larynx is not clearly examined. This negates the obligation to examine all tissues along the airway for possible pathologic condition or locus of foreign bodies, previously undiscovered, that would be missed.

A complete endoscopic approach should be accomplished by practitioners dealing with the problems described in the box below. First, a rigid straight blade laryngoscope should be used to examine the oral, oropharyngeal, laryngopharyngeal, and laryngeal structures. Next, the bronchoscope should be inserted through or alongside the laryngoscope under direct extraluminal vision. After the larynx is traversed, the rigid laryngoscope is withdrawn and direct endobronchoscopic vision is aided by telescope for further insertion of the bronchoscope, particularly of the soft posterior wall of the trachea.

PROBLEM INTUBATIONS WITH INDIRECT LARYNGOSCOPY RECOMMENDED

Laryngeal tumors	Arthritis (airway or neck)
Myopathy or myositis	Collagen vascular disease (neck or
Neck masses	pharynx)
Old tracheostomy	Cicatricial burns or pemphigoid
Foreign body	Swallowing dysfunction
Radiation therapy	Congenital abnormalities
Fixed neck	Unstable bridge work
Temporomandibular joint disease	Vocal fold paralysis
Mallampati Classes 3 and 4	Radical neck dissection
Diabetic "stiff joint" syndrome	Unstable neck fractures
Morbidly obese patients	Mandibular hypoplasia

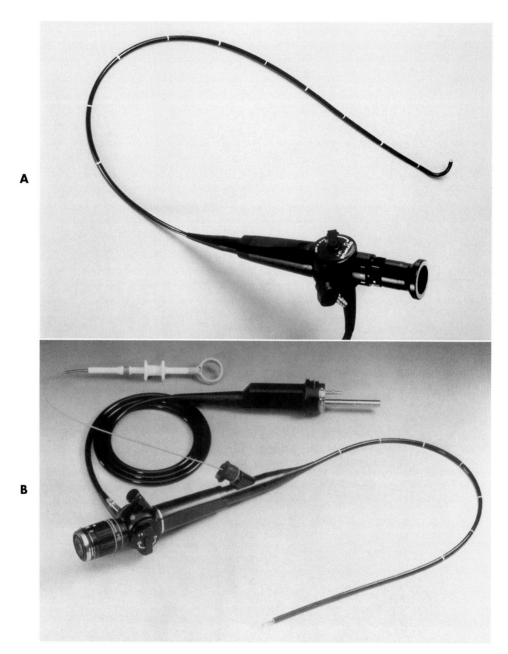

FIG. 7-6   Fiberoptic endoscopes. **A,** Olympus flexible intubating endoscope (**A** Courtesy the Olympus Corporation, Tokyo, Japan). **B,** Olympus fiberoptic bronchoscope with biopsy/oxygenation side port.

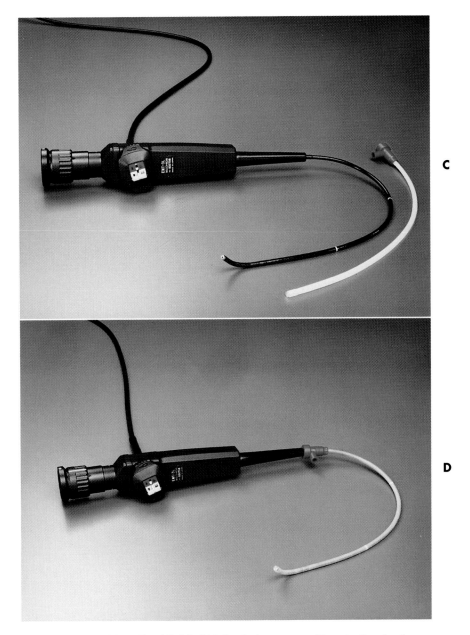

FIG. 7-6, cont'd. C and **D,** Machida intubation scopes with protective sheaths.

FIBEROPTIC ENDOSCOPE*

The development of the fiberoptic endoscopes has opened up a new era in airway management (Fig. 7-6).

Diagnostic indications for the use of the fiberoptic endoscope include sampling of airway secretions, assessment of airway patency, preoperative and postoperative laryngeal evaluation, assessment of airway damage after smoke or steam inhalation, endotracheal intubation, determination of the locus of double-lumen endotracheal tubes, evaluation of the nasopharynx, and other pulmonary applications.

The instrument has a particular application following smoke inhalation (see Chapter 13 for a further discussion of the fiberoptic bronchoscope in management of burns).

The care of the fiberoptic instrument deserves special emphasis. **The fiberoptic bundles must never be bent to an extreme nor should they be struck or compressed against anything. It is imperative to never apply forces of torsion to the instrument** (Fig. 7-7).

Emphasis should be given to immediately flushing the suction channel and washing the outside of the fiberoptic scope. It is also suggested to pass a brush as soon as possible to mechanically clear mucus and blood and to prevent blood clot and debris from plugging the suction or biopsy channel.[7] Keep in mind that these channels must be kept clear for suction or insufflation of oxygen. The outside of the fiberscope also requires some attention. The physician should not force it through a small-sized endotracheal tube because this wrinkles the outer protective coating of the bronchoscope (Fig. 7-8) and may permanently damage the exterior. Similarly, as soon as the fiberscope is removed from the patient, it should be washed off in cold water, then in a soapy solution followed by a second rinse in cold water.

Maintenance cannot be overemphasized because the cost of most fiberscopes is in the range of $4000 to $9000. Repairs are costly and a significant factor in the consideration of health care costs.

---

*The Olympus BF3C10 pediatric and the BF20 adult bronchoscope attached to an Olympus OTV-F2 camera, projecting onto a Sony television screen and attached to a video cassette recorder for tape recording have been used. These instruments have added markings to indicate depth of insertion. (Courtesy of the Olympus Corporation, Tokyo. Hiroyuki Furihata, Manager, Endoscope Section of Product Development and Akio Nakada, Design Engineer, Research & Development.) Special attention to the needs of the clinic and this book has been provided by Mr. Jay Beatus, Olympic America, Inc., NY.

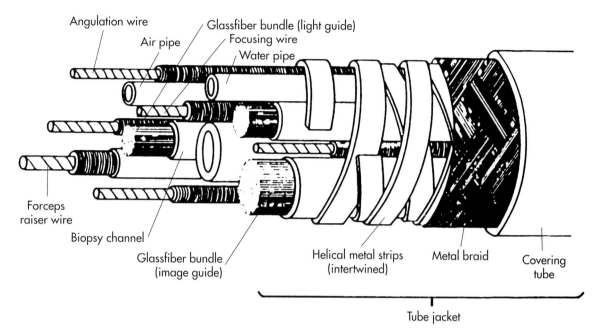

Angulation wire
Air pipe
Glassfiber bundle (light guide)
Focusing wire
Water pipe
Forceps raiser wire
Biopsy channel
Glassfiber bundle (image guide)
Helical metal strips (intertwined)
Metal braid
Covering tube
Tube jacket

FIG. 7-7   Complexity of fiberoptics, which can lead to damage during mishandling.

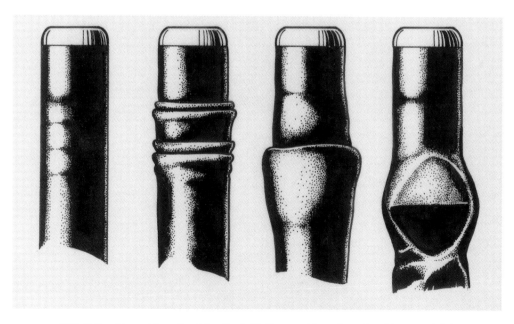

FIG. 7-8   Normal insertion tube *(far left)*. Damaged insertion tubes *(three on right)*.

REFERENCES

1. Jackson C, Jackson CL: *Bronchoscopy, esophagoscopy, and gastroscopy,* Philadelphia, 1934, WB Saunders.
2. Macintosh RR: A new laryngoscope blade *Lancet,* 1:205, 1932.
3. Cozantis DA, Nuuttila K, Merrett JD et al: Influence of laryngoscope design on heart rate rhythm changes during intubation, *Can Anaesth Soc J* 31:155, 1984.
4. Killian G: Meeting of the Society of Freiburg, Dec 17, 1897. *München Med Wochenschr* 45:378, 1898.
5. Jackson C, Jackson CL: *Bronchoesophagology,* Philadelphia, 1950, WB Saunders.
6. Sackner MA: Bronchofiberscopy, *Am Rev Resp Dis* 111:62, 1975.
7. Centers for Disease Control and Prevention: Guidelines on environmental control. Part I. Bethesda, Md, 1982, Department of Health and Human Services.

CHAPTER 8

Diagnostic Imaging for Evaluation and Management of the Difficult Airway

FRANK LONDY

Many evaluative approaches can be implemented with the use of radiologic techniques, but only recently have anesthesiologists seen the need for explicit upper-airway imaging. We are familiar with the classic lateral flat plate, using both soft tissue and standard (bone survey) densities, which is still a useful means of imaging the upper airway. The use of computed tomography (CT) scanning in recent years has provided a valuable new tool for upper airway imaging. Of late, magnetic resonance imaging (MRI) has contributed greatly to the diagnostic armamentarium. Recently, work by Lowe et al.[1] using digitized CT scans has made it possible to study tongue volume. This technique has potential for evaluation of other soft tissues of the upper respiratory tract.

Cephalometric analysis of the airway may give further insight into what is considered normal and abnormal.

Another new technique, somnofluoroscopy, combines cineradiographic observation of the upper airway with simultaneous polysomnography,[2] a useful tool in the diagnosis of sleep apnea.

C-arm fluoroscopy, although not new, has proved to be the most useful tool for planning and conducting endotracheal intubation in patients with upper airway problems.

COMPUTED TOMOGRAPHY AND MAGNETIC RESONANCE IMAGING

The wide acclaim of CT (Fig. 8-1, *A*)[3] and MRI (Fig. 8-1, *B*) for head and neck imaging is well deserved and well documented in the literature. With regard to preendotracheal intubation studies, however, few institutions have developed specific protocols. Using CT it has been found that 1.5- to 5-mm contiguous axial images with the gantry parallel to the vocal folds should produce optimum axial images. Viewing windows can be adjusted to further enhance the airway contrast as needed.

The greatest limitation of CT, besides cost, is that the scans are in the axial plane when the patient is in a prone or supine position. For nonradiologists these images can be cumbersome to interpret. To present an easier-to-read, more traditional sagittal view, the computer must reconstruct the axial images. This produces a lateral view of the airway but one that is generally a choppy, poorly defined image. As CT software improves, this reconstruction shortcoming will improve.

MRI offers the advantage of multiplanar views of the cartilage and soft tissues. However, it is expensive, requires a relatively long time to produce the final image, and is not available everywhere. For dynamic airway evaluation, MRI is usually not the method of choice. Other imaging options give as much or more information per patient dollar spent and are faster and easier to perform, while allowing greater flexibility in scheduling examinations (Table 8-1).

A new CT option is the three-dimensional reconstruction. This method reconstructs the CT data to produce an image that seems much like an image of a three-dimensional object photographed and projected into a two-dimensional screen. The viewer is able to turn the object to see it from any angle.

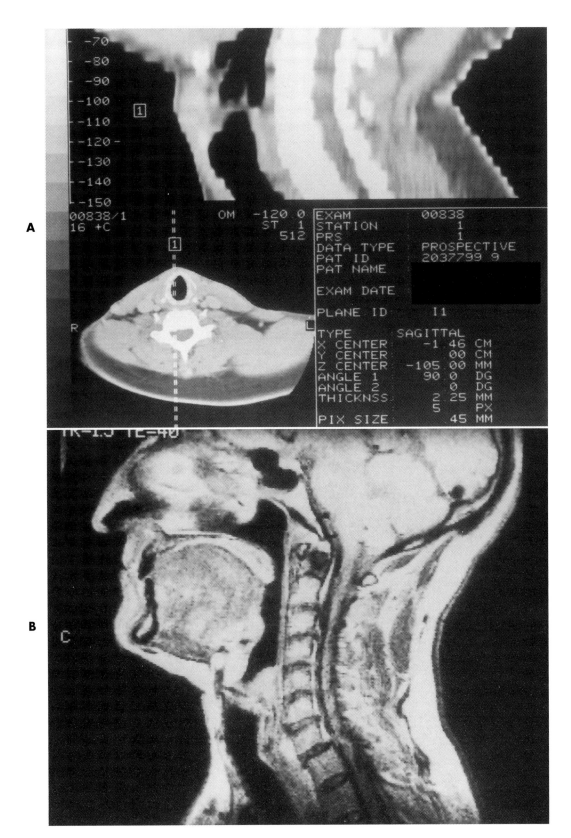

FIG. 8-1   **A,** Computed tomography (CT) scan. **B,** Magnetic resonance imaging (MRI) scan.

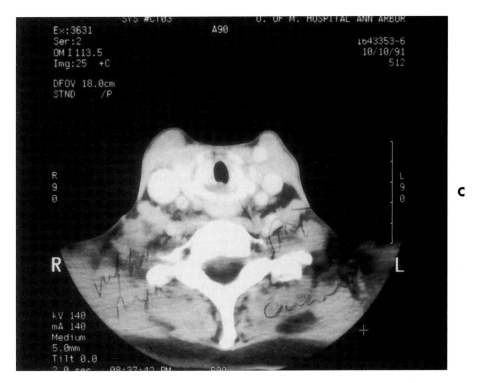

FIG. 8-1, cont'd.   C, CT of 7-mm tracheal stenosis.

Table 8-1   Costs of Various Imaging Procedures at the University of Michigan Medical Center, 1994

Procedure	Overall cost
Airway or neck CT	$ 834.00
Airway or neck MRI	1343.00
TMJ MRI	1126.00
C-arm fluorography of airway	160.00/15 min
Plain film imaging series of TMJ	156.00
Plain film imaging series of airway	111.00
Plain film imaging of cervical spine	182.00

Evaluation can usually be completed within 1 to 2 minutes of fluoroscopic time and within 15 minutes of C-arm time.
CT, Computed tomography; *MRI,* magnetic resonance imaging; *TMJ,* temporomandibular joint.

PLAIN FILM TOMOGRAPHY

Plain film tomography is a long-established modality that uses the principle of focal plane isolation through the reciprocal motion of the x-ray source and the image receptor (i.e., the film).[6] The resultant radiograph demonstrates an image that has only a narrow "layer" of the subject clearly focused. The levels nearer the x-ray tube and the film are blurred. Plain film tomography is quick and easy and does not emit a high radiation dose to the patient. Compare 135 milliroentgen (mR) per cut for plain film tomography vs. 2232 mR per cut for CT. Plain film tomography is progressively being replaced by the greater detail and definition provided by CT and MRI for imaging of tissues in the neck.

PLAIN FILM RADIOGRAPHY

Use has been made of several methods, but the greatest amount of information has been obtained from the plain film radiograph and C-arm fluorography (see the box below). The lateral soft tissue neck view is the plain film technique used most often. All plain films are taken with Kodak regular cassettes, 40-inch, nongridded, source-to-image distance, using Dupont Cromex 6 film.

This examination has been modified to meet the needs for airway studies. The greatest concern is for viewing airway configuration and not the soft tissue. The traditional method includes an exposure technique that often overpenetrates and burns away the anterior ventral border of the airway.

IMAGING WITH PLAIN FILMS

Temporomandibular joints
  Patient upright 15 to 30 degrees of angle
    as needed
  Film centered to temporomandibular joint
  Aggressive collimation
  Exposure factors
    70 kVp/8 to 10 mas
    40-inch source-to-image distance (SID)
    Radiation exposure to patient 300 mR
Airway upright
  Patient upright
  Neck in slight extension
  Mouth open
  Tongue out
  Patient's shoulders as low as possible*
  Expose during patient inspiration
  Collimate to the airway

  Center to include the nasopharynx to
    trachea
  Exposure factors
    60 kVp/2 to 5 mas
    40-inch SID
    Radiation exposure to patient 12 to 20
      mR
Imaging the cervical spine with plain films
  Collimate to cervical spine
  Center to C4 vertebra
  Radiograph in neutral†
Flexion and extension
  Exposure factors
    70 kVp/4 to 8 mas
    40-inch SID
    Radiation exposure to patient 110 mR

---

*For those patients who are unable to lower their shoulders the centering of the film should be at the level of the vocal folds. Centering higher projects the folds onto the shoulder nearest the film.

†It may be necessary to do a second film for the airway above the shadow of the mandible because of the low exposure factor. In that case center to the area not visualized on the first film to present as distortion-free an image as possible.

Table 8-2   Anatomic Location of Crucial Structures

Cartilage	Adult bony landmarks
Hyoid	C2 to C3
Thyroid	C4 to upper border, lateral wing
	C5 to lower border, lateral wing
Cricoid	C6
Trachea	C7 and below; 10 to 20 cm long, about 12+ mm diameter at approximately sixth ring becomes intrathoracic
Carina	T5 (sternal angle of Louis; second intercostal space)

A lower exposure technique yields a radiograph with much greater airway detail. To increase that detail further, the cervical spine is collimated off the film.*

Table 8-2 and Fig. 8-2 provide a guide to anatomic location of crucial structures. Plain film exposure should be obtained with the patient's mouth slightly open during inspiration and the head placed in moderate extension. Direction of the central ray is recommended to be at the level of any suspected problem areas to reduce central ray distortions. An important point that should be considered is the position of the patient during this radiographic examination. There can be a great variation in airway configuration when the patient changes from the upright to the supine position. **Radiographing a patient in only a supine or only an upright position produces a single image that can be misleading.**

---

*Collimators are x-ray beam restriction devices built into the x-ray tube housing. Beam restriction is important for two reasons: (1) it lowers the patient's radiation dose and (2) reducing the total number of x-ray photons reduces the number of photons that strike the patient, as well as scatter radiation. Scatter radiation is the major cause of the poor definition, or washed-out quality, that is sometimes seen on uncollimated films.

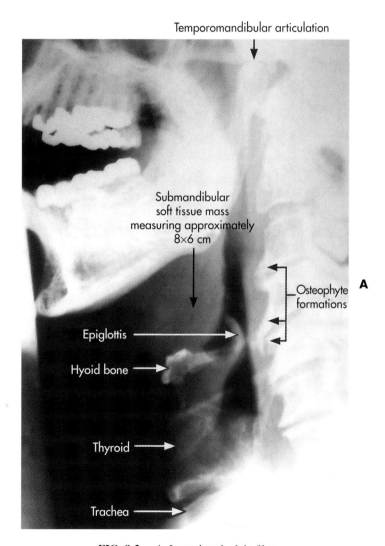

FIG. 8-2   A, Lateral neck plain film.

Continued.

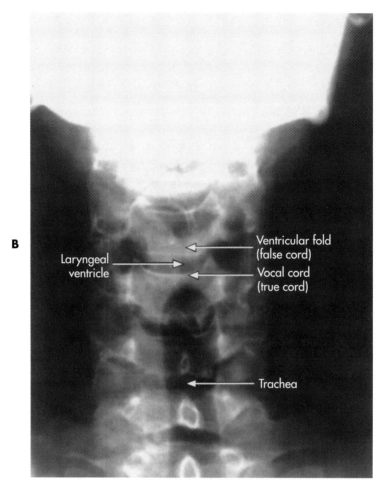

FIG. 8-2, cont'd.   B, Normal cervical spine, anteroposterior position. Laryngeal *ventricular* structures are synonymous with *vestibular* structures.

IMAGING A DYNAMIC AIRWAY IN THE ANTEROPOSTERIOR POSITION

Scout exposure and image with the following:
1. Noise reduction at a maximum
2. Image showing the base of the skull superimposed over the mandible
3. Center to the vocal folds
4. Patient's neck in slight extension; image as follows, with noise at a reduced level to prevent smearing of the image
   a. Normal respiration
   b. Deep respiration (nasal)
   c. Deep respiration (oral, mouth opened wide)
   d. Deep respiration (oral, mouth opened wide, tongue out)
   e. Cough
   f. Phonation (A, E, I, O, U)
   g. Swallowing

Because the exposure technique is light (i.e., underexposed) compared with the traditional soft tissue film, it is often necessary to take a second film of the airway above the lower border of the mandible. For this projection, standard exposure technique is used. Aggressive collimation to the region of the airway increases detail and is strongly recommended. For the anteroposterior (AP) airway, plain film standard AP soft tissue neck techniques are adequate (see the box on p. 116). When viewing lateral neck films, it must be remembered that the hyoid bone appears to transect the epiglottis.

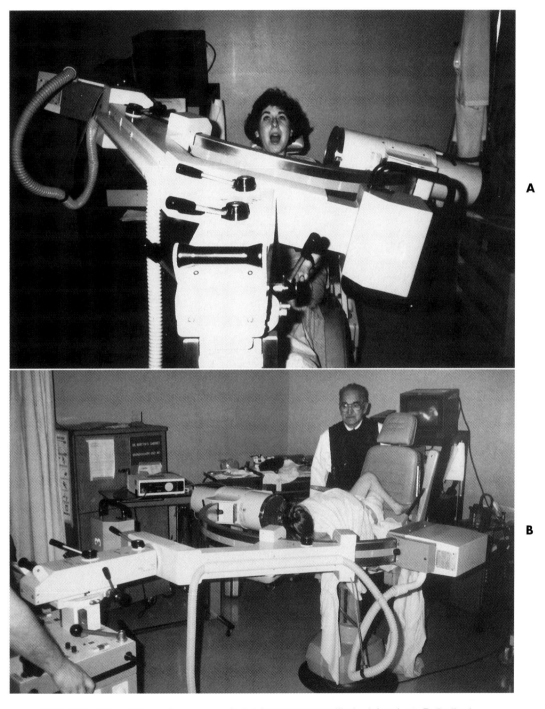

FIG. 8-3   Use of C-arm fluoroscope. **A,** Adult (temporomandibular joint view). **B,** Pediatric.

C-ARM FLUOROGRAPHY

The author has been using an extraordinarily helpful imaging option, the C-arm portable fluorography unit. It consists of an x-ray tube that is directed at an electronic image receptor (Fig. 8-3). The image is viewed with a monitor connected to the C-arm. Imaging options on the monitor cart include snapshots (still pictures) and fluorography, with or without pixel averaging (tiny dots that compose the image on the C-arm monitor). The last fluorographic image taken may be held on the screen after the x-ray beam has been turned off and until it is started again. Most C-arms also have the ability to store still images in their computer data banks for future reference. Permanent images can be obtained by recording the fluoroscopic image with a video cassette recorder, transferring still images onto x-ray film with the use of a matrix camera, or photographing the images from the monitor with a standard camera. To record fluoroscopic C-arm images, the technique outlined in the box below and at right is used.

The capabilities of the C-arm are best used with dynamic studies. The C-arm can show dynamic changes of the airway during normal respiration, deep respiration, swallowing, and tongue and jaw thrust as well as effects produced when the patient phonates, flexes, or extends the neck. Using the C-arm, the mechanics of the patient's disease or condition can be studied as they impact on the configuration of the airway and are delineated in instantaneously generated, dynamic images.

STEPS IN C-ARM FLUOROGRAPHIC IMAGING TECHNIQUES

I. Temporomandibular joint (TMJ)
   A. Scout exposure image with
      1. Patient in upright position
      2. X-ray beam in lateral position
      3. Maximum noise reduction
   B. Scout exposure to right side of TMJ image with
      1. Maximum noise reduction
      2. Angle of 15 to 30 degrees of angle as needed
   C. Scout exposure to dynamic right side of TMJ image by
      1. Decreasing noise reduction as needed to prevent smearing of image with movement
      2. Obtaining 15 to 30 degrees of angle as needed
      3. Fluorographing at least two cycles of opening and closing of patient's mouth
   D. Repeat exposures B and C above for left TMJ
II. Cervical spine
   A. Scout exposure of cervical spine image with
      1. Patient in upright position
      2. X-ray beam in lateral position
      3. Maximum noise reduction
      4. Patient's shoulders as low as possible
   B. Flexion and extension cervical spine image with
      1. Maximum noise reduction
      2. Noise reduction decreased as needed to prevent smearing of image with movement
      3. Patient's shoulders lowered as much as possible
      4. One complete cycle of flexion-extension fluorographed
III. Nasopharynx: Scout exposure image with
   A. Patient in upright position
   B. X-ray beam in lateral position
   C. Maximum noise reduction

C-arm fluoroscopy is not as valuable for fixed picture representation as is the soft tissue plain film. However, the physician can observe whether the cervical bodies move and how they move in relation to each other in flexion and extension, including the degree of potential cervical spine mobility at the time of endoscopy or intubation.

Similarly, temporomandibular joint (TMJ) motion can be quickly evaluated. By angling the x-ray beam, the physician can observe the left or right side of the TMJs separately as in standard TMJ studies. The physician may also view both TMJs simultaneously and thus evaluate bilateral TMJ motion with the assurance of uniform effort. Studies are performed with the patient in both the supine and sitting position, making it possible to quickly evaluate and compare the effects of patient positioning on airway configurations. Optimum access for intubation can be determined as the patient changes position. Every position and combination of maneuvers can be quickly evaluated for its usefulness. By using the C-arm for preintubation evaluation, the airway specialist can quickly follow up on questions as they appear, rather than ordering films, waiting for reports, and perhaps having to order more radiographs to track down problems or answer questions raised by the first set of films.

This timesaving factor should not be underestimated. Radiation exposure dosage to patients is an important consideration. It has been found that C-arm studies result in acceptable radiation ex-

---

STEPS IN C-ARM FLUOROGRAPHIC IMAGING TECHNIQUES—cont'd

IV.   Oropharynx and laryngopharynx to upper trachea
    A. Scout exposure image with
        1. Patient in upright position
        2. X-ray beam in lateral position
        3. Maximum noise reduction
        4. Patient's neck in neutral position
        5. Slight inspiration
        NOTE: It may be necessary to do two scout films; one upper (oropharynx) and one lower (laryngopharynx to trachea) because of patient size.
    B. Lateral dynamic airway image with
        1. Patient in upright position
        2. X-ray beam in lateral position
        3. Noise reduction at a reduced level to prevent smearing of image
        4. X-ray field centered so that bottom of field includes the upper trachea (If this centering does not also demonstrate oropharynx, two sets of dynamic studies should be performed; the first with the trachea at the bottom of the frame and the second with the trachea at the top of the frame.)
        5. Patient's neck in neutral position
            a. Normal respiration
            b. Deep respiration (nasal)
            c. Deep respiration (oral, mouth opened wide, tongue in)
            d. Deep respiration (oral, mouth opened wide with tongue out)
            e. Cough
            f. Phonation (A, E, I, O, U)
            g. Swallowing
        6. With patient's neck extended, image under the same dynamics as in IVB5
        7. With the patient's neck flexed, image under the same dynamics as in IVB5
    C. Lateral dynamic airway study: Follow steps IVB2 to 7 with the patient in supine position.

posure levels to the patient.* Patient radiation doses under C-arm fluoroscopy range from 300 to 450 mR/min, depending on the structures being imaged.

C-ARM–ASSISTED INTUBATION

In addition to preoperative evaluations, the C-arm is used to support those intubations that have been predetermined to be exceptionally difficult. First, the case is identified as such on the operating room daily schedule. It is then the responsibility of the radiographic technologist to have a C-arm in the operating room when the patient arrives. The patient is placed in the most advantageous position (sitting or semi-Fowler supine) on the table for intubation, as determined in the preoperative airway clinic. The technologist and the intubationist determine the placement of the C-arm to ensure that lateral and AP radiographic positions are possible and that the proper operating room table is used.[1]

The monitor cart is placed so that the radiation specialist and the intubationist can view it. During the actual intubation, the intubationist looks through the fiberoptic scope. The technologist provides a running verbal report of the image on the C-arm monitor screen (the position of the airway and the fiberscope within it). With this method the intubation team is able to use the C-arm to guide the fiberoptic scope when blood, mucus, redundant tissue, or some other obstacle has temporarily obscured direct fiberoptic visualization. In trauma patients the use of the C-arm and its ability to facilitate visualization of the airway and the fiberoptic scope within it should not be underestimated.

The C-arm indicates when the fiberoptic scope is being misdirected. From the lateral view the anteroposterior position of the scope is clearly demonstrated. The lateral view also indicates if the fiberscope is being directed off the left-right midline. Assuming that the image is a true lateral image of the airway, the tip of the fiberscope should appear square. Therefore the first indication of a rounded tip on the image alerts the intubationist that the scope is moving off midline. Confirmation of left-right positioning can be made with the anteroposterior view. Because of its structural design, the C-arm can switch from an anteroposterior to a lateral view in seconds.

C-arm–supported intubation should not be limited to a supporting role in predetermined difficult intubations; it should be employed in those cases where no difficulty has been foreseen, but intubation has been impossible using standard intubation techniques. Assuming that there is time to set up the C-arm to support an unforeseen difficult intubation (when ventilation is possible but intubation is not), it should be considered. Radiographic support often provides the missing information to intubate. Certainly, this noninvasive technique should be tried before an attempted retrograde wire intubation or a tracheotomy.

C-ARM– AND GUIDE WIRE–ASSISTED INTUBATION

The author has found that the most difficult intubations can often be easily accomplished with a guide wire via the suction or biopsy channel of the flexible endoscope, combined with the portable fluoroscope.

In a C-arm and fiberoptic guide wire intubation the patient is positioned in the same manner as that described previously. The endotracheal tube is positioned in the patient's nasal airway, and the fiberscope is passed through it. The fiberscope is then directed by C-arm image or by visualizing through the scope to be directed into the epiglottis. The shape of the epiglottis then guides the wire down to the vocal folds and into the thoracic airway. The fiberscope is then advanced along the wire, allowing the wire to direct the scope into the chest to a point just above the carina. The guide wire is then removed, and the endotracheal tube is passed along the fiberscope. As the fiberscope is removed, it is used to verify the proper location of the endotracheal tube. The tube is then secured.

The author has had 100% success with this method, and this success has been on the most difficult of patients.

---

*Population dose recommendations from the Nuclear Regulatory Commission is 500 mR/yr. NCRP report No. 116 issued March 31, 1993. The author determines patient dose in two ways: the indirect method (calculations are based on exposure factors) and the direct method (placing a film badge on the patient's neck).

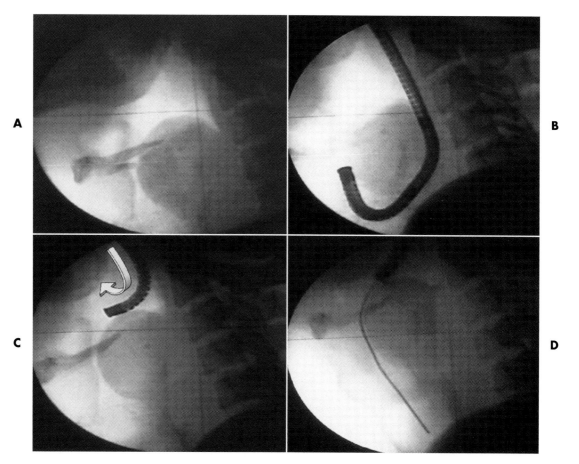

FIG. 8-4 Wire intubation (collage). **A,** Prevertebral mass at level of hyoid bone. **B,** Deflection of endoscope by mass. **C,** Cephalad deflection of endoscope. **D,** Guide wire system for fiberoptic intubation. (From Healy TEJ, Cohen PJ: Wylie & Churchill-Davidson's: A practice of anaesthesia. In Norton ML [ed]: *The difficult airway,* ed 6, Manchester, England, 1995, Edward Arnold.)

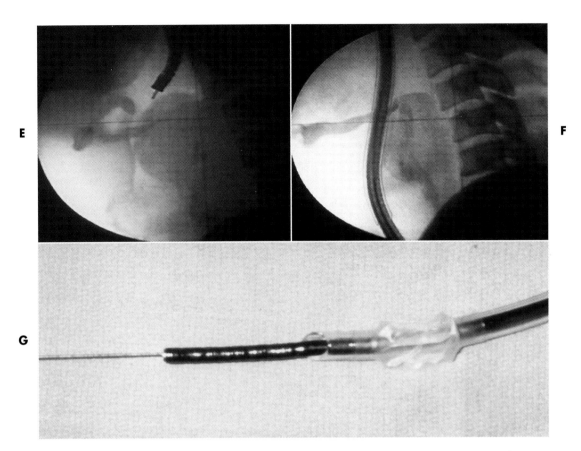

FIG. 8-4, cont'd.   **E,** Position visualizing entrance to larynx. **F,** Endotracheal tube advanced over endoscope. **G,** Note wire over which is the fiberoptic (suction or biopsy channel), over which is the softened endotracheal tube.

The use of the portable fluoroscope is most strikingly demonstrated in Fig. 8-4. A case history exemplifies its usefulness. A patient presented with a history of failed intubation. The primary diagnosis was not related to the airway. The initial view, with the patient sitting and with use of the C-arm, clarified the problem as a prevertebral mass at the level of the hyoid bone (Fig. 8-4, *A*). Using both the flexible fiberoptic endoscope and the C-arm, an attempt was made to enter the trachea (Fig. 8-4, *B*) without success. A second attempt met with similar results. However, in both cases the introitus to the laryngeal aperture could be visualized. The decision was then made to use a guide wire system (Cook Wire Guide, SF; diameter, 0.38 inches; length, 145 cm; flexible tip; straight).

The endoscope was prepared (Fig. 8-4, *D*), the endotracheal tube was preplaced, the endoscope was introduced through the lumen of the endotracheal tube, and the wire guide was inserted through the biopsy port (Fig. 8-4, *E*). The guide wire was visually inserted through the additus laryngis into the trachea, with fluoroscopic confirmation. The flexible endoscope was advanced into the trachea, and the endotracheal tube extended over the endoscope into its definitive location in the trachea.*

Limitations of the C-Arm

There are limiting factors involving the use of the C-arm and dynamic evaluations of the airway.† The C-arm has a difficult time with body parts that are small or have a wide range of densities over a small area, for example, fingers or toes. Sometimes the problem manifests itself between the airway and the cervical spine (both of which have very low density) and the cervical spine (which has a medium high density). In such cases a decision must be made about the area of greatest concern, for example, the airway configuration. In airway images the physician must realize that the cervical spine will not be well demonstrated in that individual image. The solution is to evaluate the cervical spine and the airway with separate images.

Another limited factor of the C-arm is the use of noise reduction. The problem is that the computer is unable to keep up with a dynamic image and still maintain a high degree of noise reduction. The resultant image has a smeared effect. Therefore it is necessary to use less noise reduction for the more dynamic portions of the examination. This creates a drop-off in dynamic image quality, but that drop-off does not compromise the value of the C-arm itself. This denigration is, however, noticeable.

C-arm fluoroscopy is not as valuable for fixed picture representation as is the soft tissue plain film. The C-arm image has less detail than a standard radiograph because it uses less radiation and its image density medium has vastly fewer available lines of resolution.

The mobility of the C-arm allows for its use in a clinic setting, a preoperative holding area, or in the operating room itself. Its use is strongly recommended in assessment and management of upper airway problems.

---

*Editor's note: The entire process took approximately 1½ to 2 minutes with the patient sitting upright, awake, breathing spontaneously, and using topical anesthesia only.

†The author once had difficulty imaging the airway in a patient who had a great deal of soft tissue removed during radical neck surgery. The transverse density of the patient's neck at the point of the airway was almost the same density as that of air itself. The author was unable to turn down the x-ray beam factors sufficiently to view the airway. Although the lowest setting possible was used, the anterior border of the airway was being overexposed and burned away. The solution to this problem was to increase density of the airway and lower the total amount of x-rays emitted. This was done with the use of Lucite and aluminum filters. A Lucite wedge filter was placed on the patient with the thick end of the wedge in the anterior position. This added density to the patient, with that density increasing anteriorly to the point of greatest overexposure. Aluminum filters were placed on the x-ray tube to reduce the total amount of emitted radiation. With the use of these filters an acceptable image was produced.

REFERENCES

1. Lowe AA, Gionhaku N, Takeuchi K et al: Three-dimensional CT reconstructions of tongue and airway in adult subjects with obstructive sleep apnea, *Am J Orthod Dentofacial Orthop* 90:364-373, 1986.

2. Katsantonis GP, Walsh JK: Somnofluoroscopy: its role in the selection of candidates for uvulopalatopharyngoplasty, *Otolaryngol Head Neck Surg* 94:1, 1986.

3. Ledley RS: Introduction to computerized tomography, *Comput Biol Med* 6:239-246, 1976.

CHAPTER 9

Pulmonary Function Testing in the Evaluation of Upper Airway Obstruction

FERNANDO J. MARTINEZ

Pulmonary function testing allows the relationships between air flow, lung volumes, and thoracic pressures in the evaluation of pulmonary disease to be examined and the presence of upper airway restriction to be determined. The most common tests include simple measures of expired volumes recorded with a spirometer. Flow can be expressed with a flow volume loop (see p. 127 and Fig. 9-5). Lung volumes are measured with body plethysmography or gas dilution methods. Gas transfer (diffusion capacity), maximum voluntary ventilation, respiratory muscle forces, lung compliance, and cardiopulmonary exercise testing are also available to the clinician to complete the evaluation of lung function. The role of these studies has been described elsewhere.[1] For the purpose of this chapter (evaluating the upper airway), flow volume loops are examined in the greatest detail.

PHYSIOLOGY OF AIRFLOW

The upper airway is usually thought to consist of the nasal passages and pharynx. To physicians, who manage patients with airway disease on a functional level, the larynx and trachea are considered components. These structures share variable compliance, which allows dynamic influences to affect airway geometry. As such, during respiration the magnitude of pressure change and resulting airflow depends not only on the force that drives airflow generated by the respiratory muscles, but also on the distribution of airway resistance along the airway and on the elasticity of the walls of the airway.[2] In this manner, greater resistance will have predictable effects on airflow. For example, using the effect of endotracheal tubes on airflow (Fig. 9-1), it can be seen that a progressively smaller tube orifice decreases flow resulting from any driving pressure.[3] With a 6-mm orifice, the physician can see that progressive increase in driving pressure leads to little increase in airflow. Such an opening is considered a *critical orifice*. Recent work examining the effect of driving pressure on airflow through cadaveric larynges with a varied aperture has shown that an aperture of less than 0.5 cm^2 is associated with a significant increase in resistance during normal breathing. An aperture greater than 0.67 cm^2 was not associated with increased resistance, using the pressures generated during normal breathing.[4] As such, the degree of cross-sectional compromise in airway lumen has significant impact on airflow.

The elasticity of the upper airway also has significant impact on airflow during respiration. The airway outside the thorax (extrathoracic airway) is at atmospheric pressure (Fig. 9-2). During inspiration, negative intratracheal pressures are associated with a transmural pressure change across the airway, such that it tends to collapse. During expiration the opposite effect occurs in the extrathoracic portion of the airway. However, the airway within the thorax (intrathoracic airway), is surrounded by pleural pressures and thus responds differently. During forced expiration the transmural pressure tends to collapse this intrathoracic portion of the trachea. It would be expected that the location of an abnormality along the length of the upper airway would have varying effects on airflow.

Special acknowledgement goes to Frank S. Becker, M.D., for aid in reproduction of the figures.

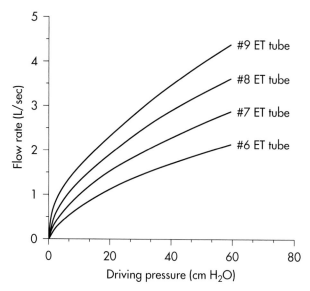

FIG. 9-1 Airflow vs. driving pressure across endotracheal *(ET)* tubes of varying diameters.

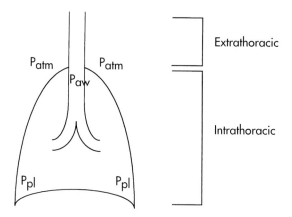

FIG. 9-2 Schematic of lung showing intrapleural pressure *(P$_{pl}$)* within thorax, atmospheric pressure *(P$_{atm}$)*, and mean airway pressure *(P$_{aw}$)*. Extrathoracic and intrathoracic portions of upper airway are identified.

The nature of the lesion in the upper airway also affects the airflow resulting from respiratory maneuvers. *Variable obstructions* are those in which airway geometry varies with transmural pressure. This includes vocal fold paralysis (extrathoracic airway) and tracheomalacia (intrathoracic airway). The aperture diameters of variable lesions depend on their locations in the airway as a result of the different transmural pressures (Fig. 9-3).

A variable intrathoracic lesion is expected to affect flow during expiration, whereas a similar lesion in the extrathoracic airway affects flow during inspiration. Regardless of its location in the airway, a lesion whose geometry is little affected by transmural pressure changes (for example, a "fixed" lesion such as a fibrotic or malignant tracheal stricture) affects both inspiratory and expiratory flow.

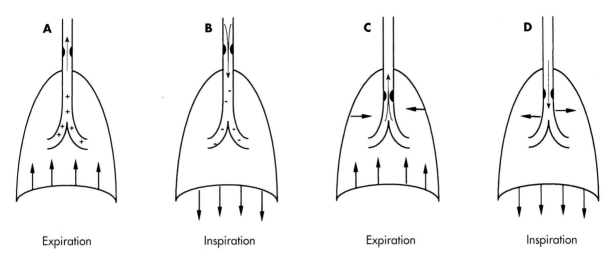

FIG. 9-3   Effect of variable, extrathoracic obstruction (**A** and **B**) expected to have greater effect on airflow during inspiration (**B**). Opposite is seen in variable, intrathoracic obstruction (**C** and **D**) in which greater diminution in airflow is seen during expiration (**D**).

Flow Volume Loops

Measures of flow may be useful in establishing abnormalities within the upper airway if the principles described previously are used. Flow volume loops express flow during expiration and inspiration as a function of lung volume. They are usually measured using a spirometer, which measures volume directly, or with a pneumotachograph, which integrates the flow to calculate volume. The divisions of lung volume that can be measured with a spirometer are illustrated in Fig. 9-4. Tidal volume (Vt) represents the volume moved during quiet, spontaneous respiration. A maximal inspiratory maneuver inflates the lungs to total lung capacity (TLC). A complete expiratory maneuver exhales the vital capacity (VC)—forced vital capacity (FVC) if forcefully expired or slow vital capacity (SVC) if slowly expired. The remaining volume in the lung after a full expiration, which cannot be measured with a spirometer, is the residual volume (RV).

Spirometric data as the airflow during a maximum inspiration from RV to TLC and airflow during maximum expiration from TLC to RV is known as the *flow volume loop* and is illustrated in Fig. 9-5. It is evident from examining this tracing that maximum expiratory flow is achieved during the first 25% of the vital capacity; this peak expiratory flow rate (PEFR) depends mainly on the effort of the subject and the resistance in the upper airway. Obstruction of expiratory flow with an upper airway lesion is demonstrated by decreases in PEFR. Diffuse airway obstruction, as is seen with emphysema, produces a typical abnormality in the flow volume loop (Fig. 9-5, *B*). Restrictive lung diseases (e.g., pulmonary fibrosis), which decrease lung volumes (VC and TLC) are associated with "narrowed" loops (Fig. 9-5, *C*).

Understanding the flow volume loop allows the physiologic principles described previously to be applied to the diagnosis of upper airway obstructions. Greater degrees of obstruction should result in progressive abnormalities of inspiratory flow, expiratory flow, or both. When normal subjects perform maximum inspiratory and expiratory efforts while breathing through progressively smaller external orifices (simulating progressively worse fixed lesions because the geometry of the orifice is independent of transmural pressure), it leads to the type of flow volume loops shown in Fig. 9-6. This figure also illustrates the effect of a fixed lesion on expiratory flow in that both inspiratory and expiratory flows are reduced during maximum respiratory maneuvers.

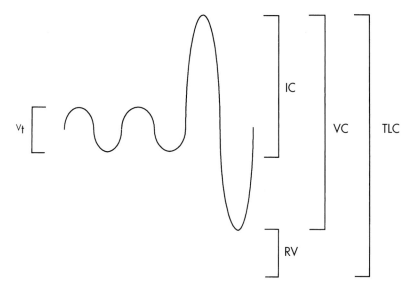

FIG. 9-4   Divisions of lung volume. These include tidal volume *(v_t)*, vital capacity *(VC)*, inspiratory capacity *(IC)*, and total lung capacity *(TLC)*. Residual volume *(RV)* cannot be measured with a simple spirometer.

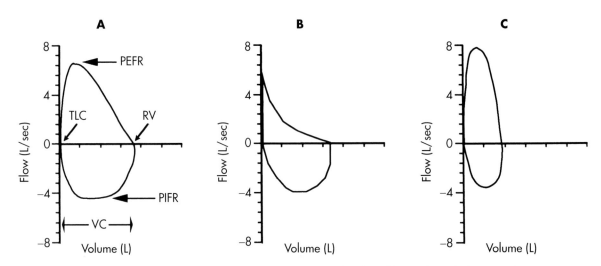

FIG. 9-5   Expiratory flow and inspiratory flow expressed as function of lung volume during a maximum maneuver (maximum flow volume loop [MFVL]). Peak expiratory flow rate *(PEFR)*, peak inspiratory flow rate *(PIFR)*, vital capacity *(VC)*, and residual volume *(RV)* shown in MFVL from a normal individual **(A)**. *TLC*, Total lung capacity. **B,** MFVL from an individual with chronic airflow obstruction revealing decreased expiratory flows. **C,** MFVL from an individual with idiopathic pulmonary fibrosis showing preserved PEFR but decreased VC.

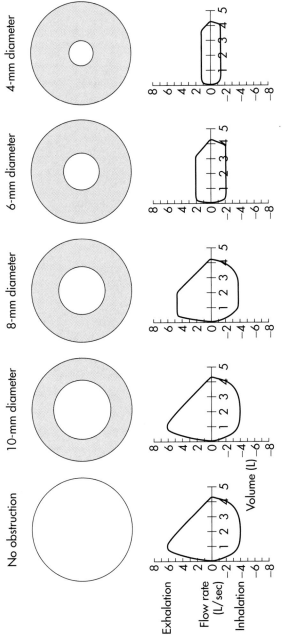

FIG. 9-6   Maximum flow volume loop from a normal individual performing maximum maneuvers through progressively smaller orifices.

The location of a variable obstruction is expected to yield specific abnormalities of inspiratory or expiratory flow, as proven in the work of Miller and Hyatt.[5] Fig. 9-7 illustrates the changes expected in a patient with a variable, extrathoracic obstruction who had preservation of expiratory flow but a decrease in inspiratory flow. The extrathoracic airway tends to alter its geometry during inspiration. A patient with variable, intrathoracic obstruction is expected to show opposite types of changes. Expiratory flow is preferentially decreased as the susceptible area of the upper airway shows the greatest alteration in geometry compared with the transmural changes seen during expiration. Fig. 9-8 shows the flow volume loop of an elderly man with a tracheal chondrosarcoma and severe tracheomalacia at the site of the tumor within the intrathoracic portion of the trachea.[6]

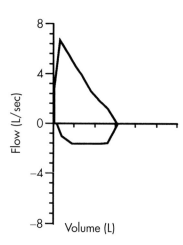

FIG. 9-7   Maximum flow volume loop from 26-year-old woman with mild asthma, hoarseness, and inspiratory stridor with voluntary hyperventilation. Inspiratory limb reveals plateau with decreased peak inspiratory flow rate typical of variable, extrathoracic obstruction. Laryngoscopy confirmed unilateral vocal cord paralysis.

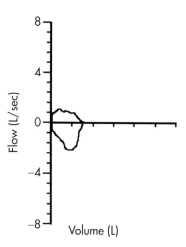

FIG. 9-8   Maximum flow volume loop from 72-year-old man with several years of progressive dyspnea, stridor during resting respiration, and enlarging paratracheal mass. Truncation of expiratory limb with decreased peak expiratory flow rate is typical of variable intrathoracic obstruction. Bronchoscopy confirmed high-grade, midtracheal obstruction. At thoracotomy, large tracheal chondrosarcoma was resected with 3-cm segment of tracheomalacia.

A patient with variable lesions in both intrathoracic and extrathoracic locations shows diminution of inspiratory and expiratory flows, thereby simulating a fixed obstruction. Such a case is illustrated in Fig. 9-9, where the flow volume loop is shown from a middle-aged woman with vocal fold paralysis (variable extrathoracic obstruction) and intrathoracic tracheomalacia (variable intrathoracic obstruction) many years after tracheostomy for severe poliomyelitis.[7]

There are limitations to the use of flow volume loops. In patients with severe chronic airway obstruction (CAO), the flow volume loop shows significant alteration caused by the peripheral airflow obstructions (see Fig. 9-5, *B*), and superimposed upper airway lesions may be missed.[8] Fig. 9-10 shows the flow volume loop of an elderly female with severe CAO months after prolonged mechanical ventilation through a tracheostomy for respiratory failure. The flow volume loops show the typical changes of CAO (compare with Fig. 9-5, *B*) and are not suggestive of upper airway obstruc-

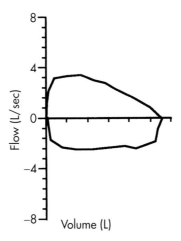

FIG. 9-9   Maximum flow volume loop from 51-year-old woman years after severe poliomyelitis, requiring tracheostomy and prolonged negative pressure ventilation with iron lung. Progressive dyspnea on exertion and stridor during exercise led to diagnosis of vocal cord paralysis (variable extrathoracic obstruction decreasing inspiratory flow) and midtracheal malacia (variable intrathoracic obstruction decreasing expiratory flow).

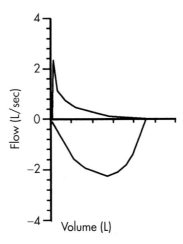

FIG. 9-10   Maximum flow volume loop (MFVL) from 63-year-old woman with severe chronic airway obstruction (CAO) 12 months after prolonged respiratory failure following exploratory laparotomy. Expiratory limb typical of CAO (compare with Fig. 9-5, *B*). Because of increased breathlessness and difficulty raising sputum, tracheal tomography was ordered and revealed high-grade (3 to 4 mm) midtracheal stenosis. Tracheal resection resulted in symptomatic improvement but no change in MFVL.

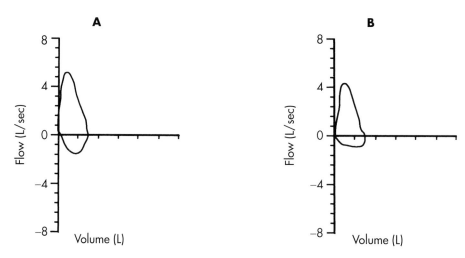

FIG. 9-11   Maximum flow volume loop (MFVL) from 65-year-old woman years after tracheal surgery for tracheal stenosis. Complaint of dyspnea during neck hyperextension led to examination with flow volume loop analysis. **A,** Relatively normal MFVL with neck in normal position. **B,** Confirmation of dramatic decrease in inspiratory flows with neck hyperextension. Tracheal tomography confirmed extrathoracic tracheomalacia with significant alteration in tracheal geometry with changes in neck position.

tion, although tracheal tomography confirmed severe intrathoracic tracheal narrowing. Changes also occur in tracheal geometry with varying neck position. Melissinos and Mead[9] recently demonstrated that, in a majority of normal subjects, expiratory flows during maximum flow volume loop maneuvers show increased expiratory flows and changes in tracheal geometry on radiography with neck hyperextension. This may have clinical utility. **Patients complaining of breathlessness with neck hyperextension reveal marked inspiratory flow limitation with flow volume loops performed with neck hyperextension compared with normal neck position** (Fig. 9-11). Extrathoracic tracheomalacia was confirmed in these cases.

Alternate Diagnostic Studies

Flow volume loop analysis is, by far, the simplest, cheapest, and most useful physiologic study in the diagnosis of upper airway obstructions. Additional studies are available in difficult situations. Changes in flows while the patient breathes a low-density gas (e.g., helium, which decreases airway resistance because of the lower gas density) have been suggested to have use in diagnosing upper airway obstructions in patients with underlying CAO.[10-12] Such a case has been recently described of a 57-year-old man with severe asthma.[11] A flow volume loop using room air and an 80% helium/20% oxygen gas mixture is shown in Fig. 9-12, *A*. There is a clear increase in expiratory flows with helium spirometry. The patient in Fig. 9-12, *A* was subsequently shown to have high-grade intrathoracic tracheal obstruction by papilloma and to experience a gratifying clinical and physiologic result with laser therapy (Fig. 9-12, *B*).

Measurement of airway resistance and exercise response with measurement of breath-by-breath flow volume loops may also aid in particularly difficult cases,[7] although their availability is limited.

CONCLUSION

Upper airway disease has predictable effects on airflow during maximum respiratory maneuvers. Understanding the use of flow volume loop analysis should provide information on the nature (variable vs. fixed), location (intrathoracic vs. extrathoracic), and approximate degree of airway narrowing in the majority of patients. The simplicity, reproducibility, low cost, and wide availability of spirometers makes flow volume loop analysis the optimum physiologic, diagnostic tool in the initial evaluation and follow-up of patients with upper airway disease.

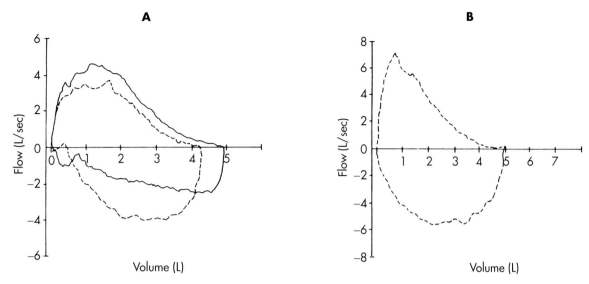

FIG. 9-12   Maximum flow volume loop (MFVL) in 57-year-old man with asthma who complained of progressive breathlessness and noisy respiration at night despite aggressive medications. **A,** MFVL performed on room air *(dashed line)* and using a 80% helium/20% oxygen gas mixture *(solid line).* Increased expiratory flow is demonstrated. Bronchoscopy confirmed high-grade tracheal obstruction by papilloma. Laser excision resulted in resolution of symptoms. **B,** MFVL after surgery.

REFERENCES

1. Clausen J: *Pulmonary function testing, guidelines and controversies: equipment, methods and normal values,* Philadelphia, 1982, WB Saunders.
2. Olson L, Fouke J, Hoekje P, et al: A biomechanical view of upper airway obstruction. In Mathew O, Sant' Abrogio G (eds): *Respiratory function of the upper airway,* New York, 1988, Marcel Dekker.
3. Eschenbacher WL: Pulmonary function tests for extrathoracic obstruction. In Norton ML, Brown ACD (eds): *Atlas of the difficult airway,* St Louis, 1991, Mosby.
4. Templer J, Von Doersten P, Quigley P, et al: Laryngeal airway resistance: the relationships of airflow, pressure, and aperture, *Arch Otolaryngol Head Neck Surg* 117:867-870, 1991.
5. Miller R, Hyatt R: Obstructing lesions of the larynx and trachea: clinical and physiologic characteristics, *Mayo Clin Proc* 44:145-161, 1969.
6. Leach KR, Martinez FJ, Morelock JW, et al: Dyspnea and tracheal mass in an elderly man, *Chest* 105:1555-1556, 1994.
7. Knobil K, Becker F, Harper P, et al: Dyspnea in a patient years after severe poliomyelitis: the role of cardiopulmonary exercise testing, *Chest* 105: 777-781, 1994.
8. Gelb A, Tashkin D, Epstein J, et al: Nd-YAG laser surgery for severe tracheal stenosis physiologically and clinically masked by severe diffuse obstructive pulmonary disease, *Chest* 91:166-170, 1987.
9. Melissinos CG, Mead J: Maximum expiratory flow changes induced by longitudinal tension on trachea in normal subjects, *J Appl Physiol: Respirat Environ Exercise Physiol* 43:537-544, 1977.
10. Lavelle T, Rotman H, Weg J: Isoflow-volume curves in the diagnosis of upper airway obstruction, *Am Rev Resp Dis* 117:845-852, 1978.
11. Pickering R, Martinez F: PFT Corner #41: helium flow-volume loop in an asthmatic patient, *Resp Care* 36:1157-1159, 1991.
12. Robertson D, Swinburn C, Stone T, et al: Effects of an external resistance on maximum flow in chronic obstructive lung disease: implications for recognition of coincident upper airway obstruction, *Thorax* 44:461-468, 1989.

CHAPTER 10

Fiberoptic Views

VIJAYALAKSHMI U. PATIL

The fiberoptic endoscope has been used extensively for diagnostic and therapeutic procedures in the fields of anesthesia and critical care medicine since the 1970s, and, with the laryngoscope, has become an indispensable part of the anesthesiologist's armamentarium. The techniques are well established and are expected in the management of difficult airway.

Flexible fiberoptic endoscopes allow the visualization of airway structures, an option beyond the capabilities of rigid laryngoscopies and bronchoscopies. The principles and descriptions of the components of fiberoptic scopes and their care have been described in detail elsewhere.[1-7] Because the endoscopes are delicate and expensive instruments, the manufacturers' instructions should be followed to minimize damage.

Anatomic structures viewed through the fiberoptic scopes differ from those viewed under direct rigid laryngoscopes. The view through the fiberoptic scope is small and can become distorted by secretions, blood, and fogging of the lens. In anesthetized patients the structures of the oral cavity are more lax and may collapse into the oral cavity. This can cause the manipulation of the endoscope toward the glottis to be difficult. The extension of the neck and retraction of the mandible allow the base of the tongue to be pulled away from the pharynx for better visualization of the larynx.

Endoscopic procedures are facilitated with the use of ancillary equipment such as nasal airways, bite blocks, intubating airways, endoscopic masks, and tongue retractors. Endoscopic airways serve to maintain the endoscope in the midline and lift the base of the tongue from the posterior pharyngeal wall, allowing easy suctioning of the secretions and blood from the oral cavity.[8-10] Bite blocks and intubating airways prevent the patient from biting on the scope. Endoscopic masks ensure uninterrupted ventilation and provide more time for visualizing the airway and performing endoscopic procedures in patients under general anesthesia.

Endoscopic procedures performed on patients with pathologic conditions of the airway should include the use of increased inspired oxygen concentration through a nasal cannula or through the operating channel of the endoscope. The flow of 2 to 3 L of oxygen through the scope keeps the secretions away from the lens and provides a high concentration of inspired oxygen to the patient. Local anesthetics can be instilled through the operating channel of the suction port of the endoscope to anesthetize the reactive airway during the procedure.

Equipment for emergency airway access must be readily available when performing procedures on patients with difficult airways. This includes devices such as jet ventilators, a cricothyroidotomy catheter, and a tracheotomy set. Functioning fiberoptic endoscopes, light sources, ancillary equipment, and local anesthetic agents should be kept readily available for use in elective and emergency situations. After use the equipment should be cleaned, making sure that all elements are functioning and that there is no damage.

Initial experience with fiberoptic endoscopes may be gained on an intubation mannequin, which provides ideal conditions for practicing the handling and maneuvering of the endoscope with-

Special credit is given to Olympus America, Inc., Lake Success, NY, and especially, Mr. Jay Beatus, for provision of fiberoptic views and instrumentation support.

out the worries about time and the patient's condition. One can become familiar with different endoscopic techniques through videotapes of procedures performed on actual patients. After gaining sufficient knowledge and experience with handling the instruments, the physician should perform the techniques on patients with normal airway anatomies followed by patients with difficult airways.

The endoscopic procedures can be effectively performed with the use of local anesthesia, sedation, or general anesthesia (with or without a muscle relaxant). Endoscopic procedures are usually performed with the patient in the supine position. Alternatively, the endoscopist may face the patient. Some patients may need to be placed in a semi-Fowler position because of an underlying medical condition. Depending on the patient's condition and underlying pathologic condition, the examination of the airway and the procedures can be performed through the mouth, the nose, or the tracheotomy stoma in adult and pediatric patients.

Antisialagogues should be administered preoperatively when fiberoptic endoscopy is planned unless the patient's condition contraindicates doing so. To reduce bleeding, a vasoconstrictor should be applied to the nasal passage before introducing the endoscope through the nose. Ample time must be allowed for the local anesthetics, decongestants, and antisialagogues to take effect. The sedatives should be titrated slowly to permit patients to respond to verbal commands. It is easier to visualize the larynx and thread the endotracheal tube during nasotracheal intubation because of the natural curve adopted by the endoscope during its passage through the nasopharynx and pharynx. During orotracheal intubation the endoscope forms an acute angle in the pharynx to expose the larynx, resulting in difficulty when threading the endotracheal tube over the scope. This is overcome by applying constant jaw thrust, withdrawing the endotracheal tube 1 or 2 cm, and rotating it medially as the tube is being advanced. A distorted or reactive airway, secretions, bleeding, or an uncooperative patient can reduce the success rate of endoscopic procedures.

The lens should be focused on printed letters before insertion into the patient. If the view is unclear despite focusing the lens, it may be covered with secretions or blood, may be against the mucosal structure, or may need to be defogged. In patients with anticipated difficult airways, it is advisable to attempt intubation with fiberoptic endoscopy rather than with conventional methods, which may result in tissue trauma, bleeding, and edema, thereby obscuring the structure. By paying attention to details, the success rate of fiberoptic endoscopic procedures can be increased.

The most common complaint of the beginning endoscopist is complete redness and "white-out" seen through the scope. The most frequent causes of this are the failure of the scope to remain in the midline or the endoscope being positioned so that is faces the mucosal tissue (i.e., pharyngeal wall, pyriform fossa, buckle mucosa, or esophagus). If the position of the endoscope cannot be brought to the midline by lateral rotation or altering the depth of the endoscope, it is better to withdraw the scope, defog the lens, and reinsert the endoscope into the patient.

Fiberoptic endoscopes are versatile instruments in the management of difficult airway. Tracheal intubation is successfully performed with minimal trauma and stress to a patient[11] when the conventional rigid laryngoscopic tracheal intubation is impossible or contraindicated (trauma or pathologic condition in the head and neck). Accurate positioning of the endotracheal tube can be confirmed in the operating room and intensive care unit.[12,13] Retrograde intubation is assisted by passing the guide wire through the operating channel or the suction port of the fiberoptic scopes and advancing the scope into the trachea under direct vision.[14] Proper positioning of the laryngeal mask airway against the glottis is assessed by passing the fiberscope through the mask.[15] Fiberscopes are used to change the existing endotracheal tube[16,17] and tracheostomy tube and to perform tracheobronchial toilet.

Complications include tissue trauma, bleeding, and laryngospasm. In the awake patient, gagging and coughing are minimized with adequate topical anesthesia and nerve blocks to the airway. The threat of aspiration is a concern in patients with full stomachs.

Fig. 10-1 demonstrates the areas of difficult airway endoscopy. Normal structures, as seen through the endoscope, are shown in Figs. 10-2 through 10-5. Figs. 10-6 through 10-16 demonstrate various pathologic states.

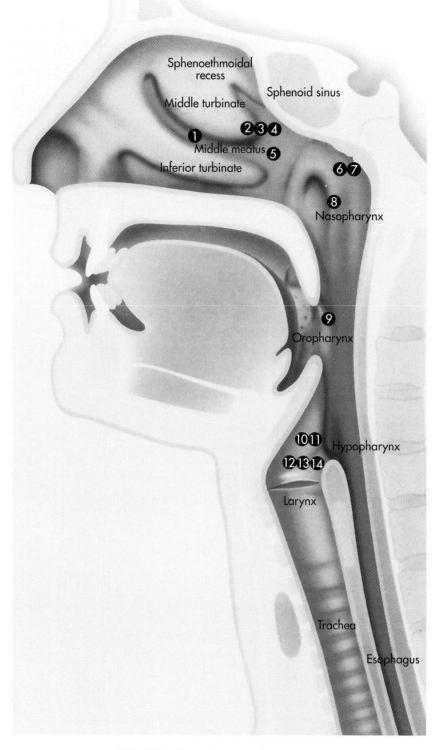

FIG. 10-1 Important areas of endoscopy.

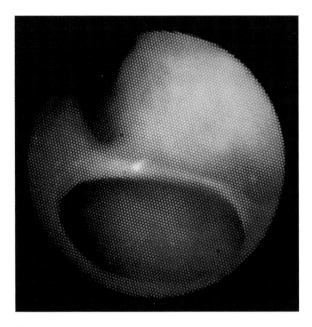

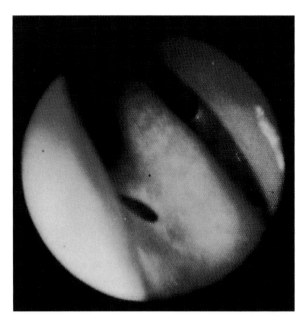

FIG. 10-2   Maxillary ostium and semilunar hiatus *(right)*.

FIG. 10-3   Superior meatus with posterior ethmoidal ostium *(right)*.

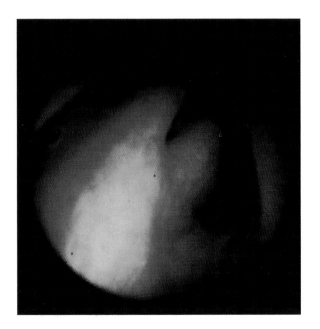

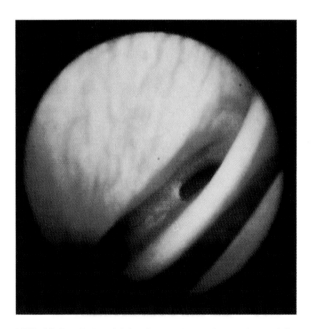

FIG. 10-4   Supreme and superior turbinates and superior meatus with ethmoidal ostia *(right)*.

FIG. 10-5   Sphenoidal ostium and superior turbinate *(left)*.

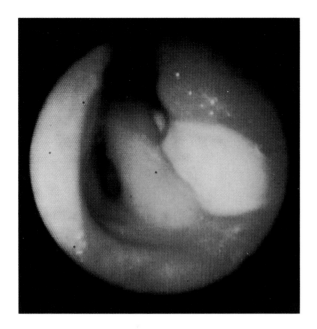

FIG. 10-6   Left choana, pus from middle meatus.

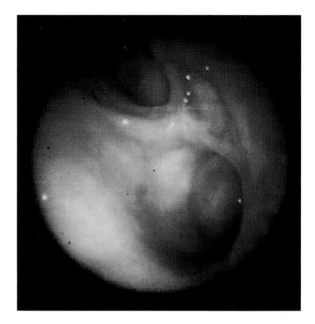

FIG. 10-7   Postoperative posterior ethmoidal cells *(right)*.

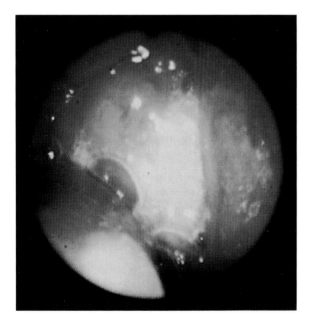

FIG. 10-8   Large adenoids obstructing choana *(right)*.

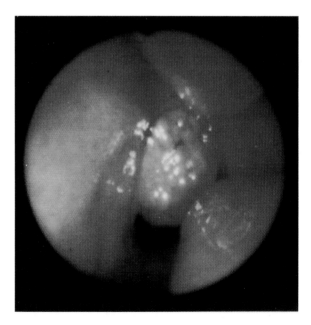

FIG. 10-9   Adenoids protruding to nasal cavity *(left)*.

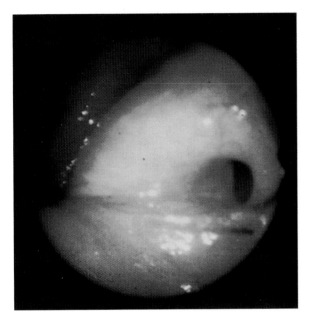

FIG. 10-10   Tubal orifice *(left).*

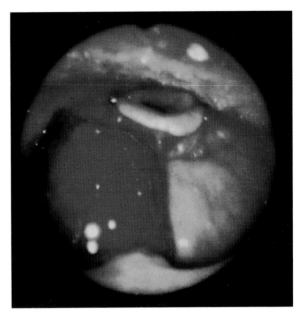

FIG. 10-11   Oropharyngeal metastasis of lung cancer.

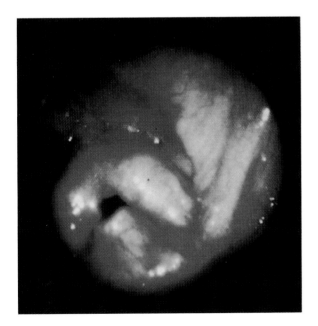

FIG. 10-12   Laryngomalacia, reflected epiglottis on inspiration.

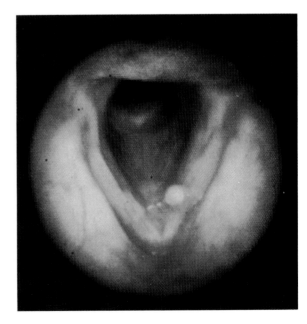

FIG. 10-13   Vocal cord polyp *(left).*

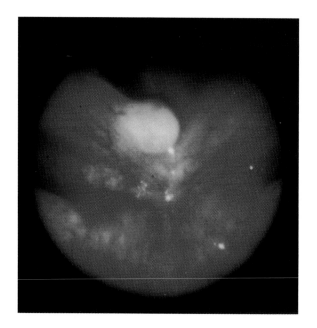

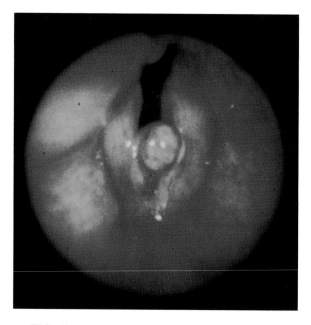

FIG. 10-14 Close view of vocal cord polyp *(right)*, anterior commissure, and ventricles.

FIG. 10-15 Vocal cord polyp *(right)* on phonation.

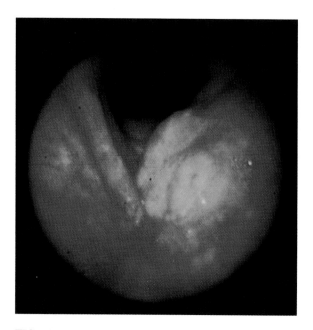

FIG. 10-16 Early stage of supraglottic cancer (left). Fiberscope reveals its precise extent.

REFERENCES

1. Berci G: *Endoscopy,* New York, 1976, Appleton-Century-Crofts.

2. Ikeda S: *Atlas of flexible bronchofiberscopy,* Baltimore and London, 1974, University Park Press.

3. Stradling P: *Diagnostic bronchoscopy,* Edinburgh, London, and New York, 1968, Churchill-Livingstone.

4. Bruce B: *Atlas of paediatric endoscopy: upper tract and oesophagus,* Oxford, Toronto, and New York, 1981, Oxford University Press.

5. Patil VU, Stehling LC, Zauder HL: *Fiberoptic endoscopy in anesthesia,* Chicago and London, 1983, Year Book Medical.

6. Ovassapian A: *Fiberoptic airway endoscopy in anesthesia and critical care,* New York, 1990, Raven Press.

7. Kitamura S: *Color atlas of clinical applications of fiberoptic bronchoscopy,* ed 2, St Louis, 1990, Mosby.

8. Patil V, Stehling LC, Zauder HL et al: Mechanical aids for fiberoptic endoscopy, *Anesthesiology,* 57:69-70, 1982.

9. Williams RT, Harrison RE: Prone tracheal intubation simplified using an airway intubator, *Can Anaesth Soc J* 28:288-289, 1981.

10. Ovassapian A: A new fiberoptic intubating airway, *Anesth Analg* 66 (suppl):132, 1987.

11. Ovassapian A, Yelich SJ, Dykes MHM et al: Blood pressure and heart rate changes during awake fiberoptic nasotracheal intubation, *Anesth Analg* 62:951-954, 1983.

12. Whitehouse AC, Klock LR: Evaluation of endotracheal tube position with the fiberoptic intubation laryngoscope, *Chest* 68:848, 1975.

13. O'Brien D, Curran J, Conroy J: Fiberoptic assessment of tracheal tube position: a comparison of tracheal tube position as estimated by fiberoptic bronchoscopy and by chest x-ray, *Anaesthesia* 40:73-76, 1985.

14. Lechman MJ, Donahoo JS, McVaugh M, III: Endotracheal intubation using percutaneous retrograde guide wire insertion followed by antegrade fiberoptic bronchoscopy, *Crit Care Med* 14:589-590, 1986.

15. Payne J: The use of the fiberoptic laryngoscope to confirm the position of the laryngeal mask, *Anaesthesia* 44:865, 1989.

16. Watson CB, Prough DS, Balestrier FJ: Bronchoscopic tube change in critically ill patients, *Crit Care Med* 8:246, 1980.

17. Rosenbaum SH, Rosenbaum LM, Cole RP: Use of the flexible fiberoptic bronchoscope to change endotracheal tube in critically ill patients, *Anesthesiology* 54:169, 1981.

CHAPTER 11

Double-Lumen and Univent Tube Insertion under Fiberoptic Control

ANDRANIK OVASSAPIAN

Endobronchial tubes and blockers are used to separate lungs and apply one-lung ventilation (OLV) during intrathoracic operations. The most common indication for OLV is to facilitate surgical exposure during intrathoracic operations (see the box on p. 143). Various kinds of endobronchial tubes and blockers have been developed for this purpose.[1,2] The Robertshaw double-lumen endobronchial tubes (DLTs) are the most commonly applied devices. This chapter covers the indications and the fiberoptic techniques used for placement of Robertshaw DLTs and Univent tube endobronchial blockers to achieve separation of the lungs.

ROBERTSHAW DOUBLE-LUMEN ENDOBRONCHIAL TUBES

The Robertshaw DLTs have a proximal and a distal or bronchial curvature to facilitate bronchial intubation. When both the bronchial cuff, located at the distal end of the bronchial tube, and the tracheal cuff, located proximal to the opening of the tracheal lumen, are inflated, a separate airway is formed for each lung. Tubes designed for intubation of the right bronchus have openings in the lateral aspect of the bronchial cuff to permit ventilation of the right upper lobe. Disposable polyvinyl chloride (PVC) tubes have larger lumina and lower resistance to gas flow than the original Carlens or White tubes that are made of red rubber. The advantages of PVC tubes include a more flexible structure, thin-walled tracheal and bronchial cuffs, and a greater inside-to-outside diameter. The PVC tubes also allow observation of the humidity of the exhaled air. The bronchial cuff is blue, which is easily identified during fiberoptic bronchoscopy.

The disposable Robertshaw right- and left-sided DLTs are available in four sizes (Table 11-1). The bronchial cuff characteristics and dimensions of slot on right-sided tubes from different manufacturers vary.

Right-Sided vs. Left-Sided Double-Lumen Endobronchial Tubes

The common practice is to intubate left mainstem bronchus using a left-sided DLT because of its high margin of safety and ease of placement.[3] Although, under most circumstances positioning of a left-sided DLT is physically possible, in some patients ventilation of the left lung is inadequate and if left lung is the dependent lung, safety of an OLV cannot be guaranteed. Under these circumstances a right-sided DLT should be used.

Others have suggested that the bronchial tube be placed in the bronchus of the operative lung because most difficulties encountered with DLTs are related to bronchial intubation and any difficulties encountered with ventilation of the operative lung will be less consequential. Intubating the bronchus of the operative side leaves the tracheal lumen vulnerable to being pushed against the tracheal wall, thus causing partial occlusion and ball valve action resulting in hyperinflation of the dependent lung.[4]

Ideally, the bronchus of the nonoperative lung can be intubated, leaving the operative bronchus free, thus eliminating the possibility of having the tube clamped or sutured in place.[5]

With the advancement of fiberoptic bronchoscopic positioning of a right-sided DLT, the technical difficulties of blind placement and the high incidence of failure have been resolved.[4]

INDICATIONS FOR SEPARATION OF THE LUNGS

Surgical
    Absolute indications
        To prevent contamination of nonoperative lung from secretions and blood
        To provide adequate ventilation in the presence of a large bronchopleural fistula
        To allow open bronchus surgery
        To avoid rupture of giant lung cyst and pneumothorax
    Relative indications
        To improve the operating field and surgical exposure
            Pulmonary resections
            Esophageal surgery
            Thoracic aortic aneurysm repair
            Other intrathoracic procedures
Nonsurgical
    Bronchopulmonary lavage
        Pulmonary alveolar proteinosis
    Differential lung ventilation
        Unilateral pulmonary insufficiency
            Severe atelectasis
            Pulmonary contusion
    Management of pulmonary hemorrhage

From Karwande SV: *Chest* 92:761-763, 1987.

Table 11-1 Characteristics of Left-Sided BronchoCath Endobronchial Tubes

Outer diameter French size (F)	Distance from bronchial tip to			Approximate equivalent inner lumen diameter*		Cuff length	
	Separation of two lumens (cm)	Upper border of tracheal cuff (cm)	Distal opening of tracheal lumen (cm)	Bronchial (mm)	Tracheal (mm)	Bronchial (cm)	Tracheal (cm)
28	33	10.6	5.6	4.5	4.5	1.2	4.5
35	33	12.9	6.7	6.0	6.0	1.4	4.5
37	33	13.0	6.7	6.5	6.5	1.4	4.5
39	33	13.5	7.1	7.0	7.0	1.4	4.5
41	33	13.8	7.1	7.4	7.4	1.4	4.7

From Karwande SV: *Chest* 92:761-763, 1987.

*The lumen is D-shaped rather than circular. Equivalent size will not be helpful for selection of fiberscope size.

Bronchial Intubation with Double-Lumen Endobronchial Tubes

Bronchial intubation with DLTs is easily achieved in anesthetized and paralyzed patients with the help of a rigid laryngoscope. The Robertshaw DLT is inserted into the trachea with the tip of the bronchial tube facing anteriorly. To achieve this position, the left-sided tube is held rotated 90 degrees clockwise and the right-sided tube is held rotated 90 degrees counterclockwise. After the tip of the bronchial tube passes the glottis, the stylet is removed and the tube is rotated 90 degrees back to its original position (left-sided DLT counterclockwise, right-sided DLT clockwise) so that the bronchial tube is pointing toward the respective bronchus.

Tracheal intubation can be achieved with a fiberscope when rigid laryngoscopy proves to be difficult or impossible. After establishing general anesthesia and muscle paralysis, the tongue is manually extended by an assistant. The fiberscope is inserted through the bronchial lumen of the DLT and advanced into the oropharynx and through the vocal cords into the trachea. The DLT is then threaded over the fiberscope into the trachea. Because of the larger size of a DLT and the distal curve, this is somewhat more difficult compared with intubation with a single-lumen endotracheal tube. To assist its passage, the tube is rotated to bring the tip of the bronchial lumen to the six o'clock position to negotiate the tip of the epiglottis and then to the twelve o'clock position to facilitate its passage into the trachea. If advancement of the DLT into the trachea results in resistance, the rigid laryngoscope is used to lift the base of the tongue and epiglottis to assist passage of the DLT over the fiberscope into the trachea.[4]

Fiberscopic Positioning of Left-Sided Robertshaw Tube

After tracheal placement of the DLT, the tracheal cuff is inflated and mechanical ventilation is begun. The fiberscope is inserted through the bronchial lumen into the left mainstem bronchus. The length, patency, and integrity of the bronchus are evaluated, and the tip of the fiberscope is positioned 10 mm above the orifice of the left upper lobe bronchus. The tracheal cuff is deflated and the tube is advanced over the fiberscope into the left mainstem bronchus until the tip of the tube is reached about 5 mm above the left upper lobe bronchial orifice. The fiberscope is then advanced beyond the bronchial lumen to visualize the orifices of the upper and lower lobe bronchi. To evaluate the position of the bronchial cuff, the fiberscope is withdrawn from the bronchial lumen and is passed down the tracheal lumen. The bronchial tube cuff should be confined inside the left mainstem bronchus, and the bronchus opening to the right mainstem bronchus should be open (Fig. 11-1).[4] If the bronchial cuff is above the carina, the tube is advanced farther, until the proximal edge of the bronchial cuff lies 3 to 5 mm inside the bronchus. The bronchial cuff is inflated with the minimum leak technique while the physician looks at it through the fiberscope.

When a left-sided DLT is correctly placed, the opening of the tracheal lumen lies 2 to 3 cm above the carina, the tip of the bronchial lumen lies above the left upper lobe bronchus orifice, and the bronchial cuff is confined inside of the left mainstem bronchus (Fig. 11-2).

A second approach may be used for positioning of the left-sided DLT. After inspection of the left bronchus, the fiberscope is pulled back, and, while it is rotated 90 degrees to the left, its tip is positioned at the level of the distal opening of the bronchial lumen (Fig. 11-3). The tracheal cuff is deflated, the tube and fiberscope are advanced together inside the left mainstem, and the tip of the bronchial tube is positioned 5 to 10 mm above the takeoff of the left upper lobe bronchus.[5] The rest of the procedure is as described under the first approach.

For fiberscopic positioning, checking the anatomy of the right bronchial tree is vital for speedy and accurate placement of right-sided DLTs.

After tracheal intubation the fiberscope is passed through the bronchial lumen into the right mainstem bronchus. The length and patency of the bronchus are evaluated. If the right mainstem bronchus is 10 mm or longer, placement of a BroncoCath right-sided DLT is possible. Two approaches may be applied.

After checking the length, patency, and integrity of the right mainstem and bronchus intermedius, the fiberscope is withdrawn inside the lumen of the bronchial tube. The fiberscope is rotated 90 degrees clockwise with its tip positioned at the proximal end of the slot in the bronchial cuff (Fig. 11-4). The tracheal cuff is deflated, and the tube and fiberscope are advanced together toward the right mainstem bronchus. The position of the tip of the fiberscope is such that the operator can see through the distal opening of the tube and through the slot of the bronchial cuff simultane-

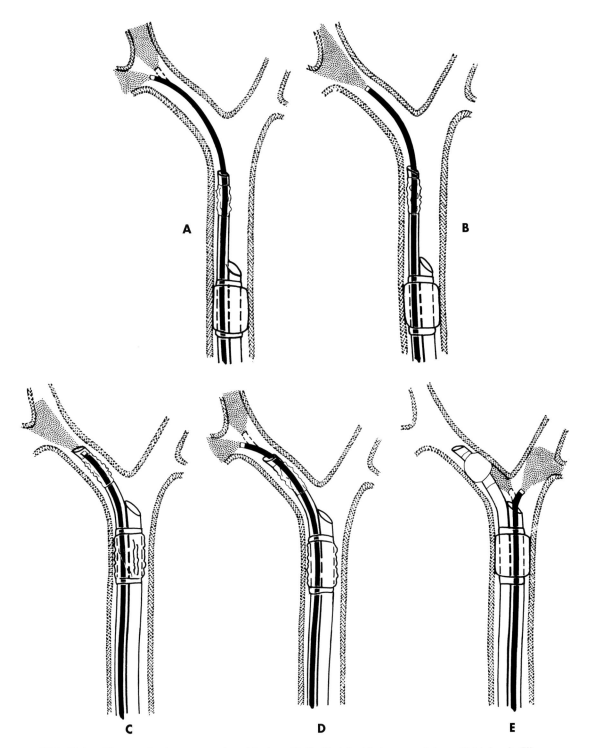

FIG. 11-1 Fiberscopic placement and positioning of left-sided double-lumen endobronchial tube. **A,** Fiberscope passed through bronchial lumen into left mainstem bronchus. Patency, length, and anatomy of left mainstem bronchus and position of orifice of left upper-lobe bronchus are evaluated. **B,** Fiberscope withdrawn and tip positioned 10 mm above origin of left upper-lobe bronchus. **C,** Tracheal cuff deflated and tube advanced over fiberscope into left mainstem bronchus until it comes into view beyond tip of fiberscope. **D,** Fiberscope advanced beyond bronchial lumen to visualize left upper-lobe bronchus. **E,** Fiberscope passed through trachea lumen to check position of bronchial cuff and opening of right mainstem bronchus. (From Ovassapian A: Fiberoptic-aided bronchial intubation. In Ovassapian A [ed]: *Fiberoptic airway endoscopy in anesthesia and critical care,* New York, 1990, Raven Press.)

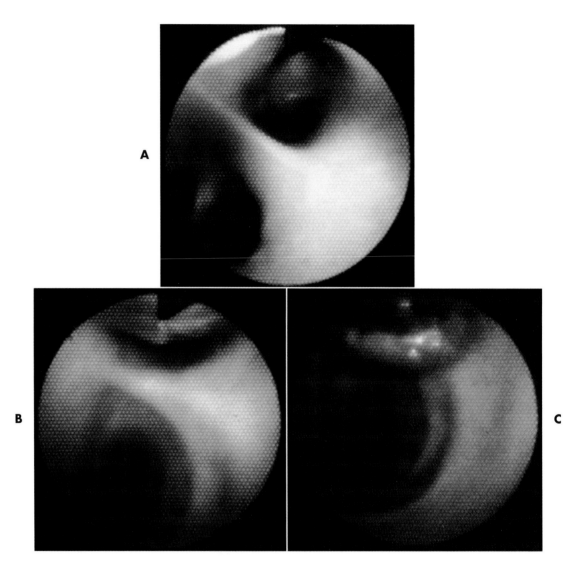

FIG. 11-2   Endoscopic view of left-sided double-lumen endobronchial tube positioning. **A,** Left upper- and lower-lobe bronchi orifices. **B,** Fiberscope inside tracheal lumen. Right mainstem bronchus open, and bronchial tube positioned in left mainstem bronchus. This represents proper positioning of endobronchial tube. **C,** Bronchial tube blue cuff herniates out of left mainstem bronchus (marginal placement). (From Ovassapian A: Fiberoptic-aided bronchial intubation. In Ovassapian A [ed]: *Fiberoptic airway endoscopy in anesthesia and critical care,* New York, 1990, Raven Press.)

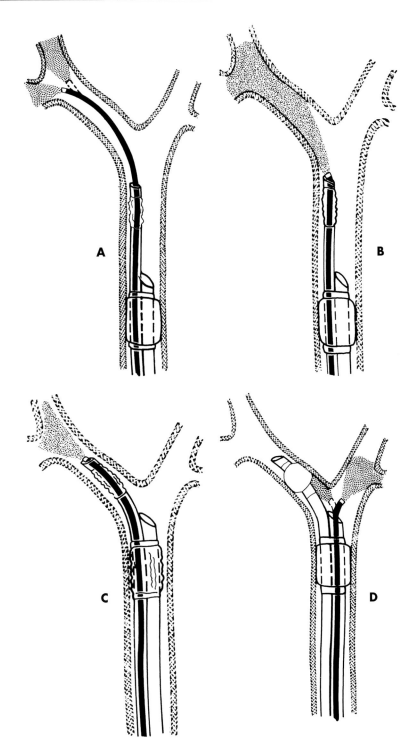

FIG. 11-3   Alternate approach to fiberscopic placement and positioning of left-sided, double-lumen endo-bronchial tube. **A,** Fiberscope passed through bronchial lumen into left mainstem bronchus. Patency, length, and anatomy of left mainstem bronchus and position of orifice of left upper-lobe bronchus are evaluated. **B,** Fiber-scope pulled back inside tube to position its tip at level of distal opening of bronchial lumen. Fiberscope posi-tioned 90 degrees rotated to left with tip angulated anteriorly toward lateral wall of trachea. **C,** Tracheal cuff de-flated. Tube and fiberscope advanced together inside left mainstem bronchus until orifice of left upper lobe comes into view. At this point, tip of fiberscope is 10 to 15 mm above left upper-lobe orifice. Tube advanced fur-ther to position distal end of tube about 5 mm above orifice of left upper-lobe bronchus. **D,** Fiberscope passed through tracheal lumen to check position of bronchial cuff and opening of right mainstem bronchus. (From Ovassapian A: Fiberoptic-aided bronchial intubation. In Ovassapian A [ed]: *Fiberoptic airway endoscopy in anesthesia and critical care,* New York, 1990, Raven Press.)

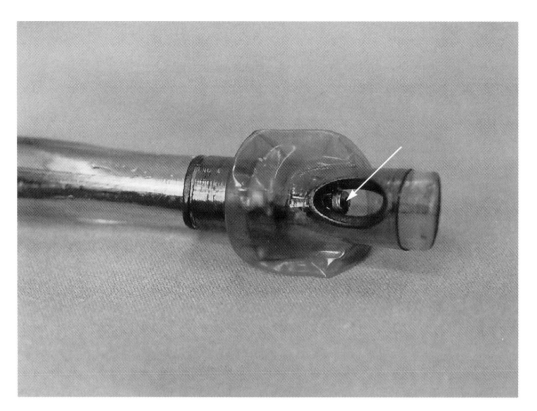

FIG. 11-4   Tip of fiberscope positioned at upper level of bronchial cuff slot. (From Ovassapian A: Fiberoptic-aided bronchial intubation. In Ovassapian A [ed]: *Fiberoptic airway endoscopy in anesthesia and critical care,* New York, 1990, Raven Press.)

ously. The tube and fiberscope are advanced into the right mainstem bronchus using the view through the distal opening of the tube and then advanced farther until the opening of the right upper-lobe orifice comes into view through the slot in the bronchial cuff. The tube is advanced until the distal edge of the slot is placed at the level of the the distal border of the orifice to the right upper-lobe bronchus. The fiberscope is then rotated counterclockwise to its neutral position and advanced beyond the distal end of the tube to visualize the right-, middle-, and lower-lobe bronchial openings. Finally, the fiberscope is inserted into the tracheal lumen to inspect the position of the bronchial cuff (Figs. 11-5 and 11-6).[6]

A second approach for positioning of the right-sided DLTs may also be applied. After visualizing the right upper-lobe bronchus with the fiberscope rotated 90 degrees to the right, the fiberscope is held stationary and its tip is returned to the neutral position. The tracheal cuff is deflated, and the tube is advanced over the fiberscope into the right bronchus until the distal end of the tip of the bronchial tube passes just beyond the tip of the fiberscope (Fig. 11-7). In this position the slot of the bronchial cuff typically lies opposite the orifice of the right upper-lobe bronchus. After confirming the proper position of the bronchial slot, the fiberscope is rotated 90 degrees counterclockwise to its neutral position and is passed beyond the tip of the bronchial tube to visualize the orifices of the right-, middle-, and lower-lobe bronchi. Finally, the fiberscope is inserted into the tracheal lumen to inspect the position of the bronchial cuff. The fiberscope is maintained in this position so that the bronchial cuff can be inflated with the minimum leak technique under visual observation.[4]

Because of the oblique design of the BronchoCath right-sided DLT bronchial cuff, placement of this tube is possible when right mainstem bronchus is as short as 10 mm. With a right-sided DLT, the upper border of the cuff is often positioned at the level of the carinal ridge and therefore is more likely to be displaced during positioning and during OLV when high airway pressures are applied.

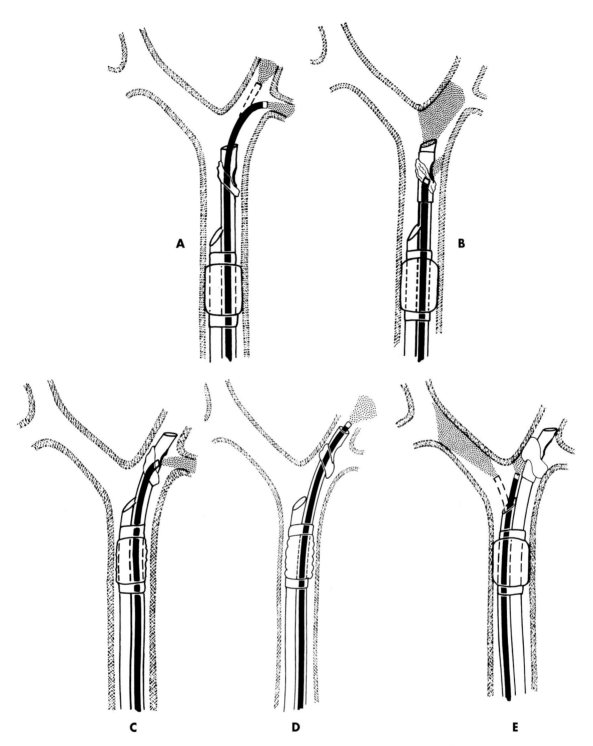

FIG. 11-5   Fiberscopic placement and positioning of right-sided double-lumen tube. **A,** Fiberscope passed through bronchial lumen into right mainstem bronchus. Patency, length, and anatomy of right mainstem bronchus evaluated. **B,** Fiberscope withdrawn inside bronchial lumen. Tip of fiberscope placed at proximal end of slot of bronchial cuff 90 degrees rotated to right and tip angulated anteriorly toward lateral wall of trachea. **C,** Tube and fiberscope are then advanced together inside right mainstem bronchus until orifice of right upper lobe comes into view through slit of bronchial cuff. **D,** Fiberscope rotated counterclockwise to its neutral position and beyond bronchial tube distal opening to verify patency of middle- and lower-lobe bronchi. **E,** Fiberscope passed through tracheal lumen to check position of bronchial cuff and opening of left mainstem bronchus. (From Ovassapian A: Fiberoptic-aided bronchial intubation. In Ovassapian A [ed]: *Fiberoptic airway endoscopy in anesthesia and critical care,* New York, 1990, Raven Press.)

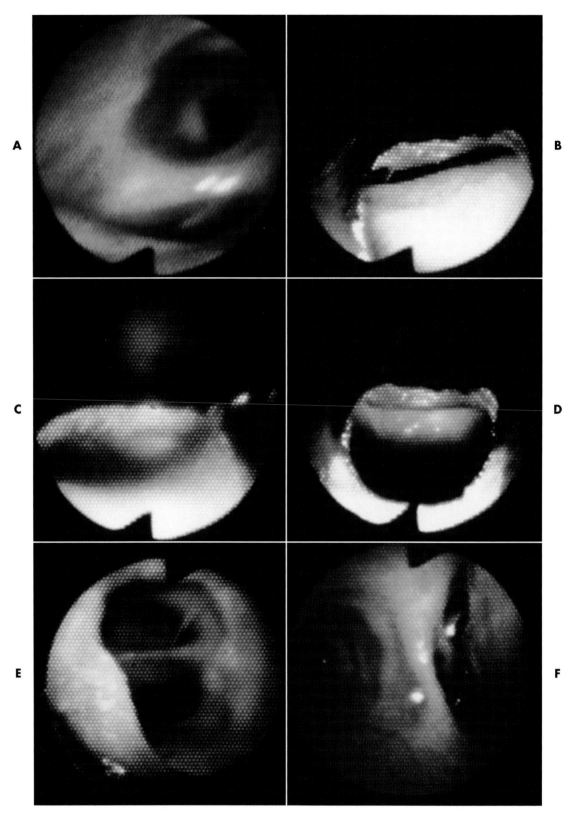

FIG. 11-6   Endoscopic view of right-sided endobronchial tube positioning. **A,** Right upper-lobe bronchus orifice and bronchus intermedius. **B,** Tip of fiberscope at upper level of bronchial cuff slot showing side opening of bronchial tube and tracheal wall. **C,** As fiberscope and tube are advanced, opening of right upper-lobe bronchus comes into view. **D,** Bronchial cuff slot positioned against right upper-lobe bronchus orifice. Distal border of orifice at level of distal border of bronchial slot. **E,** Fiberscope advanced beyond distal opening of bronchial lumen to visualize right-, middle-, and lower-lobe bronchial orifices. **F,** Fiberscope passed through tracheal lumen. Left mainstem bronchus opening is visualized, and bronchial cuff is inside right mainstem bronchus. (From Ovassapian A: Fiberoptic-aided bronchial intubation. In Ovassapian A [ed]: *Fiberoptic airway endoscopy in anesthesia and critical care,* New York, 1990, Raven Press.)

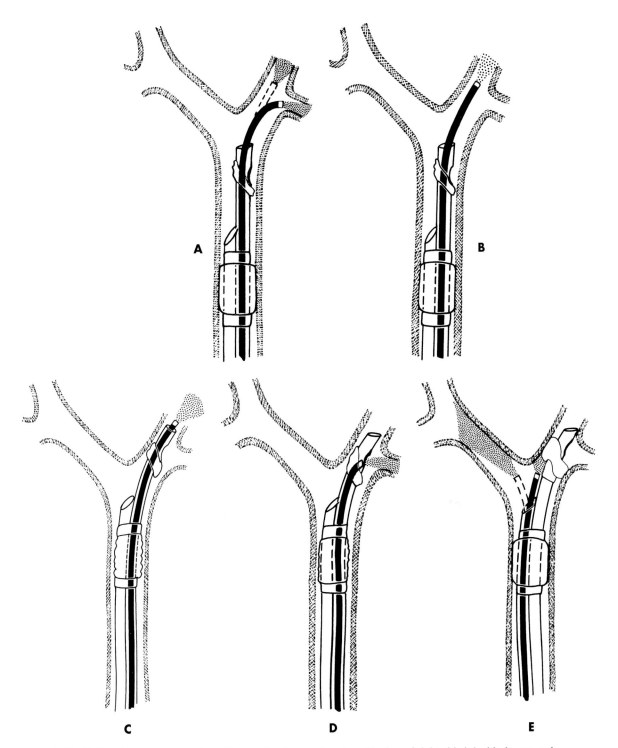

FIG. 11-7   Alternate approach to fiberscopic placement and positioning of right-sided double-lumen endo-bronchial tube. **A,** Fiberscope passed through bronchial lumen into right mainstem bronchus. Patency, length, and anatomy of right mainstem bronchus and bronchus intermedius are evaluated. The fiberscope is then rotated 90 degrees to the right and tip of fiberscope is flexed anteriorly to visualize right upper-lobe bronchus. **B,** While fiberscope is held stationary, its tip is returned to neutral position. **C,** Tracheal cuff deflated and tube advanced over fiberscope into right mainstem bronchus until it comes into view beyond tip of fiberscope. Fiberscope then advanced beyond distal lumen to visualize middle- and lower-lobe bronchi orifices. **D,** Fiberscope is withdrawn inside bronchial lumen to visualize orifice of right upper-lobe bronchus through slot of bronchial cuff. **E,** Fiberscope passed through tracheal lumen to check position of bronchial cuff and opening of left mainstem bronchus. (From Ovassapian A: *Semin Anesthesia* 6:136, 1987.)

In patients with previous total laryngectomy and permanent tracheostomy who need intrathoracic surgical intervention, DLTs may be placed through a tracheostomy stoma. Although passage of the tube through the stoma is easier than that through the mouth, the bronchial positioning needs careful attention to detail. Under these circumstances the tracheal cuff usually lies at or partially outside the tracheal stoma.

UNIVENT TUBE

The Univent tube (Fugi Systems Co., Ltd. Tokyo, Japan) was introduced by Inoue et al.[2] in 1981. It is an endotracheal tube (maintube) with a secondary channel (conduit) through its arterior wall, which accommodates a 3-mm movable balloon-tipped endobronchial blocker (Fig. 11-8). The tube cuff is made of silicone and is available in 0.5-mm internal diameter (ID) increments ranging from 6.00 to 9.00 mm ID. The external diameter of the Univent tube compared with regular endotracheal tubes is larger for comparable internal diameter size tubes. This is because of the additional space taken by the blocker and thicker wall of the Univent tube.

The 3-mm blocker is hollow inside with a lumen of 1 to 1.5 mm, which allows suctioning of secretions, oxygen delivery, or high frequency jet ventilation. It is fully retractable in the main tube and can extend up to 12 cm beyond the tip of the main tube. The blocker shaft has seven circular marks at its proximal portion. A double-circle mark lies at the entrance (proximal end) of its conduit when the blocker is fully retracted inside the main tube. The next two single circular marks are each

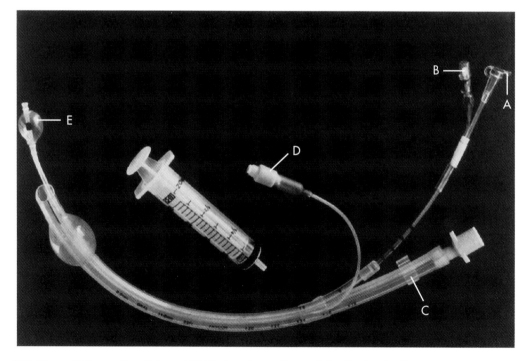

FIG. 11-8   Univent tube with bronchial blocker advanced beyond tip of maintube. *A,* Bronchial blocker plug for capping internal lumen of blocker when one-lung ventilation is not applied. This cap should not be engaged (bronchial blocker lumen open) during one-lung ventilation. *B,* Bronchial blocker inflation balloon. *C,* Hand stopper secures bronchial blocker and prevents its movement. *D,* Moveable cap on shaft of bronchial blocker to seal off leak between blocker and its conduit. *E,* Bronchial blocker cuff. (From Ovassapian A: *Semin Anesthesia* 6:136, 1987.)

3 cm apart and are followed by four other circular marks, each 1 cm apart. When the most proximal circular mark is positioned at the entrance of the blocker conduit, the tip of the blocker extends 10 cm beyond the tip of the main tube. When the blocker is advanced through the conduit as far as it can go, it passes more than 12 cm beyond the tip of the main tube. The tip of the blocker is hard and can cause tracheobronchial injury if repeated attempts are made for blind placement.[7] Dislodgement of the mold cap at the tip of the blocker has been reported.[8] The blocker cuff requires a larger volume of air to provide the seal when compared with the bronchial cuffs of DLTs. This is because of the smaller size of the blocker shaft or tube. The blocker cuff exhibits high-pressure characteristics when it is inflated to maintain a seal during OLV.[9] With the help of continuous suction through the bronchial blocker lumen, maintaining a complete collapse of the operative lung is possible by using only 3 to 5 ml of air for inflation of blocker cuff.[9]

Positioning

Before intubation of the trachea, the tracheal and blocker cuffs are tested for leaks and the blocker cuff and shaft are lubricated generously and pushed back and forth to ensure free movement of the blocker. The blocker is retracted into its conduit. After induction of general anesthesia and muscle paralysis, the Univent tube is placed inside the trachea using a rigid laryngoscope in case of difficult intubation with a fiberscope. The Univent tube is then turned 90 degrees toward the operative side (tube rotation method) to assist the passage of the blocker into the intended bronchus. The 90 degrees rotation of the main tube is necessary because the control of the direction of the blocker tip is impossible by manipulation of the blocker proximal shaft. Blind positioning of the blocker is not recommended because the blocker may not enter the intended bronchus on the first attempt, and repeated attempts for its placement may cause tracheal and bronchial injuries. Intubation of the wrong bronchus is possible, and the desired depth of insertion of the blocker cuff is difficult to judge and may require repeated evaluation of lung ventilation.

Fiberscopic-aided placement of the blocker is easy and allows for avoiding repeated attempts and possible trauma to the tracheobronchial tree. A bronchoscopy adapter is placed at the main tube adapter, and the fiberscope is advanced through the tracheal tube lumen to expose the carina. An assistant advances the blocker toward the intended bronchus. If necessary, fiberoptic manipulation is applied to direct the blocker toward the intended bronchus. Under fiberoptic observation the blocker balloon is placed at a depth that seems appropriate. For collapse of the entire lung, the balloon is positioned at the level of the upper lobe bronchus opening or a few millimeters above it. The bronchial cuff is inflated slowly under fiberoptic observation. Capping the proximal opening of the blocker conduit prevents air leak from around the blocker shaft. After verifying isolation of the lung, the balloon is deflated, leaving the blocker in place. For starting OLV, the main tube is disconnected from the anesthesia machine, the surgeon is asked to compress the lung for rapid deflation of the lung, and then the blocker cuff is inflated.

The advantages of using the Univent tube for intrathoracic operations are that it is easier and simpler to place the blocker in intended bronchus compared with proper placement of DLTs, long-term intubation is possible without tube changing, and fiberoptic bronchoscopy before or after surgery is possible through the main tube.

The main disadvantage of using the Univent tube is that of all other blockers, either OLV or separation of the lungs occurs. In some patients, isolation of the lungs is necessary from the beginning of anesthesia to avoid contamination of the lower lung; however, some patients may not tolerate OLV. The possibility of maintaining adequate ventilation by application of high-frequency jet ventilation through the blocker lumen has been suggested, but no published papers demonstrate the feasibility, ease of use, drawbacks, and possible complications of the technique.

If the Univent tube is left in place for postoperative ventilatory support, precautions should be taken to avoid accidental injury to the patient. In one patient the Univent tube was left in place, and the bronchial blocker had moved beyond the tip of the main tube. To correct air leakage around the tracheal cuff, the technician inadvertently inflated the bronchial cuff. The inflated bronchial cuff obstructed the main tube lumen, causing severe patient distress. The problem was immediately recognized by the anesthesiologist who corrected the problem by deflating the bronchial cuff before the patient was harmed.

When the patient is left intubated with a Univent tube, precautions should be taken to avoid similar accidents. The bronchial blocker should be retracted fully inside the conduit, and the shaft of the blocker should be taped to the main tube to prevent advancement of the blocker into the trachea. In addition, the bronchial blocker cap and cuff balloon pilot should be taped to prevent accidental opening of the cap, which causes a leak in the system or inflation of the blocker balloon, which causes airway obstruction. It is vital to provide inservice and training to all medical and paramedical personnel who will be managing patients with a Univent tube in place.

Success and Failure Rate of the Univent Tube

The number of papers based on clinical research in regard to the Univent tube is limited. In one report of 50 cases the Univent tube was placed satisfactorily in 90% of cases using the blind technique.[10] The bronchofiberscope was used for successful placement in five other cases. In one case, satisfactory deflation of the lung could not be achieved; in another case hypoxemia and hypercarbia resulted from partial blockade of the Univent tube by secretions. On two occasions the blocker was dislodged after the patient was positioned in a lateral decubitus position, but the blocker was repositioned with the help of a bronchofiberscope.[10]

In another series of eight, blind placement was unsuccessful on seven occasions.[7] Bronchofiberscopes were used for successful positioning of four of those seven patients. Satisfactory seal could not be achieved in three patients, and a Univent tube was replaced with a DLT.

ONE-LUNG VENTILATION

Relatively large tidal volumes (10 ml/kg) are used during OLV to avoid atelectasis. If the minute ventilation during OLV is kept the same as that during two-lung ventilation, the arterial carbon dioxide tension ($PaCO_2$) will be maintained at a level similar to that of two-lung ventilation. However, because the compliance of the dependent lung is decreased and its tidal volume is almost doubled during OLV, the peak airway pressure is increased by approximately 50% when compared with two-lung ventilation. A larger proportion of the delivered tidal volume may be wasted because of increased airway pressure and compression effect or distention of the breathing circuit. Many factors contribute to the decrease in arterial oxygen tension (PaO_2) during OLV.[4] These factors include the preoperative condition of the lungs, surgical compression of the major vessels and heart, decrease in cardiac output, effects of gravity on perfusion with the patient in the decubitus position, hypoxic vasoconstrictive reflex, and the method of ventilation.

One hundred percent inspired oxygen is recommended during OLV. However, in some patients the PaO_2 may still be suboptimal because increasing the inspired oxygen concentration is ineffective in the presence of a large shunt.

The shunted blood during OLV is measured between 20% and 35% of the cardiac output, which is less than would be expected from complete collapse of an entire lung. Hypoxic pulmonary vasoconstriction (HPV), the effect of gravity and hydrostatic pressure in the lateral decubitus position, and the disease of the operative lung contribute to the smaller-than-expected degree of shunted blood. HPV of a nonventilated lung increases the pulmonary vascular resistance in that lung and diverts blood flow away from the operative lung and toward the nonoperative dependent lung. The effect of gravity in the lateral decubitus position increases the distribution of blood flow to the dependent lung.

The operative lung may have decreased pulmonary blood flow if the underlying pathologic condition is extensive. High concentrations of inhalation anesthetics may inhibit HPV, increase the blood flow to the nonventilated lung, and, consequently, decrease the PaO_2. It has been shown that halothane and isoflurane cause an insignificant change in the amount of shunted blood when used in a concentration of up to 1 maximum allowable concentration (MAC). To avoid the possible inhibition of HPV from high concentrations of inhalation anesthetics and to minimize the respiratory depressant effect of high-dose narcotics, a combination of a narcotic and an inhalation anesthetic may be used for intrathoracic operations and OLV. It is critical that arterial oxygenation during OLV be monitored, either by frequent blood gas analysis or by continuous measurement of hemoglobin saturation by pulse oximetry.

VERIFYING FUNCTIONAL STATUS

Achieving separation of the lungs does not guarantee proper ventilation through each lung. The following steps are applied to evaluate the correct placement and function of a DLT:

1. With the mechanical ventilator set at a tidal volume of 10 ml/kg and at a rate of 8 breaths/min, both lungs are auscultated and chest wall movement is observed. The exhaled tidal volume and the peak and plateau airway pressures are noted, and the expiratory flow pattern and the rate of appearance of humidity in both lumens are observed.

2. The tracheal lumen connector tube is clamped, and the tracheal lumen is opened to the air. In a properly placed endobronchial tube the breath sounds and good chest wall movement should be present only on the bronchial side, and there should be no air leak around the bronchial cuff, which will escape through the tracheal lumen. Compared with two-lung ventilation, the exhaled tidal volume should show a decrease of not more than 10% to 15%, and the peak airway pressure should not increase by more than 50%. The expiratory flow pattern should remain the same.

3. The clamp is then moved to the bronchial lumen connector tube, and the bronchial lumen is opened to the air. Breath sounds should be present only on the tracheal side. Tidal volume, peak airway pressure, and expiratory flow pattern should change little from one lung to the other (Table 11-2).

4. With clear PVC tubes both lumens should fog with vapor with the same intensity during exhalation. A slow, incomplete appearance and clearance of the fog may indicate poor airflow through that lumen.

Two-lung ventilation is then resumed. **Easy, unobstructed ventilation of the nonoperative lung is critical for successful use of OLV.**

During positioning, the head of the patient is supported to minimize flexion or extension of the neck. **Neck flexion and extension may cause 2.5 cm distal or proximal movement of the endotrachial tube, leading to upper lobe obstruction (distal movement) or accidental extubation from the bronchus (proximal movement).**

In the presence of advanced lung disease or loss of lung tissue, more exaggerated change of tidal volume and airway pressure with or without any change in exhaled airflow pattern is expected when switching from two-lung ventilation to diseased-lung ventilation. When the lung is restricted as a result of empyema or the volume is acutely decreased, as occurs in acute atelectasis of one lobe or when the mainstem bronchus is obstructed, the pattern of airflow does not change when each lung

Table 11-2 Tidal Volumes and Peak Airway Pressures during One-Lung Ventilation

	Supine		Lateral	
	TV	**PAP**	**TV**	**PAP**
Left-sided tube ($N = 16$)				
Two-lung ventilation	756 ± 67	24 ± 4	760 ± 64	24 ± 4
Left-lung ventilation	700 ± 84	36 ± 4	708 ± 67	36 ± 4
Right-lung ventilation	714 ± 75	35 ± 4	715 ± 70	36 ± 4
Right-sided tube ($N = 16$)				
Two-lung ventilation	785 ± 75	23 ± 3	787 ± 84	23 ± 3
Left-lung ventilation	722 ± 67	35 ± 4	733 ± 65	34 ± 3
Right-lung ventilation	711 ± 72	34 ± 4	735 ± 63	34 ± 4

From Karwande SV: *Chest* 92:761-763, 1987.

TV, Tidal volume of 10 to 12 ml/kg; *PAP,* peak airway pressure (cm H_2O).
All values are means $\pm$ SD.

is ventilated individually. It is comparable with airflow during two-lung ventilation, whereas the tidal volume is drastically decreased and airway pressure is substantially increased.

Success and Failure Rate

In a retrospective review of 214 DLT placements, the incidence of difficult and failed tracheal intubations and improper placements of red rubber Carlens tubes has been reported to be 50%. With red rubber Robertshaw tubes it was 22.5%, but it was only 4% with PVC Robertshaw tubes.[11] OLV was abandoned in 9.6% of patients in whom the red rubber Robertshaw tubes were used and in 2% of patients in whom the PVC tubes were used. In three patients, one in each group, a single-lumen tube was substituted for a DLT because of failure to intubate the trachea.

In a prospective study using both left- and right-sided tubes (57 left, 46 right), the initial placement of the tube was unsatisfactory in 27% of patients, and in 12% of patients OLV was abandoned because correct placement of the bronchial tube could not be achieved or because of persistent hypoxemia.[12]

Black and Harrison[13] reported 11.5% difficulties in a retrospective review of 78 patients in whom red rubber Robertshaw tubes were used. However, in a prospective study of 59 cases, they reported difficulties in 37.2% of them. In 8.5% of the cases the use of DLT had to be discontinued. Clinical observation and evaluation of blindly positioned DLTs lack precision. Marginally positioned tubes could not be identified, nor could air trapping and atelectasis of the left upper lobe.

Bronchoscopic evaluation of blindly placed DLTs has shown a large number of marginally placed endobronchial tubes with the bronchial cuff above the carina.[4]

Tracheal intubation using a rigid laryngoscope was successful in 128 of 132 (22 right-sided) cases in which Robertshaw disposable DLTs were used.[4] The four failed rigid laryngoscopic tracheal intubations were successfully intubated with the aid of a fiberscope. The initial positioning of 22 right-sided tubes was successful with good separation. In one patient the tube's tracheal lumen lay against the tracheal wall, leading to difficulty in ventilating the left lung; however, after turning the patient into the right lateral decubitus position, both lungs could be ventilated well. In five patients, right, 41-F DLTs were pulled out of the bronchi during OLV, causing an air leak; the tubes were successfully repositioned in all five situations.[4] In two patients OLV was unnecessary; thus it was not used. The duration of OLV in the remaining 20 patients was 25 to 200 minutes (the average is 85 minutes).

COMPLICATIONS

Because of the size and shape of the DLTs, the incidence of difficult and failed rigid laryngoscope-aided tracheal intubation is high.[12,13] PVC tubes are easier to pass into the trachea and cause less mucosal damage than red rubber tubes.[12] Rupture of the tracheobronchial tree has been reported with both right-sided and left-sided tubes and with both red rubber and disposable tubes.

In a series of 2700 thoracotomies in which a red rubber Carlens tube was used, tracheobronchial rupture occurred in five patients.[14] The site of laceration is usually the posterior membranous wall of the trachea or a mainstem bronchus. Many factors have been suggested as the cause of tracheobronchial rupture; however, none have been studied or proved. These factors are direct trauma during intubation, use of large tubes, advancing the tube with a force or with a stylet, rapid overinflation of the bronchial cuff, and presence of a pathologic condition of the respiratory tree.[13] Suggestions made to prevent bronchial rupture include inflation of the bronchial cuff with anesthetic mixture to avoid overdistention by absorption of nitrous oxide, deflation of the bronchial cuff periodically to avoid excessive pressure buildup, and delay of inflation of the bronchial cuff until the onset of OLV. Deflation of the bronchial cuff leaves the down lung unprotected; secretions and necrotic tumor may contaminate it and cause airway obstruction.

Malpositioning of DLTs include intubation of the wrong bronchus, inadequate advancement of the tube, and insertion of the tube too far down into the intended bronchus.[13] Difficulties resulting from improperly positioned bronchial tubes include incomplete isolation of the lungs, air entry into the wrong lung, difficulty in ventilating one or both lungs, air trapping, and unsatisfactory deflation of the lung.[13] If not recognized, airway obstruction results in poor ventilation and hypoxemia, and air trapping can cause rupture of the lung and tension pneumothorax. If isolation is incomplete, soiling of the dependent lung adds to the problems of ventilation and oxygenation, and, in the presence of a bronchopleural fistula, inadequate ventilation may result.

One potentially fatal complication reported with the use of DLTs was rupture of the pulmonary artery on extubation because one of the sutures of the pulmonary artery had gone through the bronchial tube.[5] In another case the passage of an endobronchial tube in the presence of a large mediastinal mass caused displacement of the mass and obstruction of major vessels, resulting in cardiac arrest.[15]

REFERENCES

1. White GMJ: Evolution of endotracheal and endobronchial intubation, *Br J Anaesth* 32:235-246, 1960.
2. Inoue H, Shohtsu A, Ogawa J et al: New device for one-lung anesthesia: endotracheal tube with movable blocker, *J Thorac Cardiovasc Surg* 83:940-941, 1982.
3. Benumof JL, Partridge BL, Salvatierra C et al: Margin of safety in positioning modern double-lumen endotracheal tubes, *Anesthesiology* 67:729-738, 1987.
4. Ovassapian A: Fiberoptic-aided bronchial intubation. In Ovassapian A (ed): *Fiberoptic airway endoscopy in anesthesia and critical care,* New York, 1990, Raven Press.
5. Dryden GE: Circulatory collapse after pneumonectomy: an unusual complication from the use of a Carlens catheter—case report, *Anesth Analg* 56:451-452, 1977.
6. Ovassapian A: Flexible bronchoscopic positioning of right-sided, double-lumen endobronchial tube, *J Bronchology* 2:12-19, 1995.
7. MacGillivray RG: Evaluation of a new tracheal tube with a movable bronchus blocker, *Anaesthesia* 43:687-689, 1988.
8. Arai T, Hatano Y: Yet another reason to use a fiberoptic bronchoscope to properly site a double-lumen tube, *Anesthesiology* 66:581-582, 1987.
9. Hannallah MS, Benumof JL: Comparison of two techniques to inflate the bronchial cuff of the Univent tube, *Anesth Analg* 75:784-787, 1992.
10. Karwande SV: A new tube for single lung ventilation, *Chest* 92:761-763, 1987.
11. Burton NA, Watson DC, Brodsky JB et al: Advantages of a new polyvinyl chloride double-lumen tube in thoracic surgery, *Ann Thorac Surg* 36:78-84, 1983.
12. Read RC, Friday CD, Eason CN: Prospective study of the Robertshaw endobronchial catheter in thoracic surgery, *Ann Thorac Surg* 24:156-161, 1977.
13. Black AMS, Harrison GA: Difficulties with positioning Robertshaw double-lumen tubes, *Anaesth Intensive Care* 3:299-311, 1975.
14. Guernelli N, Bragaglia RB, Briccoli A et al: Tracheobronchial ruptures due to cuffed Carlens tube, *Ann Thorac Surg* 28:66-68, 1979.
15. Wells DG, Zeleer J, Padolakin W et al: Cardiac arrest from pulmonary outflow tract obstruction due to a double-lumen tube, *Anesthesiology* 66:422-428, 1987.
16. Ovassapian A: Fiber-optic aided bronchial intubation, *Semin Anesthesia* 6:133-142, 1987.

PART III

APPLIED CLINICAL PRACTICE AND CASE MATERIAL

Order and simplification are the first steps toward the mastery of a subject—the actual enemy is the unknown.

THOMAS MANN, 1924

The Magic Mountain

CHAPTER 12

Cranial, Cervical Spinal, and Other Bony Considerations in the Difficult Airway

MARTIN L. NORTON

The human body…indeed is like a ship; its bones being the
stiff-standing rigging, and the sinews the small running ropes,
that manage all the motions.

HERMAN MELVILLE (1819-1891)

Redburn, Chapter XIII

Bony areas, such as the temporomandibular joint, and problems like craniofacial dysostoses that involve disproportions or that impose mechanical limitations to airway access must be taken into account by the endoscopist. Micrognathia (small jaws) is the most striking feature in the spectrum of bony anomalies, but, as has been pointed out, maxillofacial and nasal malformations also contribute to the difficulty of establishing and maintaining an effective airway. *Micrognathia* is the term most frequently employed to describe this anomaly of the mandible, although other terms, such as *hypoplasia of the mandible, mandibular hypotrophy, congenital mandibular atresia, brachygnathia, ateliosis of the mandible,* and *hypomicrognathia* have appeared in the literature.[1]

Retrognathia (posterior displacement of the chin), a more accurate and inclusive term, refers to several conditions that can lead to backward chin displacement without an abnormally small jaw. Retroposition of the chin is a finding common to many types of jaw deformities.

A review of the various craniofacial syndromes suggests the types and frequency of the malformations contributing to a difficult airway.[2]

MICROGNATHIA

Micrognathia (sometimes erroneously called *retrognathia*) is the prime, constant body finding that signals trouble for access to the airway. It represents the most difficult problem to deal with primarily because of the attachment of the root of the tongue and the effects this and other tendinomuscular structures have on suspension of the larynx. These latter structures lie more superior in relation to the mandible (often described by the practicing endoscopist as anterior) and are thereby drawn closer to the base of the tongue.

The result is that the rigid laryngoscope blade, whether it is curved or straight, cannot readily deflect the soft tissues of the laryngopharynx. Therefore visualization of the additus laryngis and positioning of soft tissue is made extremely difficult, if not impossible.

If the horizontal ramus (extension) of the mandible is decreased in size relative to the maxilla, as it is in micrognathia, it will also be reduced relative to the length of the genioglossus and geniohyoid muscles. Consequently, these muscles must actively contract to a length much shorter than their passive length to maintain a normal-sized pharyngeal lumen.

Another point to consider when opening the mouth is the effect of Bernoulli's principle in maintaining the airway (see Chapter 1). This exposes the tongue and soft palate to atmospheric pressure. The anterior portion of the tongue relaxes, producing a dorsal motion of the belly of the genioglossus muscle and thereby decreasing the size of the posterior pharyngeal lumen. The entire transmural pressure of the pharynx is now exerted across the soft palate, moving it dorsally and narrowing the lumen of the oropharyngeal space. Classic examples are shown in Treacher Collins syndrome (Fig. 12-1), Goldenhar's syndrome (Fig. 12-2), Hallermann-Streiff-François syndrome (Fig. 12-3), and arthrogryposis multiplex syndrome (Fig. 12-4).

On initial viewing of the patient with Hallermann-Streiff-François syndrome from the front, as noted in Fig. 12-3, the most striking appearance is that of microstomia. However, the lateral view clearly demonstrates the micrognathia and a strong indication of hyoid-to-thyroid limitation. Crouzon's disease (Fig. 12-5) may or may not represent a true micrognathia because this cranial malformation may, on occasion, give the appearance of micrognathia without its actual presence.

RETROGNATHIA

Securing the airway in a patient with traumatic retrognathia, (posteroinferior displacement of the anterior segment, also known as an *Andy Gump* bimandibular fracture) must be accomplished rapidly because acute closure of the upper airway may occur. Immediate tracheostomy may be required, although an attempt should be made to relieve the situation by forcibly pulling the mandible and related glottic paraglottic soft tissues forward (ventrally and cephalad).

Text continued on p. 168.

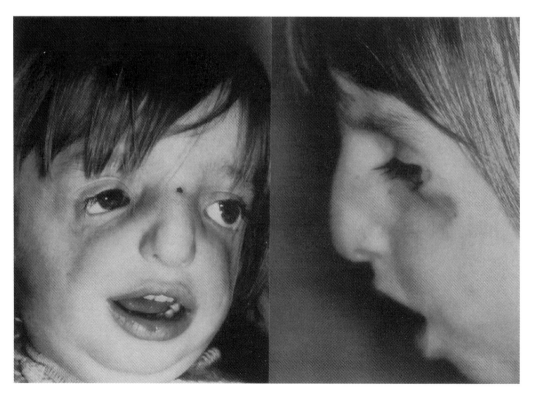

FIG. 12-1   Treacher Collins syndrome.

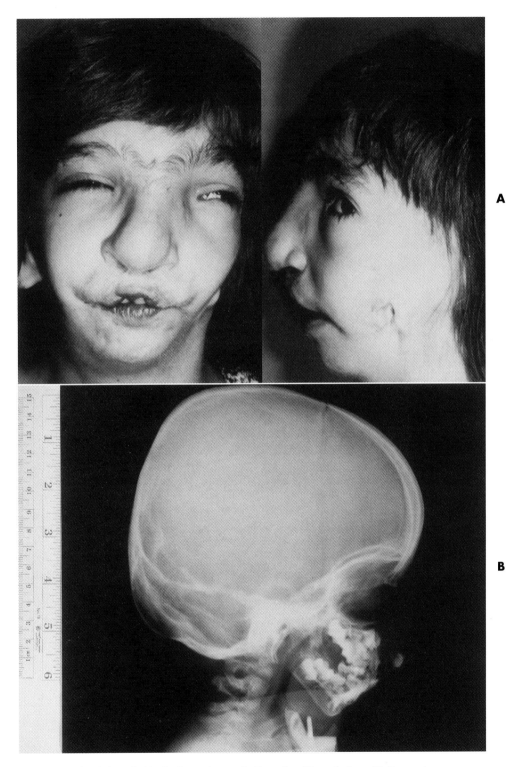

FIG. 12-2   Goldenhar's syndrome. **A,** Frontal and lateral views. **B,** X-ray view.

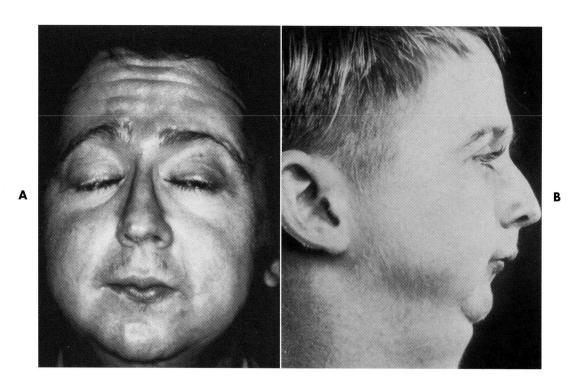

FIG. 12-3   Hallermann-Streiff-François syndrome. **A,** Frontal view. **B,** Profile view.

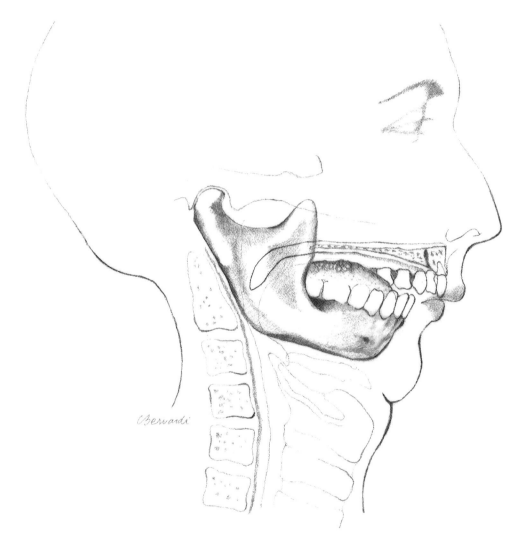

FIG. 12-3, cont'd. **C,** Underlying pathologic condition.

A

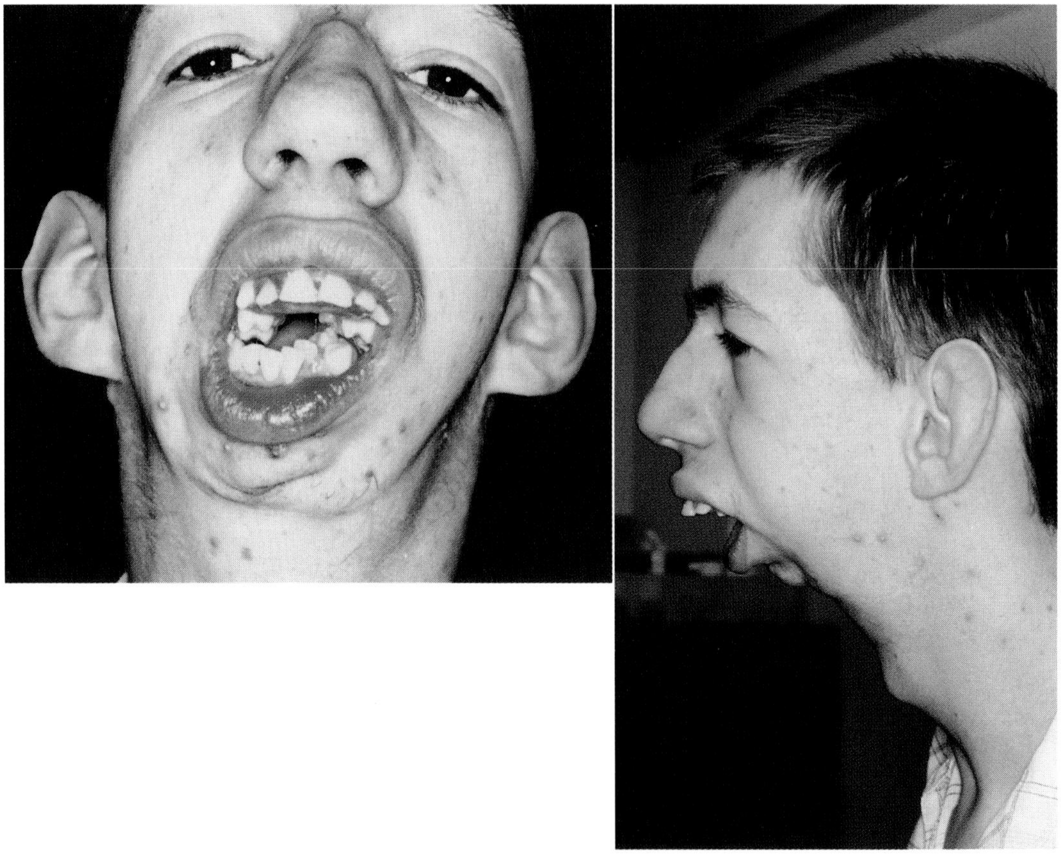

B

FIG. 12-4 Arthrogryposis multiplex syndrome. **A,** Frontal view. **B,** Profile view.

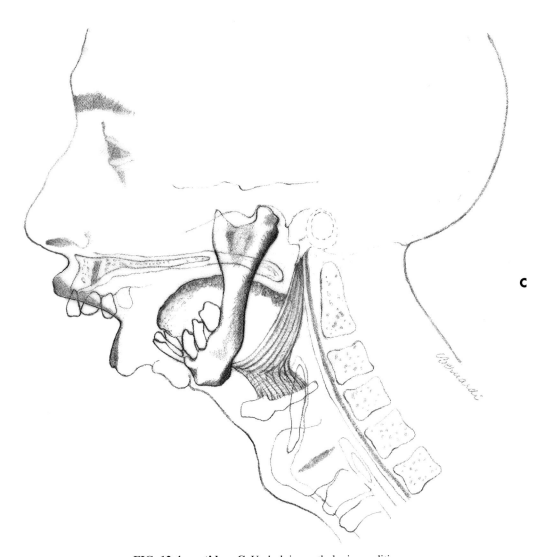

C

FIG. 12-4, cont'd. C, Underlying pathologic condition.

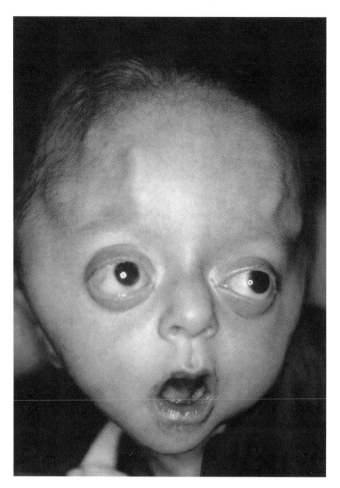

FIG. 12-5   Crouzon's disease.

FACIAL TRAUMA

Facial trauma can produce major problems in airway management. For a complete understanding of this problem, what has come to be known as the Le Fort Classification of Facial Fractures must be reviewed. Le Fort, of Lille, France, published his categorization based on studies of traumatized cadaver skulls. Although he was not fully successful in determining a clear relationship between soft tissue signs of facial trauma and demonstrable craniofacial disruption, he did describe a logical pattern of bony changes for our consideration. Guerin and Le Fort both described what is commonly known as a Le Fort I fracture (Fig. 12-6, *left*). This involves a horizontal maxillary fracture with a line above the floor of the nose across the lower third of the septum, resulting in mobilization of the palate, maxillary alveolar process, inferior third of the pterygoid plates, and parts of the palatine bones. The patient can be intubated either orally or nasally, without great difficulty.

A Le Fort II fracture (Fig. 12-6, *right*) is pyramidal, with the line extending from the junction of the thick upper part of the nasal bone and its thinner portion at the upper margin of the anterior nasal foramen. This line continues across the orbital medial wall and the lacrimal bone and below the zygomaticomaxillary suture and the lateral wall of the antrum and pterygoid plates. **The importance of a Le Fort II fracture lies in the associated risk of a concomitant fracture at the base of the skull. Considerations of cerebral spinal fluid leakage and risks of C1-C2 base of skull manipulation are extant** and must be appreciated when choosing either nasal or oral intubation.

Le Fort III fractures (Fig. 12-7) run parallel with the base of the skull, effectively separating the midfacial skeleton from the cranial base. A Le Fort III fracture extends through the base of the nose

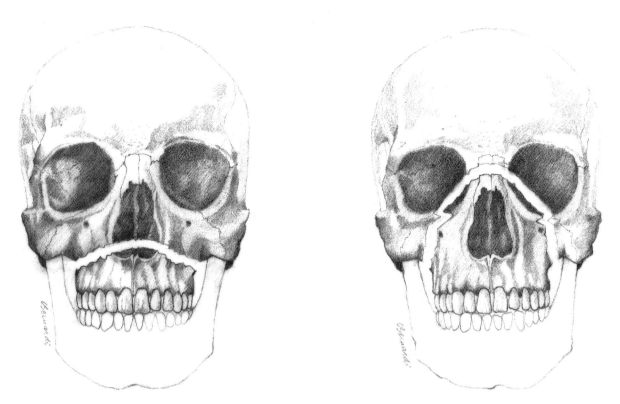

FIG. 12-6 Le Fort I fracture, transverse fracture of maxilla *(left)*. Le Fort II fracture, pyramidal fracture of maxilla *(right)*.

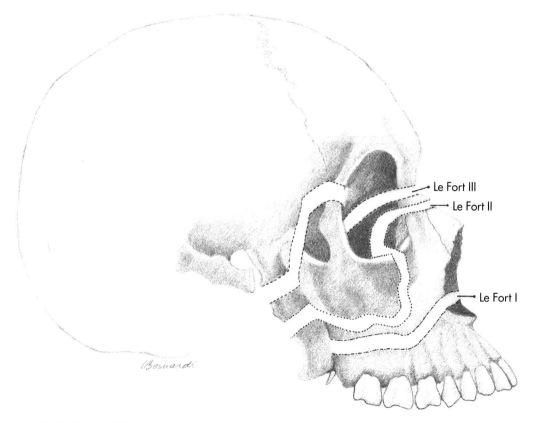

FIG. 12-7 Le Fort III complex craniofacial fracture shown with Le Fort I and II fracture sites. (Modified from Kazanjian VH, Converse JM: *The surgical treatment of facial injuries,* ed 3, Baltimore, 1974, Williams & Wilkins.)

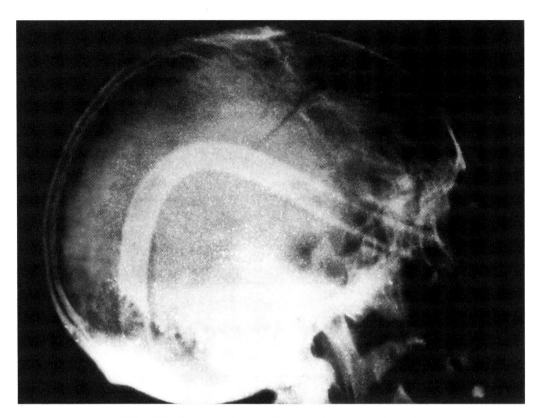

FIG. 12-8   Intracranial nasotracheal tube (computer enhanced).

and ethmoid sinus and the orbital plates and *may involve the cribriform plate.* Also involved are the lesser wings of the sphenoid, the pterygomaxillary fissure, and the sphenopalatine fossa. Extension includes progression laterally and cephalad to the frontozygomatic suture and caudad and dorsally to the pterygoid plates. The zygomatic arch is also involved. **Nasotracheal intubation is contraindicated because it may lead to endotracheal tube penetration of the cranium and its contents** (Fig. 12-8). Cerebrospinal fluid rhinorrhea is an absolute contraindication to nasotracheal intubation and ventilation by mask because of the risk of meningitis from introduction of foreign matter into the cranial vault. A further diagnostic sign of a Le Fort III fracture is the characterized "dish-face" concave deformity of the facies.

CERVICAL SPINE

The range of mobility of the cervical spine is a major factor in the ease of endoscopy and intubation, and the successful endoscopist requires a significant understanding of its biomechanics. The complexity of this area is emphasized by the fact that there are at least 23 joints or points of contact at which motion occurs from the occiput down to the first thoracic vertebrae. All have incongruous surfaces that combine sliding and rotation with some degree of flexion.

The fact that there is more mobility at the upper and lower ends of the neck than in the midcervical region makes the unit concept of motion inapplicable to the cervical vertebrae. Motion in the sagittal plane is called flexion or extension, depending on the direction of movement. Motion in the transverse plane is called rotation and motion in frontal plane lateral bending. Average ranges[2] are re-

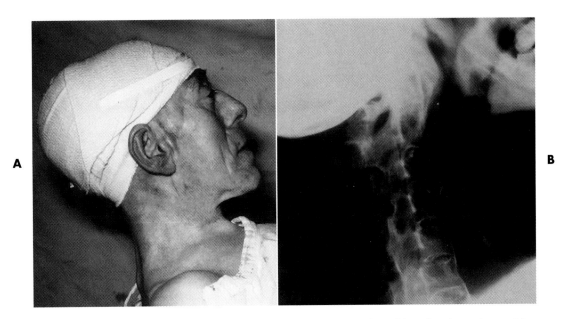

FIG. 12-9   Ankylosing spondylitis. **A,** Note fixation of cervical spine with patient in supine position. **B,** X-ray view.

ported as flexion, 70 degrees ± 10 degrees; extension, 75 degrees ± 10 degrees; rotation (right or left), 75 degrees ± 10 degrees; and lateral bending (right or left), 45 degrees ± 10 degrees. However, these studies were done on young people without disability. In older people mobility is gradually lost, starting perhaps as early as the ages of 25 to 29 years and certainly after age 55.

The greatest amount of flexion-extension occurs in the interspace between the fifth and sixth cervical vertebrae, plus or minus one vertebra. In flexion each vertebrae below the axis shifts anteriorly on the subjacent vertebrae. In extension the vertebrae shift posteriorly. This produces a diagonal inclination. The atlantoaxis atlas can rotate on the axis approximately 45 degrees in either direction. The remaining 30 degrees of rotation occur between the lower cervical vertebrae.[3] Nonradiologic measurements of this motion suggest that a gravity goniometer or protractor is the most convenient, although certainly not the most exact, instrument for estimating the flexion-extension position of the relatively spherical head.

The positional movement of the atlantoaxial axis must be considered when preparing the patient for endoscopy, especially in the supine position.

Striking cervical spinal problems are found in osteoarthritis (ankylosing spondylitis, Fig. 12-9; see also the cases at the end of the chapter, juvenile rheumatoid arthritis, and Klippel-Feil syndrome [Fig. 12-10]). Atlantoaxial instability (Fig. 12-11) represents another problem in the cervical area. This latter problem is primarily, but not solely, found in women over the age of 40 who have rheumatoid arthritis and have been on corticosteroids for a long period.[4] A serious complication is subluxation of the atlantoaxial joint that may lead to compression of the spinal cord by the odontoid process.

This joint should also be considered in patients with varying types of dwarfism because of the high incidence of cervical spinal maldevelopment. Another odontoid process problem is found in patients with osteoporosis, specifically Paget's disease. With osteoporotic concerns and changes from Paget's disease in the odontoid process, hyperextension can produce fractures of the odontoid and subsequent cervical cord trauma during extension. **The common practice of manually manipulating the head to maximal hyperextension for endoscopy is particularly hazardous.**

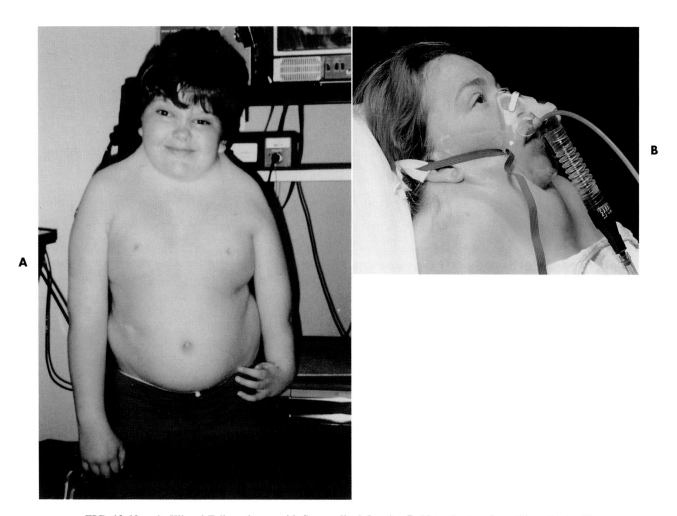

FIG. 12-10   A, Klippel-Feil syndrome with Sprengel's deformity. **B,** Note short neck on this patient with Klippel-Feil syndrome. (Courtesy Dr. A.C.D. Brown, Ann Arbor, Mich.)

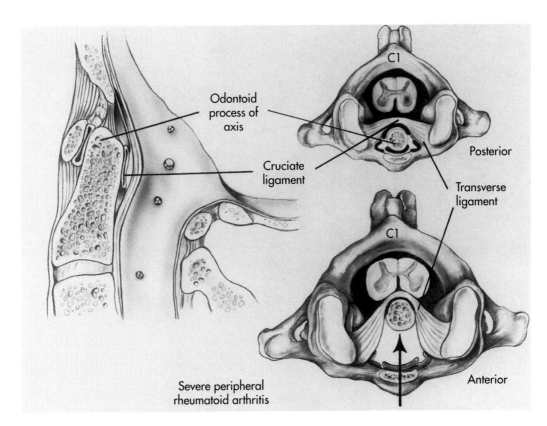

FIG. 12-11   Atlantoaxial instability.

A 60-year-old patient had been told that he would not survive surgery because of cervical spinal difficulties affecting his trachea. His primary diagnosis was listed as rheumatoid arthritis, and his neck had progressed to a twisted position approximately 20 years ago (Fig. 12-12). He also had serious soft tissue complications along with his bony abnormalities, including tracheal torsion, vascular torsion, and visual problems.

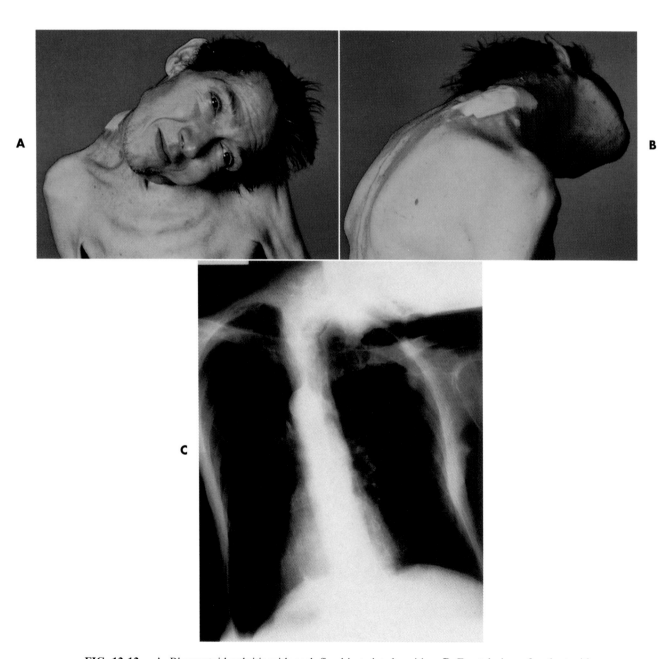

FIG. 12-12   A, Rheumatoid arthritis with neck fixed in twisted position. **B,** Frontal view of patient with rheumatoid arthritis and twisted neck. **C,** X-ray view of rheumatoid arthritis and twisted cervical spine.

CASE 12-1   *CERVICAL SPINAL FUSION*

A particularly striking example of positional movement risk presented in one patient (Fig. 12-13).[5] This patient was sent for management of a proposed total hip replacement with the notation that he could not open his mouth widely. The latter was true. However, when his x-rays were reviewed, it was noted that C1 and C2 vertebrae were fused, C2 and C3 moved relatively normally, the transverse processes of C3 to C5 were totally fused, and there was a marked laxity of ligaments in the C5-C6 interspace. In fact, there was serious hypermobility at C5 and C6, which presented the hazard of trauma to the spinal cord on movement of the head to the traditional position for endotracheal intubation. This case demonstrates the need to *comprehensively* examine any patient presenting with any of the indications of airway access problems.

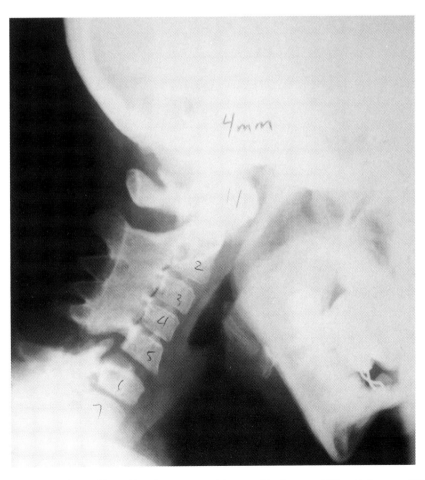

FIG. 12-13   Patient with positional movement risk caused by hypermobility at interspace C5-C6.

CASE 12-2   *CERVICAL VERTEBRAL CURVATURE AND CENTRAL CORE MYOPATHY*

A 7-year-old child was brought to surgery for correction of cervical vertebral curvatures (Fig. 12-14). Although a tracheostomy could easily be accomplished, the desire was to avoid one at all costs. The concern was the probability that, on straightening the neck, the trachea would retract under the sternal angle of Louis, posing an extreme risk that the site would be substernal with the potential for superior mediastinal infection.

The lesson to be learned from this case is the recognition of the risk of tracheostomy and the use of several combined techniques as a substitute for it.

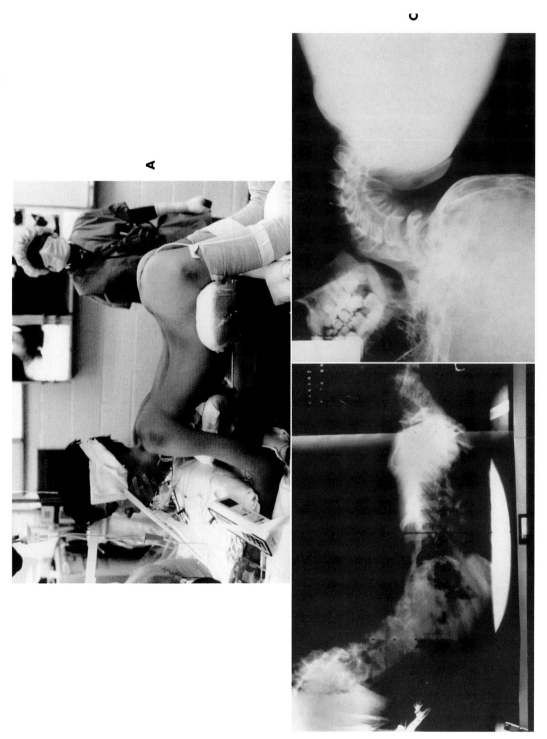

FIG. 12-14   Central core myopathy. **A,** Patient face down. **B,** Spinal x-ray films. **C,** Cervical x-ray film.

REFERENCES

1. Randall P: The Robin sequence: micrognathia and glossoptosis with airway obstruction. In McCarthy JG (ed): *Plastic surgery,* vol 4, *Cleft lip & palate and craniofacial abnormalities,* Philadelphia, 1990, WB Saunders.
2. Norton ML, Brown ACDB: *Atlas of the difficult airway,* Chicago, 1991, Mosby.
3. Kottke FJ, Mundale MO: Range of mobility of the cervical spine, *Arch Phys Med* 40:379-382, 1959.
4. Fielding JW: Cineroentgenography of the normal cervical spine, *J Bone Joint Surg* 39A:1280, 1957.
5. Norton ML, Ghanma NA: Atlantoaxial instability revisited: an alert for endoscopists, *Ann Otol Rhinol Laryngol* 87:554-557, 1978.

CHAPTER 13

Soft Tissue Considerations in the Difficult Airway

MARTIN L. NORTON

Discussion of soft tissue concerns during airway intubation includes conditions both directly and indirectly asserting influences on the airway.

MACROGLOSSIA AND GLOSSOPTOSIS

Macroglossia and glossoptosis are two syndromes that have a major influence on the ability to visualize the larynx and other structures of the oropharynx, esophagopharynx, and laryngopharynx. *Macroglossia* refers to an enlargement of the tongue, whereas *glossoptosis* is a downward and backward displacement of the tongue to the point of close approximation of the basal tongue to the posterior pharyngeal wall. Among many diseases or syndromes that manifest this feature are dwarfism, hemangiopericytoma (Fig. 13-1), Down's syndrome, lymphangioma, cretinism, and amyloidosis.

It is important to note that these syndromes may take many forms (e.g., the tongue in amyloidosis may be enlarged, and it may also become stiffened and *firm to palpation* as well as being obstructive). In all of these syndromes physicians are obligated to conceptualize the function of the tongue in relation to the oropharyngeal structures and mechanisms of swallowing and respiration. Similarly, an achondroplastic dwarf may appear perfectly normal externally and indeed have an esthetically beautiful face, but a complete examination frequently reveals glossoptosis.

ACQUIRED SOFT TISSUE PROBLEMS

Two other examples of specific soft tissue problems encroaching on the airway are best visualized from a computed tomography (CT) scan of the airway. The first example (Fig. 13-2, *A*) is presented as a postsurgical problem. A carcinoma of the floor of the mouth had been excised widely, with the tongue sutured to the floor of the mouth over the defect. When the patient was first seen, she was unable to advance her tongue and the basal portion lay posterior. The consequences included fixation of the epiglottis, an obvious consequence in view of the anatomic relationship of the epiglottis and the tongue. The extent of the problem was more clearly elucidated after the lateral view of a flat plate of the airway was reviewed (Fig. 13-2, *B*). Here it was noted that the base of the tongue was clearly delineated with the wings of the hyoid in direct and close approximation to the base of the tongue. This produced a situation that most anesthesiologists call "anterior larynx" but which is more correctly called "superior larynx." A differing viewpoint was noted, presented by Sivardjan and Fink,[1] in which they find the hyoid bone and epiglottis shifted anteriorly. However, the patients they cited were all in the supine position with extended necks. The dynamic fluoroscopic studies show a shift cephalad (superiorly) *with change in position* from the upright (sitting) position to the supine position. It was submitted that the differences observed by Sivardjan and Fink were more related to collapse of the ventral (anterior) structures because of the loss of the suspensory mechanism secondary to general anesthesia and muscle relaxation. Further review of the pathway that the endotracheal tube would have to traverse demonstrated a Z-shaped channel. This patient also had keloid formation scars of the neck, which limited head motion.

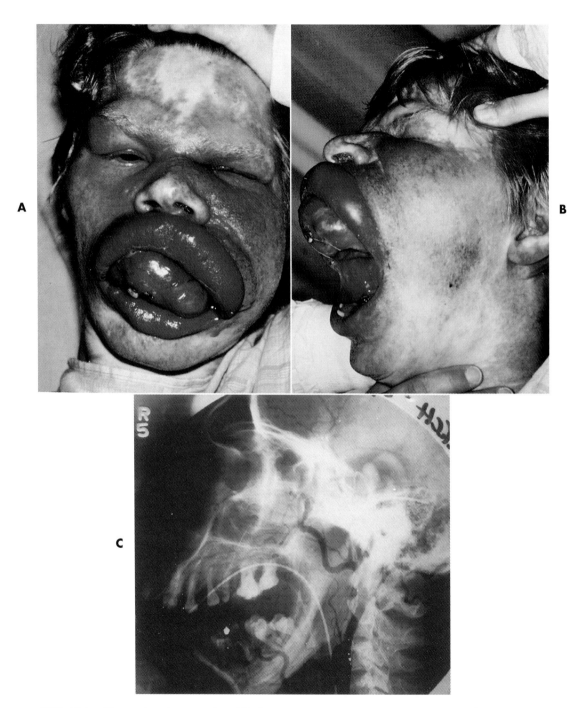

FIG. 13-1 Hemangiopericytoma. **A** and **B,** Sturge-Weber syndrome with dilantin effect. **C,** Composite at time of thromboembolization.

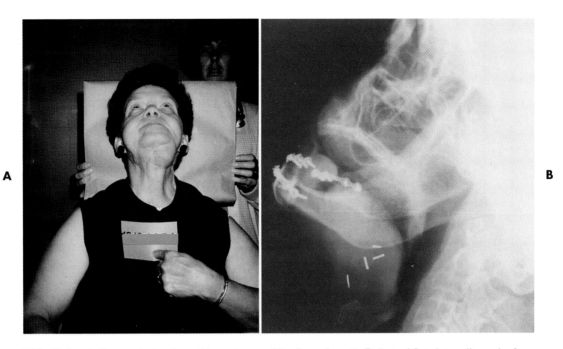

FIG. 13-2   **A,** Postsurgical patient with carcinoma of the floor of mouth. **B,** Lateral flat plate radiograph of patient in **A** (Note clips).

After fiberoptic transnasal intubation, a very strong reflex pattern with a Müller 4 test was noted. This response was so severe that, at times, it was impossible to advance the fiberscope or the nasotracheal tube. The advance was synchronized while the awake patient was encouraged to exert deep respiratory efforts.

Another patient presented with a mass of the neck under the right angle of the ramus of the mandible. Upon further examination, it was noted that the mass encroached upon the airway at the level of the pharynx. Digital palpation indicated that there was an extension behind the last molar tooth and in the posterior pharynx to the midline and down the pharynx along the midline to the point that the epiglottis was able to be touched. It was interesting to note that the patient had no gag reflex on palpation over this area. The left side of the midline was totally free of the mass to palpation, and the gag reflex was very active. Review of the CT scan (Fig. 13-3) confirmed the clinical impression and provided support for the conclusion that access to the airway by the oral route was possible using a left-handed Macintosh blade with an intubation guide (Norton Teflon or Eschmann woven) for insertion of the endotracheal tube.

Trismus, by definition, is muscle spasm *usually associated with pain.* It may have many causes, including displacement of a fractured zygomatic process, infection, or hematoma. It is often relieved with the use of anesthetic and muscle relaxants. If the condition is chronic, there is associated masseter muscle fibrosis that will not respond to muscle relaxant or other pharmacologic agents.

Soft tissue neck trauma mandates the clinician to look for signs and symptoms of spinal cord compression and dislocation or fracture of the vertebrae.

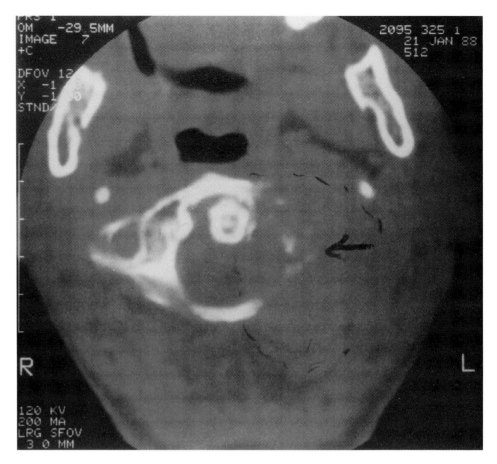

FIG. 13-3 Computed tomography scan of patient with neck mass under right angle of ramus of mandible.

NEUROFIBROMATOSIS AND MUMPS

Fig. 13-4 shows a case of extensive neurofibromatosis in a child. The problem in this case is mechanical in a space-occupying context.

Parotiditis (mumps), besides its soft tissue-occupying component, produces pain referred to the temporomandibular joint and ear canal with trismus.

NEUROMUSCULAR DISORDERS

Occasionally other disease processes present airway considerations. Chapter 12 discusses a case of central core myopathy with continuous hyperlordosis (see Fig. 12-14). It underlines the fact that late diagnosis of neurologic and myopathic disorders may have far reaching effects on the bony development of the patient which, in this case, radically affects access to the airway.

In that case, access to the airway was obtained by a retrograde wire technique. The wire was passed through the membrane between the cricoid and first tracheal cartilage. It was visualized through the mouth and partially pulled out through the mouth to enable the fiberoptic endoscope (on which a suitable endotracheal tube had been threaded) to be, itself, threaded onto the wire. Then, using the wire as a guide (not a stylet), the fiberoptic endoscope was advanced visually into the trachea, and the endotracheal tube was then moved into position.

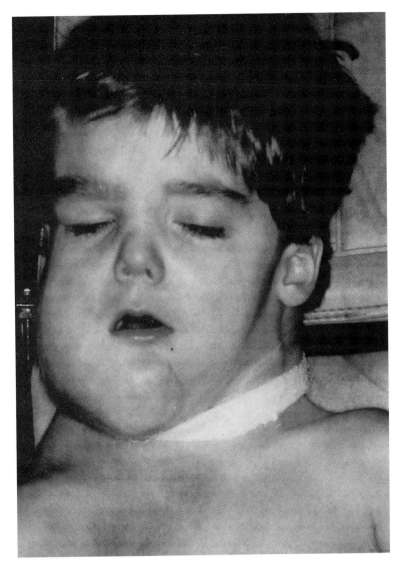

FIG. 13-4   Patient with neurofibromatosis.

MISCELLANEOUS SOFT TISSUE PROBLEMS

The endoscopist is often faced with soft tissue problems not immediately related to the airway. Examples of these are lesions affecting movement of the neck. One patient presented with pain in the neck, head positioning as in torticollis, and a tingling sensation in the hands upon rotation of the head but not manifest on flexion-extension. A review of her CT scan at the level of C1-C2 demonstrated an extrinsic mass eroding the ramus of the body of the C1 vertebrae and extending into the epidural space. Based on visual examination the endoscopist could not have suspected the hazard of standard rigid blade endoscopy merely by the external appearance of the patient. **The maneuver used by many endoscopists, placing one hand under the chin with the other pushing downward on the top of the head, risked driving the odontoid process up into the medulla oblongata because of the weakening of the structural integrity of C1 vertebra.**

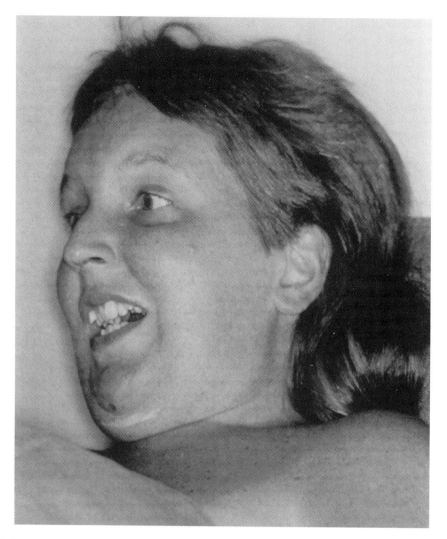

FIG. 13-5 Patient with fibrofascial myositis ossificans progressiva. Note maximal mouth opening with cervical spinal fixation.

This particular problem may also occur with other pathologic processes involving the dens such as fractures, Paget's disease, extreme osteoporosis, and most frequently in patients with platybasia (a softening of the skull bones resulting in the floor of the posterior cranial fossa bulging upward in the region of the foramen magnum).

Thus it is incumbent upon the endoscopist not to use this maneuver routinely for positioning the patient for rigid blade laryngoscopy. **Habits in and of themselves can sometimes lead to disaster!**

A rare condition, fibrofascial myositis ossificans progressiva (FMOP) (Fig. 13-5), presented an unusual problem. This disease of unknown origin consists of bone formation within muscles. It starts as an interstitial fibromyositis in which osteoid and cartilage formations develop in the connective tissue, enclosing intact muscle fibers. With progression, limitation of movement, contractures, deformities, scoliosis, rigidity of the spine, abnormal posture, and limited expansion of the thorax occur. (The condition should be differentiated from calcinosis universalis in which there are calcium deposits in the skin, subcutaneous tissues, and connective tissue sheaths around muscles that usually occur in relation to scleroderma or polymyositis; however, this differentiation is, by no means, clear cut.)

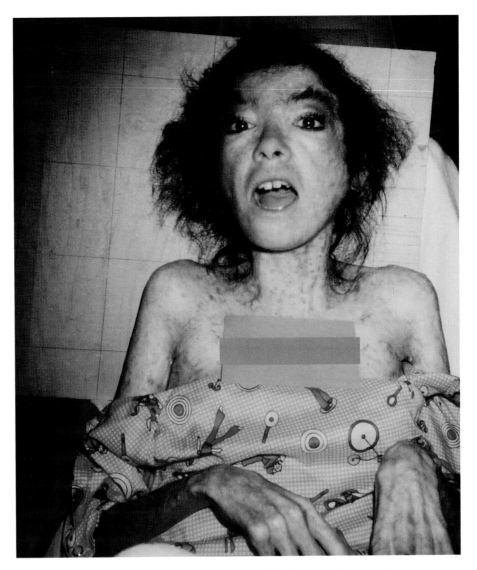

FIG. 13-6   Patient with dermatomyositis with calcinois universalis.

Both FMOP and calcinosis universalis patients often have no movement of skeletal musculature. One patient could only move her fingers, lips, and eyelids and had limited function of the
tongue. Her pharyngeal musculature was progressively weakening, although it still was possible for
her to use them to suck nutritive fluids through a straw. She was presented for consideration of airway access to allow teeth to be removed for placement of that straw. She had limited motion at the
temporomandibular joint and her apnea muscles were significantly invaded and rigid. Still, she could
communicate, she could work from an adapted electrically controlled wheel chair, and she was men-
tally alert and functioning at a high intellectual level, although obviously euphoric.

Airway access through the oropharynx was almost impossible, and the route available was determined to be through the nasotracheal pathway. It is important to note that she manifested a Müller 2
test that confirmed the limitation of pharyngeal muscle activity.

An analogous patient, with a combined diagnosis of dermatomyositis and calcinosis universalis
(Fig. 13-6), manifested similar signs and symptoms, but because of the added problem of dermatomyositis also provided an extremely difficult intravenous access problem. However, this latter patient
showed no sign of bony cervical limitation but only hardening of the cervical soft tissues resulting
from the calcinosis. In addition, her nasotracheal access route was patent.

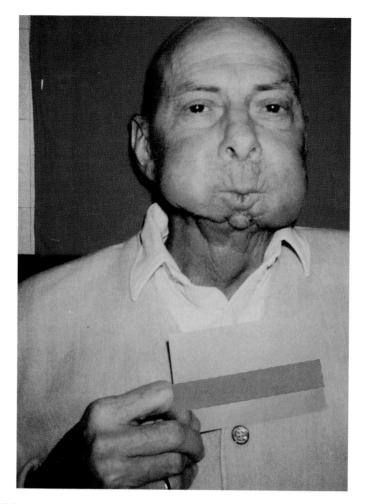

FIG. 13-7   Patient after glossectomy, mandibulectomy, radical neck surgery, and radiation.

Major complexities to be addressed are the postglossectomy, postradical neck surgery, postradiation situation, particularly when there is a degree of induration, fixation of the tongue, and approximation of the hyoid bone to the base of the tongue or plastic flap substituting as the floor of the mouth (Fig. 13-7). Access to the airway is limited by the lack of compressibility of the tongue, extreme angulation required in the posterior pharyngeal area to approach the additus laryngis, and potential post endoscopy or intubation edema causing further obstruction. This is the case even though radiographs taken with the patient awake and sitting demonstrate a patent airway.

Oral access is extremely limited, and nasofiberoptic access may prove to be the only noninvasive approach. The degree of postradiation induration, concomitant inflammation with submucosal fibrositis, and distortion of the normal anatomy can be extreme, even leading to total airway obstruction. Failure to perform a complete evaluation, which includes fiberoptic visualization of all structures including the trachea and dynamic C-arm fluoroscopic studies in the sitting and supine positions with deep breathing and swallowing maneuvers, can lead to dangerously erroneous conclusions regarding management.

Of equal, if not greater, consequence is the postsurgical situation (e.g., after biopsy of the base of tongue, manipulation of the pharyngeal tissues for rigid blade access or other purposes, and postintubation laryngeal edema). The "better part of valor" often is to recommend an awake tracheostomy or at most monitored, light sedation anesthesia. This, however, does not obviate the need for thorough

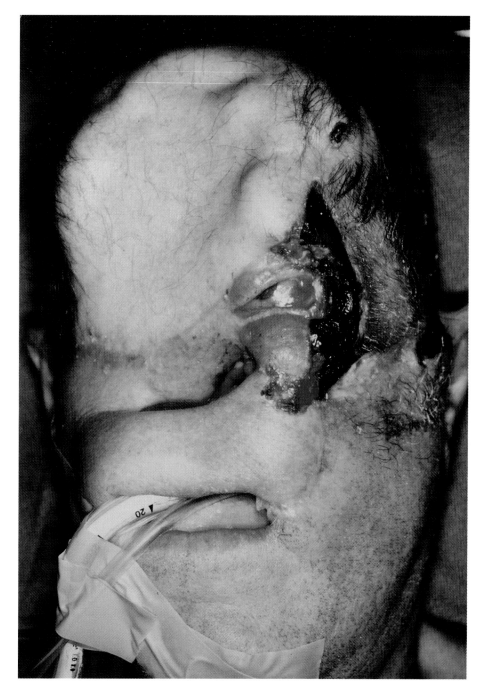

FIG. 13-8   Patient with basal cell carcinomatosis.

examination, including soft tissue radiology, and direct fiberoptic observation of tissues of the pharynx and larynx to support the clinical decision.

Appearances, however, can sometimes by deceiving. A disastrous-appearing patient with massive soft and hard tissue destruction secondary to basal cell carcinomatosis is shown in Fig. 13-8. This was in fact only an apparent airway access situation because the tissue destruction and concomitant plastic surgical amelioration permitted easy access by pushing soft tissue aside.

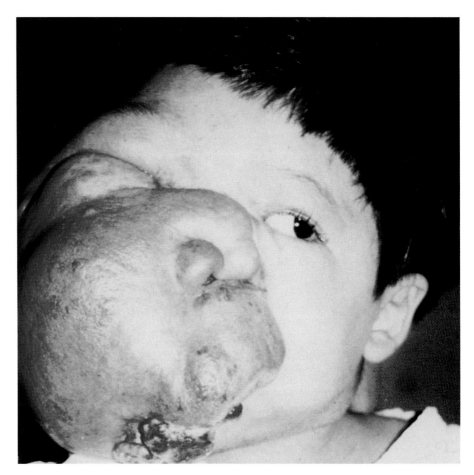

FIG. 13-9   Kasabach-Merritt syndrome. (Courtesy Dr. P. Sirivanasandha, Ramathibodi Hospital, Bangkok, Thailand.)

The patient with Kasabach-Merritt syndrome (thrombopenia hemangioma syndrome) (Fig. 13-9) demonstrates spectacularly the level of complication presented for airway access.

SLEEP APNEA

A clear understanding of the different classes of apnea is essential when treating apnea patients. *Central apnea* refers to cessation of nasal and oral airflow with concomitant cessation of respiratory effort. The source of this disorder lies in pathophysiology of the central nervous system. *Obstructive apnea* is defined as blockage of nasal and oral airflow despite continuing respiratory effort, and it is generally caused by anatomic abnormalities in the upper respiratory tract. *Mixed apnea* has both central and obstructive components, with the obstructive part usually following the central.

Originally mixed apnea was believed to occur only in obese patients, most vividly represented by the famous character in the Dickens novel after whom the Pickwickian syndrome was named. It is now known that a number of other types manifest similar airway obstruction. The mechanism itself is caused by backward movement of the tongue and collapse of the pharyngeal walls (glossoptosis) (Fig. 13-10), attributable to interference with the dynamic phasic contraction of the pharyngeal and hypopharyngeal muscles. This may also be caused by greatly enlarged tonsils or adenoids, macroglossia, or assorted other factors, including the anesthetic sleep state.

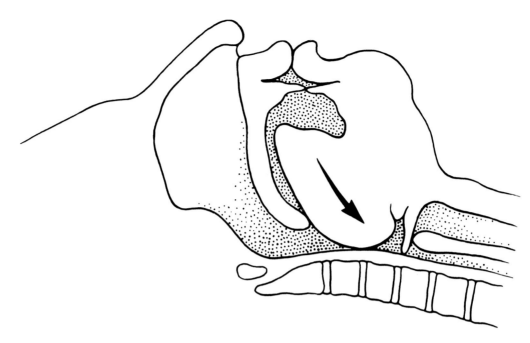

FIG. 13-10   Glossoptosis. Glossoptotic tongue placement *(arrow).*

Mixed syndromes can be diagnosed from signs and symptoms of chronic sleep deprivation, daytime somnolence, chronic fatigue, loud snoring, morning headaches, and often, personality disturbances.

Prudence dictates that all sleep disturbances not be called by the title, *sleep apnea.* There must be diagnostic signs and symptoms, first confirmed visually and then by classic techniques in the sleep laboratory. A respiratory pause indicates a cessation of airflow of less than 10 seconds duration. A sleep apneic episode involves a cessation of airflow of more than 10 seconds duration. The sleep apnea syndrome is diagnosed by at least 30 episodes of true apnea during a 7-hour period, although apnea patients may have as many as several hundred episodes during the night. The apnea index is the mean number of apneas per hour of sleep as calculated for each individual patient being observed. This is particularly important if active intervention is contemplated to correct the syndrome.

Sleep apnea is interesting because it illuminates some of the airway problems that are encountered in sleeping patients. First, it must be remembered that this is a syndrome rather than a specific disease. Sorting out the etiologic factors is crucial to an understanding and logical plan for management. Etiologic factors may include neurologic, anatomic, or pathofunctional soft tissue (i.e., mechanical) considerations.

A cause of breathing disturbance not often recognized is that related to nasal obstruction. Exactly why oropharyngeal airway obstruction occurs when the nose is occluded is postulated by reports by Blakely and Mahowald[2] and Cole and Haight.[3] It appears possible that nasal obstruction causes a reflex change in the tone of the pharyngeal musculature. Pharyngeal constriction may represent a compensatory attempt to increase total airway resistance when the nasal passage is limited. This constriction may be caused by loss of abductor tone, increased adductor tone, or hypotonia of all pharyngeal muscles. It must also be recognized that mouth breathing appears to be a learned or, at least, a later developmental progression. Newborn infants are nose breathers, and neonates who have obstructions to the nasal passages (choanal atresia) pass on to an unfortunate demise. (The latter situation is the basic reason for inserting a catheter through the nares of newborn infants at birth to check for any obstruction and to suck out thick mucoid or meconium collections functionally obstructing the nasal passages.)

Similar obstructions have been demonstrated in patients with micrognathia, often complicated by glossoptosis (as in Pierre Robin syndrome).

Patterns of hypoventilation accentuated by sleep can also develop during the course of disorders of the brain stem as well as in a number of patients with chronic muscular or neuromuscular diseases. They represent a potential cause of asphyxial coma in susceptible subjects.

These patients are at potential risk for airway obstruction, frequently unexpected and often catastrophic, during the induction and recovery phases of anesthesia. They should be induced for and recovered from anesthesia in the sitting position whenever possible to minimize the collapse of pharyngeal wall soft tissue and to take advantage of the suspensory supports of the laryngotrachea. The safer, albeit more conservative, approach is to anticipate sudden airway obstruction in all of these patients and to opt for elective, sedated, but spontaneously ventilating, endotracheal intubation in the sitting position. The physician must also be alerted to the rarer abnormalities occurring in association with subacute medullary disease or after surgical damage to the respiratory reticulospinal projection. These occur during the course of ventrolateral upper cervical cord section, which is designed to interrupt afferent spinothalamic projections.

An excellent review of mortality in obstructive sleep apnea patients by Jiang and associates[4] suggests the potential risk factors to be faced with anesthesia-induced sleep apnea. Other studies from sleep apnea clinics include the works of Thorpy and others.[5] The obvious reason for not having documented mortality figures for the anesthesia situation is that the anesthesiologist pays specific attention to early establishment of the airway. However, while sedating the patient to that anesthesia level compatible with inserting one form or the other of artificial airway, the physician tends to superimpose the obstructive component of apnea on the central form. The anesthesiologist's propensity for rapid inductions and immediate endotracheal intubation (often more for convenience than patient needs) can induce problems in the recovery period or whenever the endotracheal tube is removed because of each of the earlier observed tissue changes. In other situations the sedated patient has obstructive ventilatory manifestations after premedication or on anesthesia induction.

A particularly revealing diagnostic procedure is Müller's maneuver with fiberoptic endoscopy in the awake patient as described by Borowiecki and others.[6] This consists of forced inspiratory effort with the mouth and the nose closed and may be extended to describe a variety of mechanisms of pharyngeal collapse involving different portions of the pharynx in a population of patients with craniofacial anomalies.

This technique has been modified for patients who are unable to cooperate readily by having the procedure done in the sitting and then in the reclining position and by having the motion of the airway observed both with a Müller attempt and with swallowing at different levels. Using this method the fiberscope should be inserted to the level of viewing the epiglottis, the maneuver exercised, the fiberscope withdrawn to the base of the tongue where papillae may be visualized, and then the whole series of steps repeated. Noting the distance of the tip of the epiglottis from the posterior pharynx and the motion of the pharyngeal walls are intrinsic parts of this procedure, revealing the site of pharyngeal collapse. This can be repeated at several levels as indicated. Conventional grading is recorded to wit:

1+: Minimal movement of the components of the pharynx toward the center
2+: Movement toward the center, decreasing the cross-sectional area by 50%
3+: Movement toward the center, decreasing the cross-sectional area by 75%
4+: Inward movement, totally obstructing the airway

OBESITY

Perhaps the most frequently observed airway problem is that found in obese patients. A weight of 20% over ideal or twice the predicted weight for age, sex, body build, and height is considered morbid obesity. All physicians recognize that the morbidly obese individual presents ventilatory risks. Not as many are aware that even the "relatively" obese have similar hazards. Endomorphism even without morbid obesity (i.e., abdominal mass overshadowing thoracic bulk, all anatomic regions notable for softness and roundness, and hands and feet relatively small) can signal trouble.

Frequently the patient with a short, thick neck and a large tongue represents an intubation and endoscopic challenge. The bulk weight of soft tissues and tongue can, themselves, cause supraglottic obstruction during sleep and induction of anesthesia. During preoperative examination of the patient, the mobility of the neck and its range of motion should be carefully delineated. The physician must be alert to consider complicating etiologic conditions such as Cushing's syndrome, myxedema, hyperinsulinism, suprasellar hypothalamic lesions, Stein-Leventhal syndrome, and the classic Pickwickian syndrome. Similarly, physicians are all aware of the mechanical instrumentation difficulties experienced when performing an endoscopy on a patient with a massive chest, particularly endomorphic females. Many endoscopists consider the obese patient as a mandatory awake intubation situation. Certainly, as discussed previously, the sitting position is preferable from many viewpoints.

Less often recognized is the relationship of a high-arched palate, narrow posterior dentition (intermaxillary space), and a narrow anterior central dental arch to endoscopic access and airway patency. This, coupled with the fact that hypotonus of the muscle of the floor of the mouth occurs unusually rapidly during anesthetic induction in obese patients, explains the frequency of soft tissue obstruction in some patients during the induction phase of anesthetic management. Of particular note is the finding of Safar, Escarraga, and Chang[7] of a significantly high prevalence of airway obstruction in obese patients when their necks were extended. Interestingly, a phenomenon of polyarthritis with migratory arthralgia than can involve all joints, and particularly the neck, is often observed. Additionally, it must be recognized that the problem of hypoventilation manifest in all pathologically overweight patients. Tracheotomy has been shown to restore normal $PaCO_2$, as have nasopharyngeal airways.

The major importance of postural changes on lung function should be noted. Functional residual capacity (FRC) decreases as the patient changes from the erect to the Trendelenburg position. This results in findings of hypoxemia, marked reduction in expiratory reserve volume, maximum volume ventilation, and functional residual capacity despite only a slight reduction in vital capacity. These are associated with a progressive rapid increase in the work of breathing and compensatory decrease of tidal volume while the respiratory rate increases, resulting in decreased ventilation to the already underventilated, dependent portions of the lungs, which then become atelectatic (thus increasing the shunting of arteriovenous blood) and early peripheral airway closure. Add to this the commonly observed thoracolumbar lordosis, limitation of rib movement, inability to raise the lower sternum, and preexistent upper airway mechanical obstructive processes, and we have the all-too-often seen ventilatory and respiratory catastrophe of the obese patient.

These combined hazards explain the tendency of anesthesiologists to do awake intubations when faced with an obese patient.

MULTIPLE SYMMETRIC LIPOMATOSIS

A patient with multiple symmetric lipomatosis falls into a slightly different category of obesity syndromes. This unusual disease is characterized by the formation of multiple, nonencapsulated lipomas with a predilection for the nape of the neck and the supraclavicular and the deltoid regions and produces an extraordinary bull-necked appearance (Madelung collar or neck) (Fig. 13-11). The danger in this situation, besides the massive truncal appearance of the patient, is that the lipomas tend to infiltrate along fascial planes and can cause life-threatening tracheal, laryngeal, and particularly, mediastinal compression. The supine position, even with moderate sedation and certainly general anesthesia in the supine position before splinting the upper airway, can add to the danger.

Access to the airway is crucial! Positioning of the patient for either diagnostic or surgical intervention requires serious thought. Additionally, consideration must be given to debulking the lipomas around the airway and in the mediastinum to avert the compression of vital structures. When dealing with these patients, hypertriglyceridemia, hyperuricemia, hyperinsulinemia, and renal tubular acidosis must be ruled out. These lipomas can develop anywhere, similar to von Recklinghausen's disease (see Fig. 13-4).

TUBERCULOSIS

The advent of acquired immunodeficiency syndrome (AIDS) has been accompanied by a dramatic resurgence of tuberculosis. The most difficult problem with this historic scourge is its resistance to most pharmacologic agents currently used.

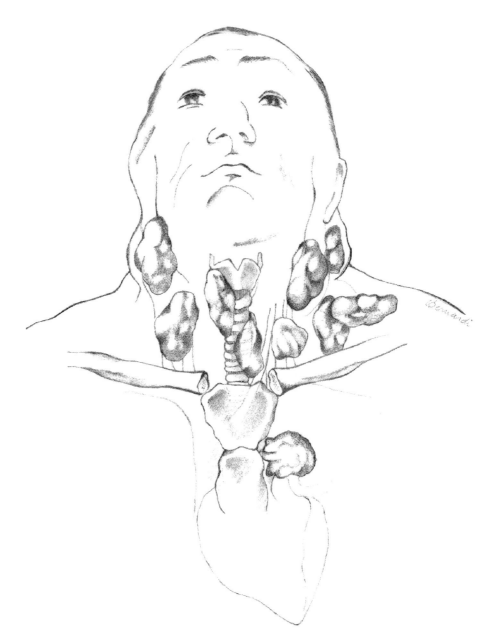

FIG. 13-11   Multiple symmetric lipomatosis.

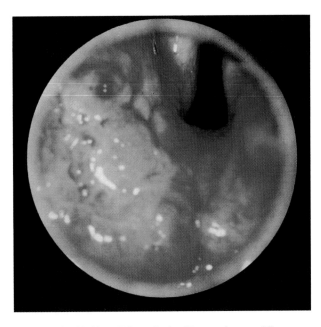

FIG. 13-12   Tuberculosis of larynx (arytenoid).

Clinical manifestations in the airway commonly involve the posterior structures of the larynx. Fig. 13-12 demonstrates the characteristic lesion involving the arytenoid and aryepiglottic fold. There may be diffuse swelling or a localized irregular mass, depending on whether the pathologic process is acute, exudative, or chronically productive.[8] Pulmonary tuberculosis is closely associated and may be the primary source.

If laryngeal tuberculosis is not recognized and treated early, the larynx goes through the stages of ulceration, true edema, perichondritis, chondral necrosis, stenosis, and impending asphyxia.

The epiglottis and the aryepiglottic folds are the usual locations of the lesion. In almost all cases the pharynx is invaded by a similar process at a later stage of the disease.

CROUP AND SUPRAGLOTTITIS

Croup remains a serious problem in clinical practice. This condition is found in both pediatric and adult medical practice. Repeated studies have demonstrated that 0.25 ml/5 kg body weight of 2.25% racemic epinephrine in normal saline by intermittent positive pressure breathing (IPPB) administration has salutary results.[9-11] If endotracheal intubation is anticipated, this regimen should be instituted preoperatively and continued in the postextubation period. Best results appear when dexamethasone is administered concurrently. Therapeutic results achieved using dexamethasone alone are not impressive.[12]

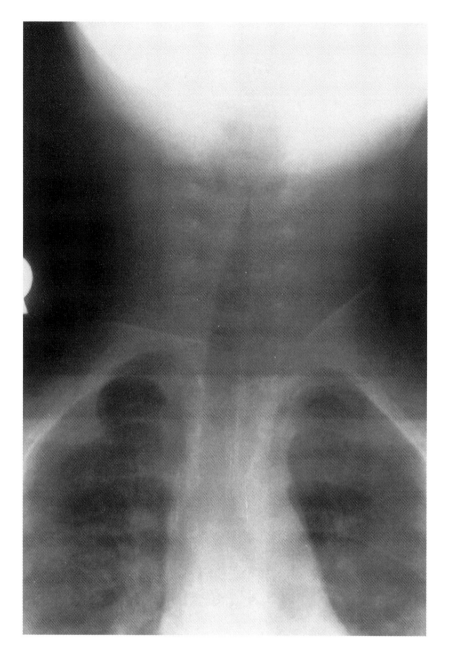

FIG. 13-13   "Steeple sign" in supraglottitis.

Endoscopy and endotracheal intubation in the croup patient can be a real *tour de force*. The diagnosis is established by a history of sore throat, sounds of a croupy cough, and anteroposterior radiographic confirmation of the "steeple sign" (Fig. 13-13). The patient must be kept in the sitting position and the airway assured before full anesthetic management. All upper airway tissues will be very friable as well. The laryngoscope blade should closely approximate the tongue and should be lubricated thoroughly. The endotracheal tube should be small enough to permit a slight leak.

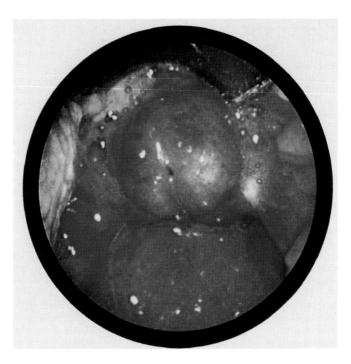

FIG. 13-14   "Trap-door" appearance in fulminating supraglottitis.

Supraglottitis is the classic "trap-door" obstruction circumstance, often presenting as an acute, fulminating emergency (Fig. 13-14). The diagnosis can be made from the history of upper respiratory infection, inspiratory stridor, sore throat, sensation of a "golf ball" on swallowing, patient in a bolt-upright sitting position, anxious facies, and, in rare cases, x-ray finding of a massive epiglottitis and often of a swollen uvula (i.e., the "thumb sign" [Fig. 13-15]). If the clinical diagnosis suggests epiglottitis, delaying intervention for an x-ray scan can lead to catastrophe.

Epiglottitis is the ultimate in airway emergencies, and every effort must be expended to get the patient to the operating room emergently and to control the airway. Diagnostic x-ray scans, blood and urine studies, or other tests must not be the cause of delay. The danger of forcing the patient into the supine position to effectuate anesthesia induction and intubation of the laryngotrachea should be particularly noted. The most skilled intubationist should be in attendance, and a tracheostomy set should be opened. The surgeon should be scrubbed and ready to perform an emergent tracheostomy.

Table 13-1 emphasizes various important aspects of croup and supraglottitis.[13-16]

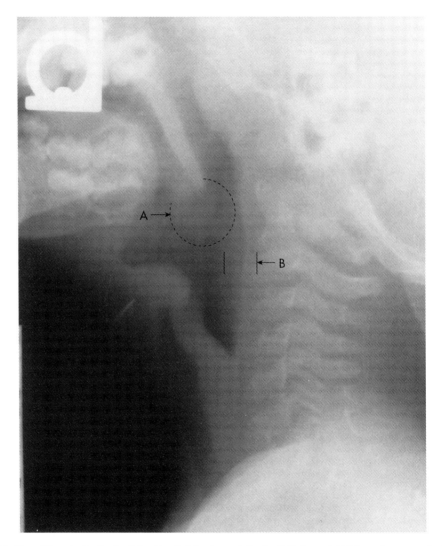

FIG. 13-15   "Thumb sign" of epiglottitis. *A,* Massive epiglottis. *B,* Inflamed (thickened) prevertebral tissue.

Table 13-1 Important Aspects of Croup and Epiglottitis*

Aspect	Croup	Epiglottitis
Age	Children <3 years	Children 3-6 years Adults
Pathologic condition	Laryngotracheobronchitis	Supraglottitis Epiglottitis
Etiology	Viral†	Bacterial
History and examination	24-28 hours, mild URTI Inspiratory stridor, barking cough, breathing with marked effort Oxygen saturation decreases with exhaustion	6-12 hours, severe URTI Inspiratory stridor, expiratory snore, unable to swallow Breathing with marked care, often in "sniffing position" Oxygen saturation decreases with coexistent bronchopneumonia and abruptly if acute obstruction occurs
Special investigations	Not particularly useful Blood film (lymphocytosis) Lateral neck x-ray ("steeple sign")	Not recommended (adds little, may delay intervention) Lateral neck x-ray ("thumb sign")
Management	Handle patient gently, anxiety and fear can worsen situation; treat obstruction medically initially (oxygen, hydration, nebulized epinephrine, IV steroids); airway intervention required if patient is hypoxemic (despite oxygen therapy) or exhausted (rising $PaCO_2$ and pulse rate) or if obstruction is not stabilizing. Intubation hints: inhalation induction prolonged, ability to identify glottis not hampered, use of one tube size smaller than age calculated, and intubate orally, suction trachea, and change to nasotracheal tube Extubate when leakage occurs around endotracheal tube for 2-5 days and secretions are diminished.	Handle patient gently, anxiety and fear can worsen situation; airway intervention *urgent* (obstruction may occur suddenly, unpredictably, and with rapid oxygen desaturation); transfer patient to operating room (summon anesthesiologist or surgeon); do not unnecessarily disturb child (e.g., placing IV positioning before induction of anesthesia); nebulized epinephrine in adults may improve airway before induction (it is more likely to scare a child). Intubation hints: always an inhaled induction, avoid traumatizing airway, induce in position of greatest patient comfort (usually sitting), move patient to supine position when asleep (cPAP may improve airway at this stage) and gently assist ventilatory effort, and ability to identify glottis may be hampered. If so, try pressure on thorax to create air bubbles in glottis and consider tracheotomy. Oral styletted tube, suction trachea, change to nasal tube (same size for age); if not epiglottitis, swab epiglottis with patient awake and treat medically, as in croup. Extubate Children: when fever is resolved. Adults: when leak is demonstrable around endotracheal tube (2-5 days).

Courtesy Dr. Philip Cornish.

*More extensive descriptions may be found elsewhere.[13-15] This table emphasizes various important aspects of croup and epiglottitis.

†Recent increases in the incidence of papillomatous disease and sexually transmitted disease of the upper airway raise the possibility of more unusual and complex etiologies.

URTI, Upper respiratory tract infection; *PaCO₂*, arterial partial pressure of carbon dioxide; *cPAP*, continuous positive airway pressure.

AIRWAY MANAGEMENT IN THE BURNED PATIENT

Airway management in the burned patient requires skill and experience in intubation as well as knowledge of the natural history and course of burn injury.[17] Indications for endotracheal intubation in the burned patient are listed in Table 13-2. Many patients are prematurely intubated because they present with soot on their faces. Other patients are at risk for airway obstruction because of swelling of soft tissues during the resuscitation phase of their injury. Because of physician inexperience, some patients may go without intubation to the point where it is no longer possible.

Carbonaceous sputum has been used as a sign of inhalation injury in the burned patient. This is a weak sign. The most definite thing that can be said about this finding is that the patient has inhaled carbonaceous air, which may occur as the result of a great many causes. Of much more concern are findings of facial burns, pharyngeal burns, or singed nasal hairs. **Hoarseness and or stridor are particularly ominous signs and indicate the need for immediate therapy.**

People who have inhaled steam represent extremely difficult airway access as a result of massive edema. This is usually manifested primarily in the nasal and oropharyngeal tissues as well as in the neck and facial soft tissues.

On the other hand, lye and other caustic chemical burns are usually limited to the oropharynx and pharyngoesophagus, although areas such as the piriform sinuses and vestibular folds of the larynx may be affected. There is also a real danger of adhesion of a swollen tongue to the posterior pharynx. Further down the tracheobronchial tract, casts may form as a result of dehydration and mouth breathing or secondary to nonhumidified endotracheal tube ventilation and poor tracheobronchial toilet. This may be aggravated by suppression of surfactant and lysosomes.

Regularly scheduled inhalation of nebulized racemic epinephrine may reduce upper airway swelling sufficiently to avoid endotracheal intubation, but such patients must be monitored closely and intubated promptly if signs of impending airway obstruction do not quickly abate or if they worsen. Methods of intubation may include direct laryngoscopic visualization, blind nasal, flexible fiberoptic visualization of the vocal folds, and trachea (via oral or nasal routes) and rigid bronchoscopy. Adequate suction is critical for all forms of intubation, but particularly so when using fiberoptic endoscopes. Secretions tend to be thick and tinged by the inhaled products of combustion. They easily obscure visualization and are frequently difficult to remove through the endoscope.

Table 13-2   Indications for Endotracheal Intubation in the Burned Patient*

Absolute	Relative (requires physician judgment)	Unlikely
Hoarseness and stridor not responding *promptly* to racemic epinephrine aerosol treatment	Singed nasal hairs and facial burns	No hoarseness or stridor
Oral burns	Injury occurred in a closed space	No singed nasal hairs, no facial or oral burns
Arterial blood gases inappropriate for FiO_2	Large burn for age and previous medical history	Injury did not occur in a closed space
Depressed level of consciousness such that patient is unable to protect own airway	—	—
Carboxyhemoglobin >10 in the presence of depressed level of consciousness	—	Patient alert and appropriate

*All criteria and relative and physician judgment must always supersede any published list of criteria. Criteria from the absolute list should always take precedence over any other criteria in the relative or unlikely lists. Similarly, criteria from the relative indications list should supersede any criteria present from the unlikely category.

Another important consideration is tissue edema. Edema caused by direct tissue injury to the face, pharynx, and lungs as well as generalized edema is of significance. Properly resuscitated burned patients also develop edema in any tissues that are still viable (i.e., areas of superficial [partial thickness] burns or in areas underneath more completely burned tissues). Edema may develop in tissues distant from burned areas such as the face, pharynx, and larynx. At this time soft tissue edema may be at its worst and intubation the most difficult (Fig. 13-16). Compromise of the upper airway by edema may result in a totally inaccessible airway. The edema may become so intense that an expeditious tracheostomy may be technically impossible. This is a particularly important consideration in patients suffering from burns involving greater than 20% of their total body surface area, where fluid requirements begin at 4.2 L/day in the mythical 70-kg patient and increase with the patient's weight and percentage of body area burned.

Frequently a judgment about intubation must be made early in the course of treatment, while the airway is still asymptomatic. **Failure to intubate within the first 24 hours of burn injury may preclude intubation at a later time. During the first 24 hours soft tissue swelling may become so extensive that range of motion of the cervical spine and temporomandibular joints may be limited by the surrounding tissues.** This is usually accompanied by soft tissue edema about the face and neck and can prove a deadly combination. Edema about the head and neck may be minimized by placing the patient in a 30 degree, head-up position whenever possible to facilitate lymphatic and venous drainage.

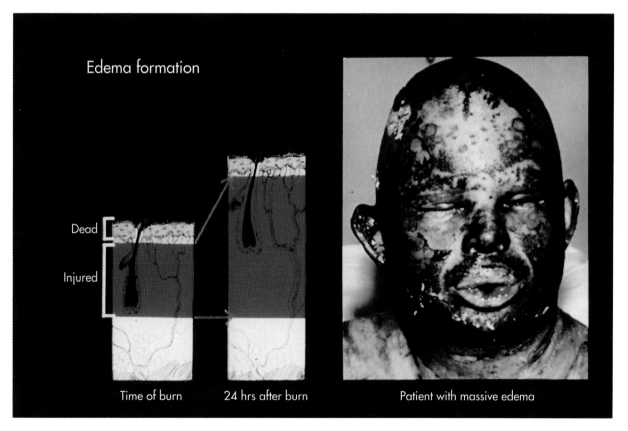

FIG. 13-16   Edema formation.

Another consideration is the seriousness of the overall injury to the patient. Burns involving greater than 50% of the body surface area, even in otherwise healthy patients, often require endotracheal intubation during the first week after injury, at a time when intubation may be difficult or impossible. It is therefore essential to anticipate the need for endotracheal intubation before this time. Causes of respiratory failure may include sepsis, resulting in increased metabolic demands and alterations in the level of consciousness, inhalation injury, or inability to compensate for the increased metabolic demands of the burn injury itself. **The most common time for pulmonary interstitial inhalation injury to be manifest is on the third postinjury day, when tissue edema is at its maximum.** Surgery for escharotomy (Fig. 13-17) or wound debridement is frequently performed during this time, and intubation becomes necessary because of competition with surgeons for the airway, intraoperative positioning (prone, extreme lateral, etc.), and technical demands of massive transfusion or managing hemodynamic instability.

In addition, young (less than 2 years) or elderly patients or patients with underlying medical diseases suffer increased morbidity and mortality from burns of lesser severity and frequently develop respiratory failure soon after injury, *even when the upper airway is not directly involved.*

Intubation is generally accomplished in a routine fashion through the oral route with a laryngoscope. However, several things about burned patients warrant discussion. First, there are the psychologic aspects of approaching a disfigured human being and the smell of burned tissue, both of which must be ignored. Second, these patients frequently have a significant quantity of oral secretions. Third, the various topical agents used for wound treatment make the skin slippery.

Securing endotracheal tubes should routinely be done with ties of either cloth or intravenous extension tubing. These may be secured over the ears, taking care to leave a sufficient amount of slack so that tissue necrosis is not induced and venous drainage from the head through the internal and external jugular veins is not occluded, thus avoiding cerebral edema. Endotracheal tubes should not be secured to anything else, such as nasogastric tubes. This prevents a confused patient from removing all tubes just by catching hold of one. Frequent adjustments in the securing ties are necessary to accommodate changes in soft tissue edema.

The use of fiberoptic equipment in either nasal or oral intubation is a necessary skill for those managing the airways of burned patients. The adage that says to use this modality when needed, before laryngoscopy or blind instrumentation, is particularly true in this setting. Secretions, burned nasopharyngeal tissue, and edema make endoscopy difficult, and the addition of laryngoscope-induced bleeding further reduces the chances of a successful intubation.

The instrument has particular application following smoke inhalation. It has been established that patients with severe laryngeal edema following smoke inhalation will eventually require intubation.[18] Proper endoscopic evaluation assists in choosing between endotracheal intubation and tracheostomy.

Technical Approaches to Management of Soft Tissue Problems

Use of the flexible fiberoptic endoscope has contributed to the safety of the patient. Another aid is the ventilating laryngoscope using Venturi (jet) principles to enrich the gas at the additus laryngis during intubation attempts and thus extend the time the anesthesiologist needs to locate and intubate the larynx. The concept is also based on a premise, not fully demonstrated, that with proper application the jet gas can be insufflated into the laryngotracheal route by bouncing off the posterior pharynx. Unfortunately, this may result in gas being propelled into the esophagus and down to the stomach. However, inadvertent gastric dilation can readily be remedied by prompt insertion of a nasogastric or orogastric tube as soon as airway control has been assured. Of course the physician must always keep in mind the risk of regurgitation; consequently, the semi-Fowler's position will be of assistance as will ready availability of adequate suction devices.

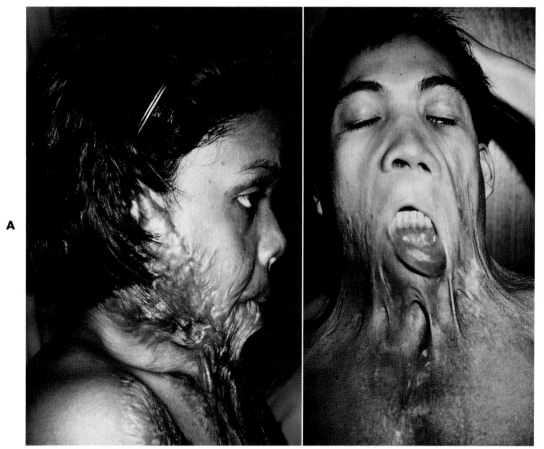

FIG. 13-17 Cicatrix. Two extreme examples limiting cervical motion and airway access. **A,** Patient attempted self-immolation. **B,** Pilot burned in airplane crash. (Courtesy Dr. Sirivanasandha, Ramathibodi Hospital, Bangkok, Thailand.)

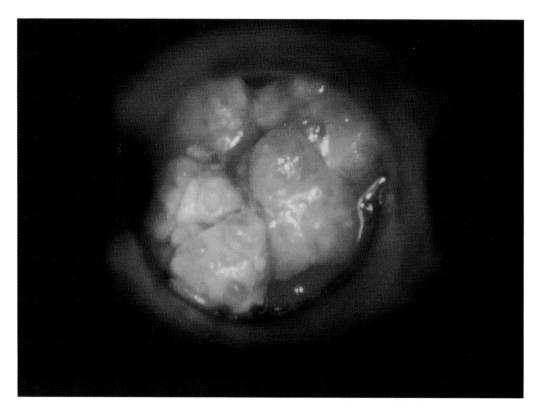

FIG. 13-18   Laryngeal papillomatosis.

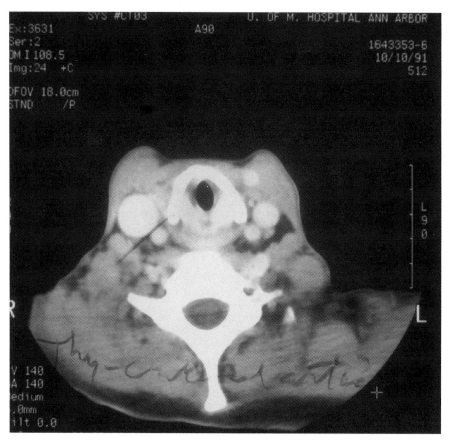

FIG. 13-19   Tracheal stenosis.

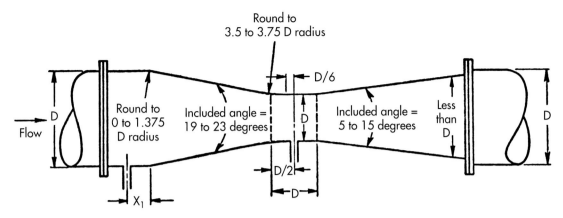

FIG. 13-20   Design of vena contracta portion of injector needle. (From Spink LK: *Principles and practice of flow meter engineering,* ed 8, Foxboro, Mass, 1958, Foxboro.)

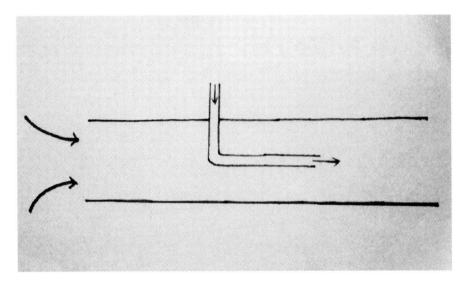

FIG. 13-21   Simplified diagram representing application of Venturi needle to airway.

Lasers. The use of lasers in the airway, with or without obstructive airway lesions, presents special problems in certain circumstances (e.g., juvenile papillomatosis [Fig. 13-18], tracheal stenosis [Fig. 13-19], or webs). In some situations visualization of the target falls within the difficult airway sphere. In lasers the need for instrumental access, often obstructed by the presence of an endotracheal tube, makes surgery difficult. Finally, the use of traditional airway management techniques, such as endotracheal tubes, in the presence of laser energy risks catastrophic injury from resultant fire.

Venturi ventilation. In 1797 Giovanni B. Venturi described a specially streamlined tubular constriction system to minimize energy losses in fluid flowing through the tube, while minimizing the fall in pressure in the constriction, in accordance with Bernoulli's principle, which defined the relationship between changes in pressure and speed of gas flows in 1738 (see Chapter 1). These physical principles are applied to Venturi or jet ventilation of the respiratory tract. The critical factor lies in the design of the vena contracta portion of the injector needle (Fig. 13-20) and production of negative flow pressure behind and beside the egress port of the needle. A simplified diagram represents the application to the airway (Fig. 13-21).

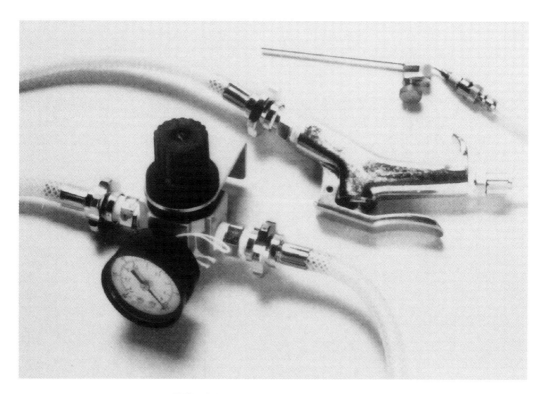

FIG. 13-22   Jet Venturi delivery system.

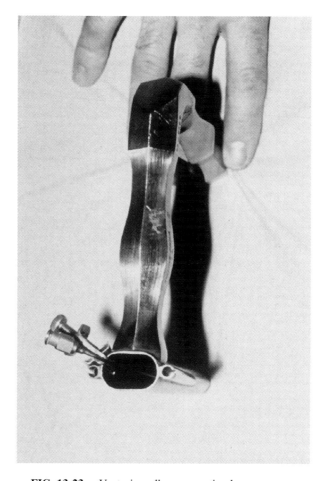

FIG. 13-23   Venturi needle on operating laryngoscope.

The objective of Venturi ventilation is to produce a forceful jet of gas or oxygen through the vena contracta of the Venturi tube and then entrain air from behind (i.e., the ingress port of the laryngoscope), which is then transmitted as increased volume and pressure down the tracheobronchial tree for purposes of patient ventilation. This obviates the need for presence of an endotracheal tube during laser surgery of the respiratory tract from the larynx to and including the major bronchi. Furthermore, because light waves are not inhibited by the gas transmitted, vision is not impeded during the process.

The use of Venturi ventilation in laser surgery of the aerodigestive tract has been described. The advantage of the aerodigestive system in laser surgery is removal of a hydrocarbon base (endotracheal tube) required for propagation of a flame (combustion), thus improving safety during laser surgery.[19]

Jet Venturi instrumentation includes a high-pressure oxygen source, a jet needle, an all-or-nothing trigger, and a pressure-reducing valve (Fig. 13-22). With this system the jet needle can be placed on any operating laryngoscope (Fig. 13-23). The design of the needle is crucial (Fig. 13-24). The tip should be located in the middle third of the laryngoscope lumen for optimum effect.[20]

This approach requires intravenous anesthesia for maintenance during the Venturi phase. With the advent of the rapid-acting Propofol, we have an almost ideal anesthetic, but the use of a rapid-act-

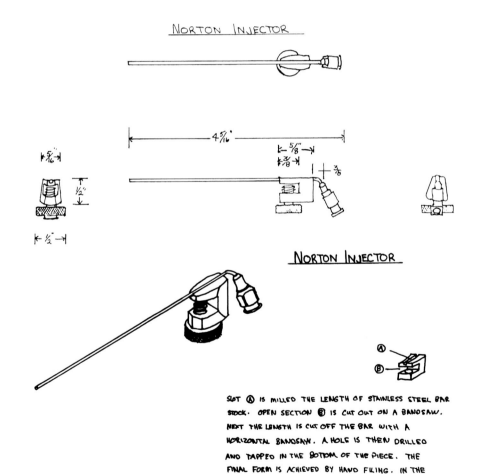

FIG. 13-24 Design of Venturi needle.

ing muscle relaxant with short duration is still required. Monitoring is best accomplished by pulse oximetry, electrocardiography, automatic blood pressure cuff sequencing, and watching the chest motion. The prime concern is progressive hypertension during the time the patient is on suspension laryngoscopy. This can be treated with labetalol or with another antihypertension agent.

Another suggested approach to reducing flammability has been reducing oxygen concentration delivered. With the advent of on-line arterial oxygen concentration and transcutaneous oxygen saturation devices, this can be achieved. There are several factors to be kept in mind. First is the avoidance of hypoxia.

Patients who require airway surgery have a tenuous oxygen and carbon dioxide balance. They are the very individuals requiring higher-than-usual oxygen concentration delivery! Their needs must not be secondary to the risk of airway fires. Thus other ways to manage the problem are used. First the combustible substrate such as the endotracheal tube or the flammable anesthetic such as nitrous oxide can be removed, replacing them with nonflammable alternatives such as Venturi ventilation and intravenous anesthesia. Next combustion can be suppressed by the addition of helium to the gas mixture in the respiratory tract. This also requires close monitoring by pulse oximetry (saturation) and arterial oxygen (concentration). The prime concern must be to provide the patient with requisite oxygen requirements.

CASE 13-1 *CERVICAL SPINAL TORSION WITH RHEUMATOID ARTHRITIS WITH LARYNGOSPASM AND OTHER SOFT TISSUE COMPLICATIONS*

A 60-year-old man was referred to us with cervical spinal rheumatoid arthritis and cervical soft tissue torsion (see Fig. 12-12). At the time of initial airway evaluation, he was in a circular bed, in cervical traction, using a halo. His head was positioned with his right ear on the shoulder, and he was looking over his right shoulder. He had all the indications of far-advanced rheumatoid arthritis. His airway was patent and, other than clinical rotation, appeared cachectic.

After sternocleidomastoid section, there was marked improvement in head positioning. However, progressive audible airway obstruction with tracheal tug developed during the period between surgery and when he was seen in the Difficult Airway Clinic.

C-arm fluoroscopy showed evidence of airway rotation, rheumatoid arthritic C2-C6 fusion, and obstruction at the level of the vocal and vestibular folds. Direct laryngoscopy indicated available access to the larynx, but the larynx could not be visualized beyond the basal tongue airway. Fiberoptic endoscopy through the left nasal route was normal down to the level of the epiglottis. The piriform sinuses were normal bilaterally. However, the long epiglottis moved little with swallowing, cough, or phonation. The tip remained in close approximation to the pharyngeal wall. The arytenoids moved little (arthritic fixation), although the aryepiglottic folds were sharp. The vestibular folds were significantly thickened and covered with mycotic-appearing flaps. The vocal folds were blunted and markedly thickened, including the anterior commissure. Vocal fold motion was symmetric; however, the motion was essentially a bilateral bowing of minimum aperture.

The recommendation was that the patient undergo early tracheostomy to relieve his airway obstruction. It was also suggested that his elective surgery be deferred for 7 to 14 days to allow maturation of the stoma. An armored (wired or anodal) endotracheal tube should be inserted for surgery, and this should be securely sutured in place and solidly anchored to limit chances of extubation when the patient was turned to the prone position.

Soon after his evaluation, the patient coughed on some secretions, developed laryngospasm, became somnolent, and required ventilatory resuscitation. A left nasotracheal tube was inserted to a level just above the vocal folds but could not be inserted into the trachea. The patient was ventilated with 100% oxygen and returned to conscious alertness. The ear, nose, and throat (ENT) team was called on an *emergent* basis but with verbal communication with the patient, and an emergency tracheostomy was performed. The patient was taken to the recovery room in excellent condition.

Following tracheostomy and cervical osteotomies followed by traction, the patient developed nausea, nystagmus, and extreme rotatory vertigo. This was controlled pharmacologically. The visual nystagmus required eye muscle exercises. Postoperative management continued for 60 days.

Reconstructing the hospital history of events, the following has been concluded:

1. Long-standing, gradual cervical torsion led to anatomic adaptation of the visual apparatus, as well as the trachea and carotid arteries and veins.

2. Abruptly changing this adaptation through sternocleidomastoid muscle section and cervical traction led to severe torsion obstruction of the trachea, cervical arterial, and venous systems. The error committed lies in failing to properly plan for *staged* surgical positional changes *after* first permitting complete evaluation and airway control as originally scheduled.

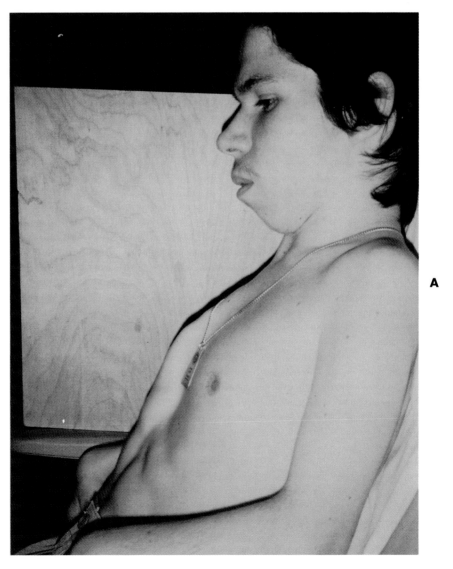

A

FIG. 13-25   **A,** Juvenile rheumatoid arthritis with mucopolysaccharidosis.

Continued.

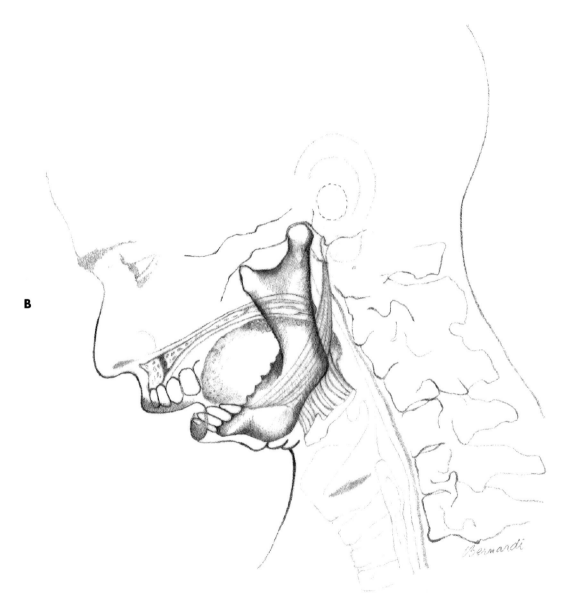

FIG. 13-25, cont'd.   B, Underlying oropharyngeal pathologic condition.

CASE 13-2   *MUCOPOLYSACCHARIDOSIS WITH OBSTRUCTIVE AIRWAY DISEASE AND JUVENILE RHEUMATOID ARTHRITIS*

A 28-year-old man with type IS mucopolysaccharidosis (MPS) (Scheie's syndrome), prior aortic valve replacement, recent failure of intubation, and a clinical history of obstructive airway disease was examined in the Difficult Airway Clinic. Cardiac valve surgery and airway laser therapy were anticipated.

The patient had full dentition, but pharyngeal examination revealed Mallampati 4+ (no visualization beyond the junction of the hard or soft palate). He had a dwarfism-type body structure, pectus excavatum, arthritis of his limbs, and cervical spinal arthritis (Fig. 13-25). The right nasal passage was larger than the left but would not permit passage of the endotracheal tube. The patient reported shortness of breath on lying down, frequent awakening, and fatigue. He had been scheduled for a sleep apnea review including a study of hemodesaturation.

Electrocardiogram and pulse oximetry studies were done. Then a dynamic fluoroscopy was performed with the patient in both the sitting and supine positions and then during swallowing, deep breathing, phonating, and coughing. Review of bony structures suggested C1-C2 limitation of flexion and extension, but rotation was adequate. However, there was evident soft tissue enlargement of the prevertebral space, larynx, and tracheal lumen, which encroached on the airway and was markedly aggravated in the supine position. The infiltrate limited the larynx and included the aryepiglottic folds. The vocal folds had an irregular pattern. Flat plate soft tissue airway studies fully confirmed these findings, as did the transnasal fiberoptic laryngeal examination. All x-ray studies revealed enlargement (infiltration) of prevertebral and perilaryngeal and tracheal soft tissue areas with obstructive dynamics of the airway.

Right transnasal fiberoptic endoscopy showed lobular infiltrate at the level of the pharyngolarynx, continuing down throughout the larynx and trachea and including the aryepiglottic fold, obliterating the vestibule on that side, and extending into the trachea. This tissue was somewhat lobulated, which produced airway obstruction and dyspneic effects.

It was noted that the patient had extensive MPS (type I) airway involvement with significant, progressive airway obstruction and possible pulmonary hypertension.

The physicians recommended against awake rigid laryngoscopy because of the posterior pharyngeal infiltrate, enlargement of the tongue base, and glossoptosis. The suggested plan of action included the following:

1. Recognize the patient's airway status and its implications, coupled with significant management expertise.
2. Perform fiberoptic via right nasal intubation, awake and sitting.
3. Perform effective tracheostomy in semisitting position with light anesthesia.
4. Perform cardiac valve surgery.
5. Before discharge after cardiac surgery, while tracheostomy site is retained, the tracheostomy tube is replaced with a metal Mueller/Norton laser endotracheal tube. Then, using laser (Nd-YAG or CO_2), ablate the MPS deposits to open the airway lumen.
6. Perform postlaser surgery fiberoptic review of airway and consideration for extubation

The recommendation that cardiac valve surgery be done *before* laser surgery of the airway was predicted on the extreme vagal stimulation of suspension laryngoscopy required for laryngeal surgery and risk of postlaser edema.

REFERENCES

1. Sivardjan M, Fink BR: The position and the state of the larynx during general anesthesia and muscle paralysis, *Anesthesiology* 72:439-442, 1990.

2. Blakely BW, Mahowald MW: Nasal resistance and sleep apnea, *Laryngoscope* 97:752-754, 1987.

3. Cole P, Haight JSJ: Mechanisms of nasal obstruction in sleep, *Laryngoscopy* 94:1557-1559, 1984.

4. Jiang HE, Kryger MH, Zorick GJ et al: Mortality and apnea index in obstructive sleep apnea, *Chest* 94:9-14, 1988.

5. Thorpy MJ, Ledereich PS, Glovinsky PB et al: Nocturnal death in patients with obstructive sleep apnea, *Sleep Res* 18:316, 1989 (abstract).

6. Borowiecki B, Pollak CP, Weitzman ED et al: Fibro-optic study of pharyngeal airway during sleep in patients with hypersomnia obstructive sleep-apnea syndrome, *Laryngoscope* 88:1310-1313, 1978.

7. Safar P, Escarraga LS, Chang F: Upper airway obstruction in the unconscious patient, *J Appl Physiol* 14:760-764, 1959.

8. Bailey CM, Winde-Taylor PC: Tuberculous laryngitis: a series of 37 patients, *Laryngoscope* 91:93, 1981.

9. Fogel JM, Berg IJ, Gerber MA et al: Racemic epinephrine in the treatment of croup nebulization alone versus nebulization with intermittent positive pressure breathing, *J Pediatr* 25:1028-1031, 1982.

10. Taussig LM, Castro O, Beaudry PH et al: Treatment of laryngotracheal bronchitis (croup), *Am J Dis Chest* 129:790-793, 1975.

11. Westley CR, Cotton EK, Brooks JG: Nebulized racemic epinephrine by IPPB for the treatment of croup, *Am J Dis Chest* 132:484-487, 1978.

12. Kuusela AL, Vesidari T: A randomized, double-blind, placebo-controlled trial of dexamethasone and racemic epinephrine in the treatment of croup, *Acta Paediatr Scand* 77:99-104, 1988.

13. Duncan AW: Upper airway obstruction in children. In Oh TE (ed): *Intensive care manual,* ed 3, London, 1990, Butterworth.

14. Chow AW: Life-threatening infections of the head, neck, and upper respiratory tract. In Hall JB, Schmidt GA, Wood LD (eds): *Principles of critical care,* New York, 1992, McGraw-Hill Book.

15. King EG, Sheehan GJ, McDonnell TJ: Upper airway obstruction. In Hall JB, Schmidt GA, Wood LD (eds): *Principles of critical care,* New York, 1992, McGraw-Hill Book.

16. Butt W, Shann F, Walker C et al: Acute epiglottis: a different approach to management, *Crit Care Med* 16:43-47, 1988.

17. Roi LD, Flora JD, Jr, Davis TM et al: A severity grading chart for the burned patient, *Ann Emerg Med* 10(3):161-163, 1981.

18. Wanner A, Cutchavaree A: Early recognition of upper airway obstruction following smoke inhalation, *Am Rev Resp Dis* 108:1421-1428, 1973.

19. Norton ML, Strong MS, Vaughan C et al: Endotracheal intubation and Venturi (jet) ventilation for laser microsurgery of the larynx: *Transactions of the 56th Annual Meeting of the American Bronchoesophagological Association,* Palm Beach, Fla, April 27-28, 1976.

20. Woo P, Eurenius S: Dynamics of Venturi jet ventilation through the operating laryngoscope, *Ann Otol Rhinol Laryngol* 91:615-621, 1982.

CHAPTER 14

Oral and Maxillofacial Surgical Considerations in the Difficult Airway

R. SCOTT

The oral and maxillofacial surgery patient often presents unique challenges to airway management. Proposed surgery will include the following:

- Involve the airway itself
- Typically be performed on patients with some anatomic variation of the airway
- Often be of several hours duration
- Require postural changes in head position
- Be accompanied by hemorrhage and edema in the airway in the immediate postoperative period.

In contrast to many surgical procedures, in the oral and maxillofacial surgery patient the surgeon and anesthesiologist compete for the same anatomic turf during the duration of the case. To have matters proceed in an efficacious fashion, therefore, requires an additional degree of preoperative planning and intraoperative communication. The goals must include the following:

- Establishment of an adequate airway
- Securing of the endotracheal tube in a fashion that is guaranteed for the duration of the case despite numerous positional changes
- Adequate access to the airway for the anesthesiologist
- Sterile access to the surgical field for the surgeon
- Postoperative maintenance of the airway despite edema, hemorrhage, and possible maxillomandibular fixation

All oral and maxillofacial surgery procedures requiring general anesthesia also require intubation. This may be oral, nasal, or using a tracheostomy. In some cases, it requires changing from one route of access to another during the case.

It is paramount that the surgeon and anesthesiologist discuss these matters in detail in the preoperative period. The majority of oral and maxillofacial surgery cases require nasoendotracheal intubation. This most often involves use of a nasal tube with hose connections positioned along the forehead in the sagittal plane. The nasal Ring-Adair-Elwyn (RAE) tube is an example of a preshaped tube that facilitates this arrangement.

It is paramount that the tube itself and all connections be secured. Standard means of securing endotracheal tubes, such as taping to the nasal bridge or cheek region, may interfere with surgical access or cause dislodgement during the case from moisture secondary to saliva or blood. Firm attachment should be obtained in the frontal region.[1] The surgeon should assist the anesthesiologist in obtaining this goal, with both assuming responsibility for the effort.

A surgical towel is placed beneath the head and wrapped forward. It is secured with tape to the patient at the forehead and nape of the neck. A towel secured only to itself becomes dislodged during the case. The end of the RAE tube is positioned in the midsagittal plane to ensure that the flange of the tube is not impinging on the forehead and that the tube is not producing excessive pressure on the nasal rim. Both can lead to postoperative tissue injury and possible tissue necrosis (Fig. 14-1). The end of the tube is supported in this position by use of an additional folded surgical towel or 4 × 4 gauze, which is taped to the head towel. The tube is then secured in this position with tape that is wrapped completely around the patient's head (Fig. 14-2). The tube is then checked

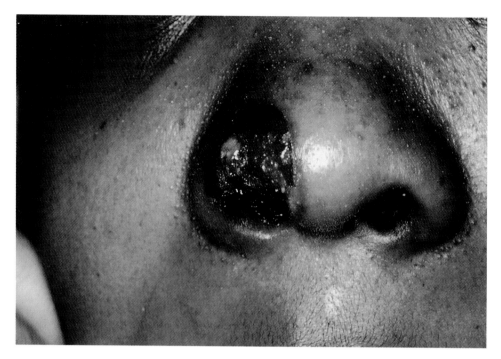

FIG. 14-1   Postoperative tissue necrosis of nose caused by undue intraoperative pressure on nasal rim.

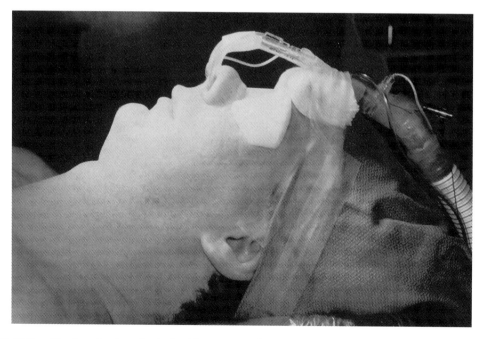

FIG. 14-2   Fixation of endotracheal tube. Note support of tube to avoid undue pressure on nasal rim and tape wrapped completely around patient's head.

for movement. Even slight in and out movement of the tube over the course of several hours contributes to postoperative pharyngeal discomfort in the patient. Additional tube stability may be obtained by securing it with a 3-0 nylon to the nasal septum. In cases of oral intubation in the primary cleft palate repair, for example, the tube can be secured with a 3-0 nylon suture placed in the base of the anterior labial mandibular vestibule.

The requirement for adequate access for both the anesthesia team and the surgical team can be accomplished in several ways. Regardless of the method used, it involves employment of various extension hoses and connectors. This, of course, introduces added variables and points of potential breakdown, as well as increased dead space and a change in requirements for adequate ventilation.[2,3] All connections must be double-checked, and the surgeon and assistants should be aware of their locations so they are not inadvertently leaned against or otherwise disturbed.

Once the airway has been established and adequately secured and access has been provided, the patient is prepared and draped. During this time a Raytec throat pack (Johnson & Johnson Medical, Inc., Arlington, Tex.) is placed. The obvious point here is that it must not be forgotten, and a definite recording of its eventual removal must be anticipated throughout the case.

Upon completion of the case the patient is extubated, either in the operating room or in the recovery room at the discretion of the anesthesiologist. Once the patient is in the recovery room, access to suction tubing with a catheter tip must be an initial priority. If the patient has been placed in maxillomandibular fixation, the anesthesiologist and recovery room nurses should be aware of the position of the maxillomandibular fixation wires and a wire cutter attached to the bedside. **A nasogastric tube should be passed on completion of the case and the gastric contents evacuated before extubation and before leaving the operating room.** Postoperative orders for an antiemetic should be written and administered in the event of postoperative nausea or emesis. The patient's head should be placed in a dependent position and suctioning through the vestibule between cheek and dentition applied.

The nasoendotracheal tube can be pulled back at the time of extubation and allowed to remain in the posterior oropharynx as an airway until it is no longer required. The use of a nasopharyngeal airway is an alternative. They should be suctioned frequently to guard against occlusion. In the pediatric patient undergoing cleft palate repair or pharyngeal flap procedures, a suture can be placed through the tip of the tongue and taped to the cheek or chest. This traction suture can then be used to pull the base of the tongue away from the posterior pharyngeal wall and support the airway. Because of postoperative edema and the nature of the surgery itself in these patients, which results in a decrease in the volume of the preoperative airway, the tongue may require some additional support while the patient is obtunded. The head of the bed should be elevated 30 degrees to help decrease edema.

A variety of types of patients will be encountered in the oral and maxillofacial surgery operating room, each with certain challenges and areas of interest for the anesthesiologist. The more common types of surgical procedures are presented below with emphasis on special airway considerations.

ORTHOGNATHIC SURGERY

Considerations for orthognathic surgery include the following:
1. Nasoendotracheal intubation may be required.
2. Hypotensive anesthesia technique may be needed.
3. The anesthesiologist must change from nasal to oral tubes in a concomitant rhinoplasty procedure.
4. Postoperative intraoral hemorrhage and edema should be expected.
5. There may be firm or elastic maxillomandibular fixation at termination of the case.
6. Patients are at special risk of tube laceration in maxillary procedures.

Orthognathic surgery involves the surgical repositioning of the maxilla, the mandible, the chin, or some combination of the three. Nasoendotracheal intubation is requested in all orthognathic patients.

Maxillary surgery may have an impact, however, in resulting hemorrhage and proximity of the endotracheal tube to the surgical field. The maxilla is an extremely well-vascularized portion of

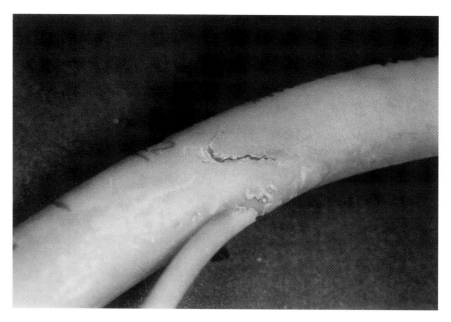

FIG. 14-3 Damaging results of close proximity of endotracheal tube to surgical field.

the human anatomy. This allows the surgeon to completely disarticulate the maxilla from the cranial base without the risk of avascular necrosis. Proximity of the nasoendotracheal tube to the surgical field poses the potential risk for tube perforation or laceration by surgical instruments (Fig. 14-3).[5,6] If adequate ventilation or cuff inflation cannot be maintained, the tube must be replaced.

Occasionally rhinoplasty is indicated in conjunction with orthognathic surgery, which necessitates the exchange of a nasal tube for an oral tube. The exchange occurs after the completion of the orthognathic surgical portion of the case in a controlled, atraumatic fashion to prevent disruption of the repositioned maxilla or mandible.

Before the mid 1980s, when transosseous wires were the standard for fixation of osteotomized bony segments, orthognathic surgery patients were placed in maxillomandibular fixation at the completion of the case. Since that time, many surgeons have converted to the use of rigid fixation of osteotomized segments. Rigid fixation involves the use of metal plates and screws to immobilize the repositioned segments of bone (Fig. 14-4). This has eliminated the need for postoperative maxillomandibular fixation, and either no interarch fixation is employed or elastic bands are used, which greatly enhances access to the oral airway in the postoperative period.

Nasogastric suctioning for the elimination of gastric contents is advised at the completion of all orthognathic cases. Extubation is at the discretion of the anesthesiologist.

TEMPOROMANDIBULAR JOINT SURGERY

Considerations for temporomandibular joint (TMJ) surgery include the following:
1. Limited or complete lack of oral access because of TMJ injury
2. Possible need for fiberoptically-guided nasoendotracheal intubation
3. Significant intraoperative rotation of the head in cases requiring bilateral surgery
4. Possible use of maxillomandibular fixation

Normal mandibular movement produces 40 to 55 mm of opening measured between the incisal edges of the maxillary and mandibular central incisors. Limitation of opening results from dysfunction of either the muscles of mastication, from disturbance of the TMJ, or both. When such dysfunction results in an opening of 30 mm or less, oral intubation becomes difficult.[8] Nasal intubation, when employing techniques other than fiberoptic intubation, may also be difficult. The surgeon may

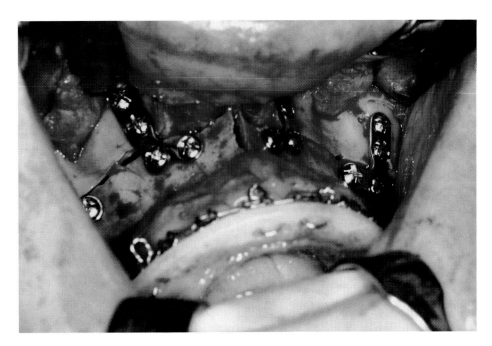

FIG. 14-4 Use of rigid fixation to secure osteotomized segments. Maxilla has been repositioned and secured with four bone plates. This often eliminates use of maxillomandibular fixation in postoperative period.

frequently request nasal intubation so that unimpeded access to the dental occlusion is available. TMJ surgery can be divided into several broad categories based on the type of pathologic condition present with definite implications for the anesthesiologist. These include the ankylosed TMJ, internal derangement of the TMJ, and myofascial pain syndrome.

True ankylosis occurs in the presence of a bony fusion. This usually involves bone formation between the mandibular condyle and the glenoid fossa. The coronoid process of the mandible may also be involved. It typically appears on conventional TMJ radiographs and is confirmed and delineated by computed tomography (CT) films (Fig. 14-5) of the region. It may be unilateral or bilateral. It is generally caused by childhood trauma to the joint, a septicemia resulting in infection, or severe inflammation of the joint.[9] Other conditions producing severe inflammation of the joint, such as juvenile rheumatoid arthritis, may result in ankylosis of the TMJ. When ankylosis occurs before completion of facial skeletal growth, there will be resultant mandibular deformity manifested by decreased vertical growth of the mandibular ramus, mandibular retrognathia, pronounced antegonial notching, and, when the ankylosis is unilateral, significant mandibular asymmetry (Fig. 14-6).[10] Maxillary growth is also affected in a compensatory fashion. The patient manifests little or no mandibular opening and grossly effected lateral and protrusive movements. When the pathologic condition is bilateral, significant postural changes of the head and neck are required during the course of operation.

Pseudoankylosis of the TMJ results when there is dense, inelastic, fibrous connective tissue in the joint, inhibiting normal range of motion. Etiologic factors are similar to those for true bony ankylosis. Growth disturbances may be present if the process occurred before completion of facial growth. These patients demonstrate some degree of opening, although the range of mandibular motion is severely limited. **Neither the true ankylosis patient nor the pseudoankylosis patient can be expected to show any improvement in opening during anesthesia induction or muscle relaxation.**

Nasoendotracheal intubation is required in the treatment of these patients. Flexible fiberoptic-guided techniques are employed.[11] Preoperative preparation for possible tracheostomy is prudent.

Patients with internal derangement of the TMJ present a distinct and different entity from the ankylosed patient. Internal derangement of the joint is a result of uncoordinated movement between the condylar head of the mandible, the glenoid fossa, and the interposed articular disk or meniscus. The meniscus has been displaced in an anterior and usually medial direction, resulting in interference

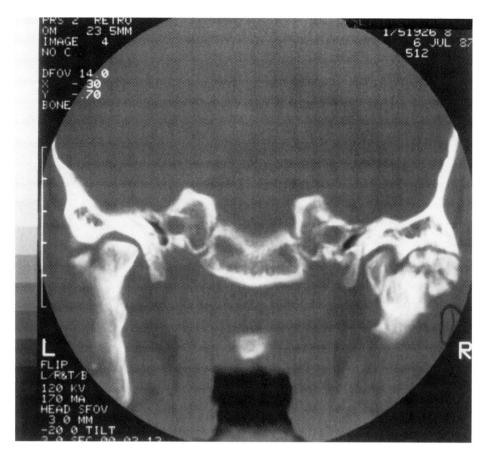

FIG. 14-5   Computed tomography scan of ankylosis of right temporomandibular joint.

with the anterior movement of the condyle required for normal opening. Rotational movement of the condyle is not affected, and these patients typically are able to open 20 to 25 mm preoperatively. The anesthesiologist, however, can expect additional opening during induction as muscle relaxation or paralysis takes effect. This typically allows for oral access but may necessitate use of Magill forceps to guide tube placement during nasoendotracheal intubation.

Patients who have myofascial pain without concomitant internal derangement are not surgical candidates. However, when internal derangement is present, the myofascial component of the disorder may contribute significantly to limited opening preoperatively because of trismus or patient guarding. Improved opening can be expected with anesthetic depth.

In these patients, postoperative edema or hemorrhage does not significantly impact on the oral airway. Mandibular opening is typically improved postoperatively. Maxillomandibular fixation is rarely employed.

There have been a number of cases of postanesthetic internal derangement of the TMJ reported where none was documented preoperatively.[12] Aggressive hyperextension of the joint during intubation may be the causative factor. For purposes of documentation, the anesthesiologist should record maximum interincisal opening measurements and any audible or palpable popping or clicking noises in the joints during the preanesthetic workup. If postoperative symptoms arise, patients should be placed on a soft-food diet, mandibular opening should be restricted, and nonsteroidal antiinflammatory agents should be prescribed. Ice applied to the TMJ region in the early postoperative period helps decrease inflammation.

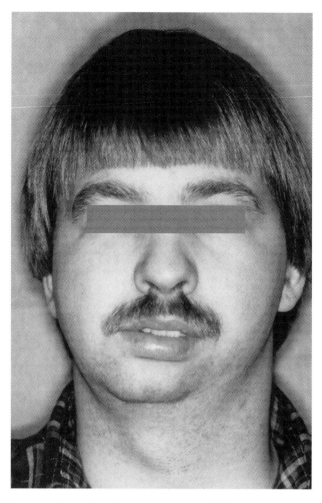

FIG. 14-6   Frontal view of patient with unilateral temporomandibular joint ankylosis on right side. Note deviation of chin to involved side.

HEAD AND NECK INFECTION

Considerations for head and neck infection include the following:
1. Limited access to the oral cavity because of trismus
2. Loss of airway in the supine position
3. Risk of perforation of pharyngeal abscess during intubation with subsequent aspiration
4. Significant postoperative edema

The most common cause of head and neck infections is odontogenic in origin. Perforation of the bony cortex and periosteum from a dental abscess allows dissemination of microbes along facial planes, thus producing "space" infections. The areas most frequently involved include the submandibular, buccal, lingual, masseter, pterygoid, and lateral pharyngeal spaces (Fig. 14-7). The surgical objective is to provide dependent drainage of the involved spaces and removal of the offending dentition.

Patency of the airway may be postural in these patients. With effort, the patient is able to maintain patency in the upright sitting or sniffing position but unable to do so in the supine position. Loss of patency is secondary to occlusion of the airway from posterior displacement of the tongue. The tongue may be elevated because of infection and edema involving the sublingual tissues. Infection that has spread to the lateral pharyngeal region can produce edema and decreased volume of the airway, precipitating loss of patency when the patient is in the supine position and the tongue moves

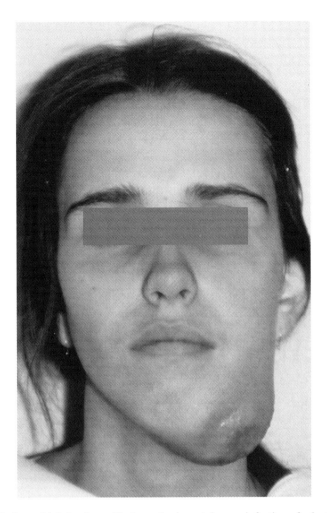

FIG. 14-7   Patient with left submandibular and submental space infection of odontogenic origin.

posteriorly. Some patients are able to maintain patency of the airway in the supine position but are unable to do so after even minute amounts of sedatives. Slight amounts of muscle relaxation or of decreased consciousness may be all that is necessary to produce obstruction secondary to tongue displacement. Accurate preoperative assessment will avoid intraoperative crisis.

Two special circumstances need to be included in this discussion. The first deals with intubation hazards; the second deals with postoperative edema. Nasal or oral intubation may be contraindicated in patients with significant lateral pharyngeal or retropharyngeal space involvement. Preoperative assessment helps determine the degree of involvement. Signs consist of draping of the soft palate and deviation of the uvula to the opposite side (Fig. 14-8). Draping of the soft palate is defined by an inferior displacement of soft palate and tissues that appear inflamed and edematous. There is often elevation of the tongue and dysphagia present. Preoperative lateral cephalograms or lateral soft tissue neck films help confirm decreased pharyngeal airway dimensions and suggest fluid accumulation. Intubation performed under circumstances of compromised visual access runs the risk of perforation of the abscess with subsequent aspiration of purulent discharge.[13] Tracheostomy should be strongly considered in such cases and may represent the treatment of choice.

The second special circumstance involves the patient with multiple space infections that are bilateral in distribution. An example is Ludwig's angina.[14-17] This involves bilateral involvement of the submandibular, sublingual, and submental spaces. It produces significant elevation of the tongue with concomitant airway embarrassment and may present as a true emergency. Because of the re-

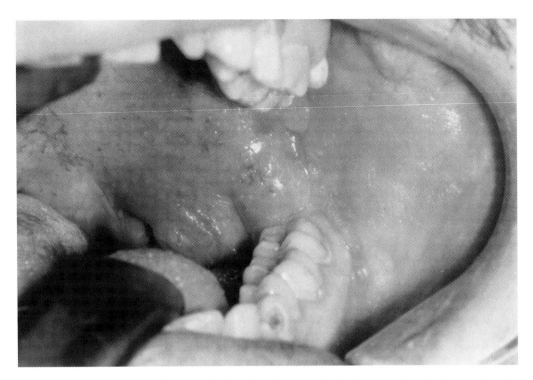

FIG. 14-8   Lateral pharyngeal space infection. Note draping of soft palate as well as limited opening. Tissues of soft palate hang down like a drape and appear inflamed and edematous. Uvula is displaced toward opposite side.

quired extensive surgical invasion of multiple spaces needed to establish drainage, postoperative edema may be anticipated to be extensive and compromise the airway. Elective tracheostomy must be considered in this circumstance.

MAXILLOFACIAL TRAUMA

Considerations for maxillofacial trauma include the following:

1. The route of intubation, which is dependent on the degree of injury
2. Possible intraoperative change of tube
3. Mandatory attention to possible cervical spine injury
4. Possible compromise of the airway when the conscious patient is placed in the supine position
5. Unaccounted for teeth or dental appliances
6. Significant postoperative edema
7. Possible employment of maxillomandibular fixation

The route of intubation in the traumatized patient is dependent on the extent of the injury and the anticipated amount of postoperative airway compromise. Blast injuries, such as shotgun wounds, severe burns, avulsive injuries of the anterior mandible and floor of mouth, and penetrating injuries of the neck, generally require tracheostomy. Much of this is caused by the significant amount of secondary edema encountered in these types of injuries. Extensive facial fractures where nasal packing and maxillomandibular fixation is used in treatment also typically requires tracheostomy (Fig. 14-9).

Patients with perioral trauma, as well as disruption of the cribriform plate such as in Le Fort II, Le Fort III, or nasoethmoidal fractures, present additional dangers regarding nasoendotracheal intubation (see Chapter 12). Such dangers include the possibility of the endotracheal tube being passed through the disrupted cribriform plate into the cranium. When doubt exists as to the feasibility of

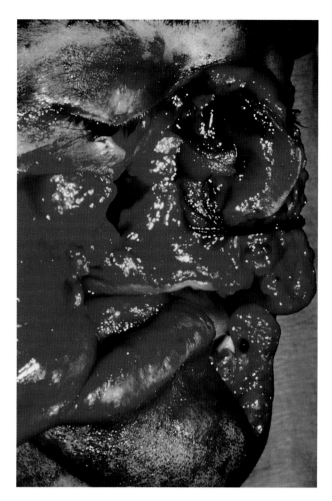

FIG. 14-9   Severe facial trauma caused by exploding truck tire. Significant involvement of both oral and nasal airway is evident. Black suture is seen in middle right portion of photograph in nose region. Just inferior to this is edentulous maxilla. Portion of mandible and displaced tooth can be seen through laceration of lower lip in lower right portion of photograph.

maintaining a patent airway postoperatively or of successfully passing a nasoendotracheal tube without added risk, tracheostomy must be employed.

Facial trauma alone does not usually require emergent surgery. Definitive treatment may be delayed for several hours or even days. This allows adequate time for appropriate work-up, adequate radiographs, fluid resuscitation, patient stabilization, and formation of an organized treatment plan.

Suspicion of cervical spinal injury must always be maintained until it is definitively ruled out. Even in isolated mandibular fracture cases a percentage of patients have C-spine injury. Cervical collars must be used, and protection against flexion, extension, and rotation of the neck must be provided. C-spine films or CT scans must show all cervical vertebrae through the level of T1 to adequately rule out injury.[18] In emergent operative situations when a cervical collar for neck immobilization is still in place, techniques for intubation must be appropriately modified.

If surgery is delayed for 48 to 72 hours, the use of corticosteroids may help limit edema. An attempt should be made to account for missing teeth, bone fragments, and dental restorations or appliances. Chest films should be examined closely to ensure that these have not been displaced into the trachea or bronchial tree. Disruption of the bronchial tree and pulmonary system should be assessed with appropriate radiologic studies. This time should also be used to discuss with the operation surgeon the intended surgical approach, amount of access required, and whether nasal packing or maxillomandibular fixation will be employed in the postoperative period (Fig. 14-10).

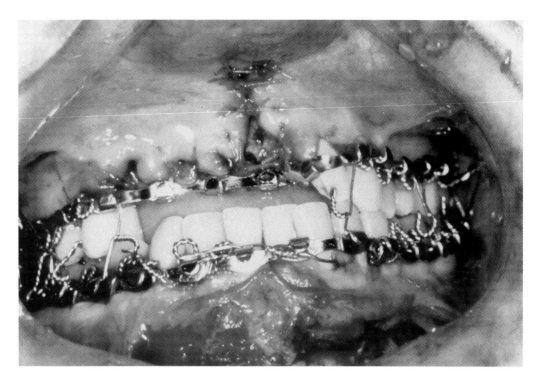

FIG. 14-10   Reduction and stabilization of fractures using maxillomandibular fixation.

In patients who have had disruption of the nasoorbitoethmoidal complex, a bicoronal flap may be used to gain access to this area. This involves an incision placed in a coronal fashion over the top of the head and subsequent retraction of tissues of the scalp and forehead superiorly and caudally to gain access to the region of the frontal sinus and underlying osseous tissue of the superior nasal region. This necessitates a change in the nasoendotracheal tube position if it was originally placed in the midline over the top of the head.

As with the infection patient, certain types of facial injury result in an airway that is dependent on posturing to maintain patency of the airway. One example is the patient, particularly the elderly edentulous patient, with bilateral displaced parasymphyseal fractures. A descriptive term used to describe this injury is *bucket-handle fracture,* based on the fact that the anterior portion of the mandible is displaced inferiorly by the pull of the digastric and suprahyoid muscles and appears to hang down like the handle on a bucket (Fig. 14-11). This injury results in lack of support for the tongue. When the patient is in the supine position, the tongue collapses posteriorly, occluding the airway. Avulsion of the anterior mandible produces similar circumstances.

When dentition is present in flail segments, temporary stabilization of segments within the maxilla or mandible, preoperatively by simple interdental wiring, is useful. In contradistinction to maxillomandibular wiring, interdental wiring stabilizes segments within an arch, either the maxillary or mandibular, and does not affect opening. Stabilization of flail segments helps control bleeding, increases patient comfort, improves oral access by temporary reduction of displaced dentoalveolar segments, and aids the anesthesiologist during intubation.

When tracheostomy is not indicated, the preferred method of intubation in the maxillofacial trauma patient is nasoendotracheal. This allows the surgeon optimal access to evaluate the dental occlusion without interference from an oral tube.

ORAL CLEFTING

Considerations for oral clefting include the following:
1. Primary repair of the hard or soft palate decreases airway volume, as does a pharyngeal flap procedure.

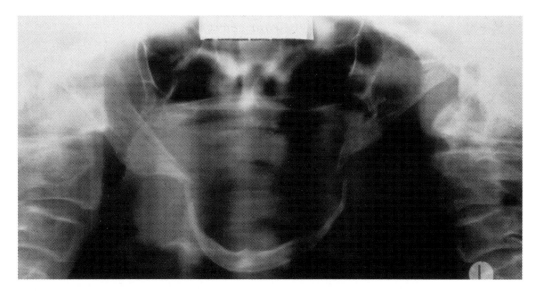

FIG. 14-11 Panoramic radiograph demonstrating bilateral fractures of atrophic, edentulous mandible. Anterior portion of mandible, seen in lower middle portion of radiograph, appears to hang down at point of bilateral fractures like a bucket handle. Lack of tongue support often results in airway embarrassment when patient is placed in supine position.

2. A surgical plan to develop a pharyngeal flap complicates nasoendotracheal intubation and extubation.
3. Oral intubation is required for primary repair of the hard and soft palate, as well as for primary lip repair.

Intubation of the child with clefting of the lip or palate does not generally present special problems to the anesthesiologist. Oral intubation is preferred for primary repairs and for pharyngoplasty and pharyngeal flap procedures. It is often a good idea to secure the tube with suture tied first around the tube and then to adjacent soft tissue, which is stable, rather than to rely on tape, which may become loosened during the surgery. As mentioned previously, this suture can be easily placed at the base of the anterior mandibular labial vestibule (Fig. 14-12). The suture is placed through mucosa and engages underlying muscle near its insertion to bone. Minimal movement of this suture occurs, even with vigorous retraction of the lip. It should be kept in mind that closure of the palate and pharyngeal flap procedures decrease the volume of the oral airway in these patients when compared with the preoperative state (Fig. 14-13). This, coupled with normal postoperative edema in the tissues, can lead to airway embarrassment from posterior movement of the tongue when the patient is in a supine position in the recovery room. The use of a traction suture in the tongue may be indicated (Fig. 14-14).

Many cleft palate patients will require additional surgery as they grow older. This may be directly related to their original deformity, or it may be unrelated. If their histories indicate that a pharyngeal flap procedure has been done previously, they should be considered as difficult airway patients. Even if the history is unclear on this point, it is good practice to examine the posterior oropharynx for evidence of flap surgery. Elevation of the soft palate with a dental mirror, tongue blade, or other appropriate instrument should be employed during the examination. The presence of a flap should indicate to the anesthesiologist that nasoendotracheal intubation, if required, will present certain difficulties. The tube must deviate from midline and pass through one of the lateral ports created by the flap. A Teflon guide may be easier to pass then a RAE tube. Once it is in the posterior oropharynx, it can serve as a guide to direct the endotracheal tube through the lateral port. Once this hurdle has been passed, intubation can proceed in a normal fashion.

An alternate technique is to use the fiberoptic scope. Retrograde transcricoid intubation may be helpful in instances where other methods, including fiberoptic laryngoscopy, have proven ineffective. An example may be in the adolescent cleft patient with transverse, vertical, and sagittal maxillary de-

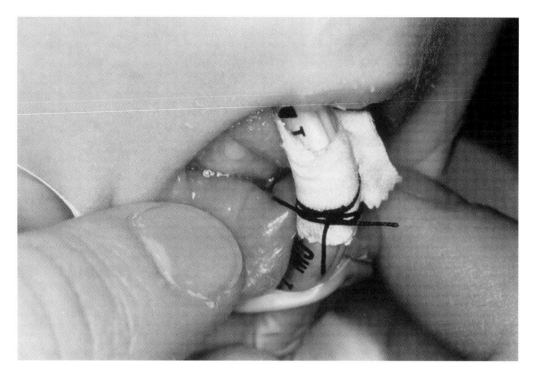

FIG. 14-12   Stabilization of oral tube in young patient with cleft palate by means of suturing in anterior mandibular vestibule. Suture extends from tube, where it has been wrapped and tied, to depth of vestibule. Portion of alveolar ridge, part of mandibular anterior tooth, and tongue are seen just superior to insertion of suture.

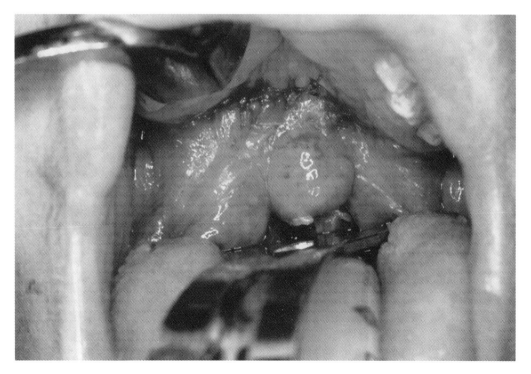

FIG. 14-13   Decreased volume of posterior oral airway is evident following pharyngeal flap procedure.

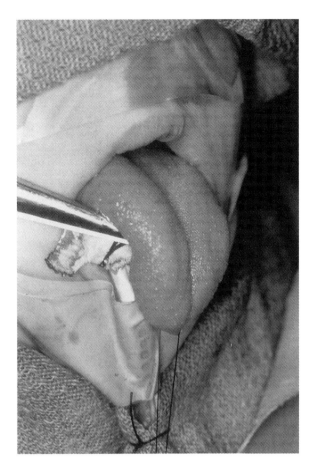

FIG. 14-14   Traction suture through anterior tongue left in during recovery provides rapid means of establishing patency, if required.

ficiency, disruption of normal nasal anatomy, scarred soft palate, and posterior-superior oral pharynx, coupled with mandibular sagittal deficiency. The technique was introduced in the early 1960s and has proven useful in such circumstances.[19,20] The technique consists of insertion of a flexible tip guide wire or a through-the-needle catheter through a puncture incision of the cricothyroid membrane. The catheter or wire is then directed superiorly past the vocal cords and into the pharynx. It can then be brought out through the mouth and joined to a catheter that has been fed through the nose and into the pharynx. It can then gently be guided past the soft palate and out the nose by withdrawing the nasal catheter. It may now serve as a guide for passing the nasoendotracheal tube. Retrograde transcrycoid intubation may also be useful in cases of significant dentofacial deformity or in patients with limited mandibular opening. As with fiberoptic-assisted intubation, tracheostomy, or other techniques to establish or maintain an airway, employment of retrograde transcrycoid intubation should be preceded by an understanding of its indications, contraindications, and potential complications.

COMPLICATIONS

Complications pertaining to airway management in the oral and maxillofacial surgery patient are varied, and several of the more common ones have already been referred to previously. These include tissue necrosis from tube pressure, corneal abrasion, intraoperative tube laceration, intraoperative disconnections, postoperative airway embarrassment, and aspiration of gastric contents. A few additional complications are worthy of mention. Dental injury during difficult intubation may occur as a result of excess force applied to the maxillary anterior dentition with the rigid laryngoscope. If the injury involves fracture of the coronal portion of the tooth or dislodgement of dental restorations, the patient should be referred to the dental service postoperatively for consultation and management. If the teeth have been loosened or avulsed, the dental service should be consulted during the case so that the teeth may be repositioned and stabilized. If not reimplanted immediately, avulsed teeth should be placed in saline solution until such time that reimplantation can proceed. Complications during difficult blind nasal intubation usually result when an inordinate amount of resistance to passage of the endotracheal tube is met with excessive application of force. Laceration of mucosal tissues accompanied by hemorrhage results. This not only leads to decreased visibility and complicates further attempts at intubation, but also may result in aspiration and postoperative pulmonary problems. Excessive force applied to advancement of the endotracheal tube in the nasal fossa may result in cleavage of the inferior turbinate with dislodgement and possible tube occlusion. Similarly, excessive force applied to advance the endotracheal tube in the posterior oropharynx may result in laceration of the mucosa of the posterior wall, creation of a false passage, and a tube positioned submucosally in the prevertebral space. This, followed by attempts at inflation, may result in cervical space emphysema and pneumomediastinum. If ventilation during the case becomes slowly but increasingly difficult following an intubation that was accompanied by excessive hemorrhage, partial tube occlusion secondary to clot formation should be suspected.

REFERENCES

1. Altemir FH: Pericranial fixation of the nasotracheal tube, *J Oral Maxillofac Surg* 44:585, 1986.
2. Fonseca RJ, Walker RV (eds): *Oral and maxillofacial trauma,* Vol II, Philadelphia, 1991, WB Saunders. 669.
3. Nunn JF: *Applied respiratory physiology,* ed 2, Boston, 1981, Butterworths.
4. Reference deleted in proofs.
5. Schwartz LB, Sordill WC, Liebers RM et al: Difficulty in removal of accidently cut endotracheal tube, *J Oral Maxillofac Surg* 40:518, 1982.
6. Fagraius L, Angelillo JC, Dolan EA: A serious anesthesia hazard during orthognathic surgery, *Anesth Analg* 59:150, 1980.
7. Reference deleted in proofs.
8. Farrar WB: Characteristics of the condylar path and internal derangements of the TMJ, *J Prosthet Dent* 39:319, 1978.
9. Topazian RG: Etiology of ankylosis of the temporomandibular joint: analysis of 44 cases, *J Oral Surg* 22:227, 1964.
10. Proffit WR, Vig KWL, Turvey TA: Early fracture of the mandibular condyles: frequently an unsuspected cause of growth disturbances, *Am J Orthod* 78:1-24, 1980.
11. Stella JP, Kageler WV, Epker BN: Fiberoptic endotracheal intubation in oral and maxillofacial surgery, *J Oral Maxillofac Surg* 44:923, 1986.
12. Taylor RC, Way WL, Hebdrickson RA: Temporomandibular joint problems in relation to the administration of general anesthesia, *J Oral Surg* 26:327, 1968.
13. Hill CM: Death following dental clearance in a patient suffering from ankylosing spondylitis: a case report with discussion on management of such problems, *Br J Oral Surg* 18:73, 1980.
14. Steinhauser P: Ludwig's angina: report of a case in a 12 year old boy, *J Oral Surg* 25:251, 1967.
15. Strauss H, Tilghmann DM: Ludwig's angina, emphysema, pulmonary infiltration, and pericarditis secondary to extraction of a tooth, *J Oral Surg* 38:223, 1980.
16. Patterson H, Kelly JH, Strone M: Ludwig's angina: an update, *Laryngoscope* 92:370, 1982.
17. Hought RT, Fitzgerald BE, Latta JE et al: Ludwig's angina: a report of two cases and review of the literature from 1945 to January 1979, *J Oral Surg* 38:849, 1980.
18. Fonseca RJ, Walker RV (eds): *Oral and maxillofacial trauma,* Philadelphia, 1991, WB Saunders.
19. Butler FS, Cirillo AA: Retrograde tracheal intubation, *Anesth Analg* 39:333-338, 1960.
20. Waters DJ: Guided blind endotracheal intubation, *Anesthesia* 18:158-162, 1963.

CHAPTER 15

Clinical Problems of the Difficult Airway in Craniofacial Surgery

S. BUCHMAN

Many surgical subspecialties have particular operations that require an individualized approach to secure and maintain the patency and control of a difficult airway, and in this regard plastic surgery is no exception. The challenge to an anesthesiologist to accommodate a plastic surgeon's requirements of an uncontaminated, unobstructed, and freely mobile operative field can be daunting and often difficult. Adequate communication and mutual understanding on both sides of the surgical drape are essential to devise an operative plan that can deliver an adequate level of anesthesia, secure a safe airway, and provide full access for the performance of a surgical procedure.

The anesthesiologist and the plastic surgeon share the airway in most craniofacial procedures. The multitude of head and neck positions used for these procedures and the frequent changes required in these positions dictate steadfast vigilance in the maintenance of an adequate airway.

Reestablishment of a lost airway takes first priority over all other aspects of any operation. Teamwork between the surgeon and the anesthesiologist is essential to recognize and quickly correct a dislodged, displaced, or dysfunctional endotracheal tube. Because the anesthesiologist is usually not at the head of the bed during most craniofacial procedures, there is an increased likelihood of an endotracheal tube mishap. Kinking, inadvertent extubation, and even severing of an endotracheal tube while doing an osteotomy may occur.

Each craniofacial procedure, as well as each craniofacial anomaly, is replete with its own unique set of characteristics. These procedures demand a carefully tailored management plan for each type of operation. By addressing the different craniofacial deformities and their individualized treatment strategies, a guide can be developed to explore the difficult airway problems encountered by the craniofacial surgeon. Many of the craniofacial procedures performed by the plastic and reconstructive surgeons are on patients in the pediatric age group. The surgical management of the craniofacial anomalies of these children often requires special considerations.

RELEVANT ANATOMY AND PRACTICAL PHYSIOLOGY

Both the size and the stability of the upper airway in the pediatric age group are decreased in comparison with the adult population. These differences confer a variation in the structural and functional components of the pediatric airway that needs to be considered when managing these patients. The smaller size of the pediatric airway leaves it susceptible to obstruction from what would otherwise seem like an insignificant amount of edema.[1] As little as 1 mm of edema in the subglottic space can cause a 40% decrease in the caliber of the upper airway. The decreased stability of the pediatric airway caused by the flexible nature of the pliable cartilage of the larynx may also predispose to collapse of the trachea and give a clinical picture of a fixed obstruction (Fig. 15-1). Many of the structural and functional differences in the upper airway of these children normalize with growth and development. Developmental delays in this patient population, however, are not uncommon.

Hypoxic episodes and apnea have been reported as a risk in premature infants after general anesthesia. Many children with craniofacial abnormalities have ongoing subtle problems with their airways. It is most important to pick these up on preoperative evaluation to allow careful preparation and avoidance of a potentially life-threatening situation upon induction. A directed and specific his-

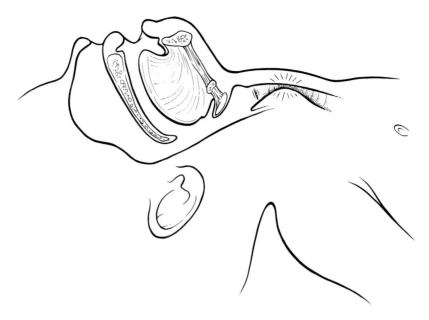

FIG. 15-1   Flexible nature of tracheal cartilage in pediatric patient can collapse.

tory and physical examination often reward the physician with the essential information necessary to prepare for an operative procedure. Careful scrutiny of a previous operative record gives the most telling clues as to the anatomy and negotiability of a patient's airway. **Scarring and anatomic variation secondary to an operative procedure can significantly alter the anatomy from the time of the last surgical intervention** (Fig. 15-2). Symptoms such as snoring, sleep problems, and inability to stay awake during the day may be telltale signs of a tendency to obstruct the upper airway or even sleep apnea (see also Chapter 13). These concerns can then be more specifically addressed by performing a monitored sleep study that may alter not only the preparation for surgery, but also the timing of surgery.[2]

Physical examination should complement and corroborate the history. Tonsillar or adenoidal hypertrophy is common in children and may distort the normal anatomy of the pharynx. An obstructive tendency can be addressed through surgical resection, if necessary, but can be better managed by sparing use of sedation preoperatively coupled with a delayed and judicious extubation. Significant findings during physical examination would also include an asymmetric or hypoplastic mandible, as well as a severe restriction in mandibular mobility (Fig. 15-3). These findings could make intubation difficult and help prepare the patient for an awake intubation, endoscopy, or even tracheostomy. **For those patients possibly undergoing nasotracheal intubation, an examination of the nose for an obstruction is mandatory.** A brief discussion with the patient as to which nostril is easier to breath through can be rewarding when a difficult intubation in a hypoplastic maxilla is required. In addition, a history of previous pharyngeal surgery and an understanding of the specific anatomy involved in a patient's pharyngeal flap or pharyngoplasty are necessary not only to allow access of intubation, but also to assure that no damage is afforded to the corrections accomplished by surgery that was previously performed (Fig. 15-4).[3]

Children with acute respiratory tract infections show an increased susceptibility to laryngospasm and airway irritability and an increase in secretions that mandate postponing surgery. Major craniofacial procedures can be lengthy endeavors, and the associated blood loss can be considerable. A significant amount of fluid is required to replace intraoperative losses and to maintain blood pressure and perfusion. A satisfactory evaluation of the patient's respiratory, renal, cardiac, and hematologic systems should be established in preparation for extensive operations. Fluid resuscitation and blood replacement can be challenging in the large craniofacial surgical procedures, especially in the pediatric age group. Blood loss can be massive and sudden. The replacement of two times the es-

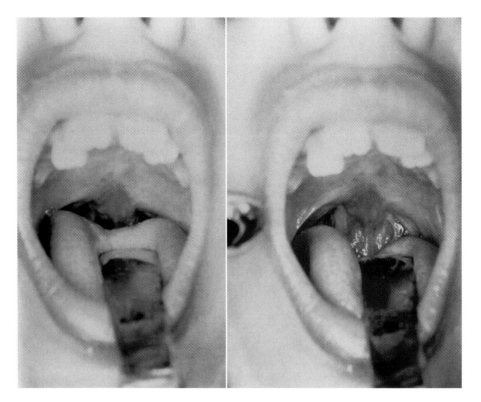

FIG. 15-2 Compromised space associated with pharyngeal flap, such as kleeblattschädel syndrome.

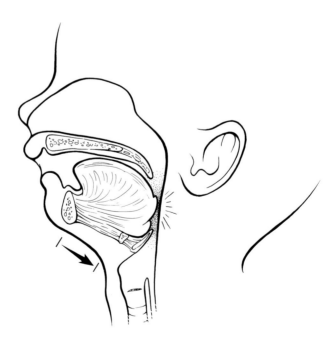

FIG. 15-3 Hypoplastic mandible could lead to difficult intubation and may require special preoperative consideration.

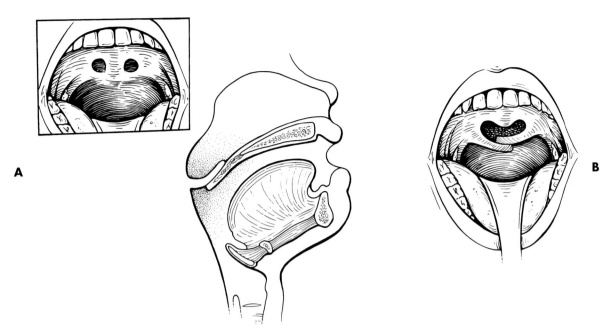

FIG. 15-4   Previous pharyngeal surgery can complicate nasotracheal intubation. **A,** Intraoral and sagittal view of posterior pharyngeal flap. **B,** Intraoral view of sphincter pharyngoplasty.

timated circulatory volume may be required, and yet the rate and amount of blood loss can be difficult to estimate. A large amount of irrigation is often used during the procedure, and a significant amount of blood stains the sheets and gowns, all contributing to the inaccuracy of blood loss estimate. Recording the amount of blood in the suction devices and weighing the blood-soaked sponges gives a working estimate of blood loss, but it is an inadequate and inaccurate measurement.

Good communication with the anesthesiologist, circulating nurse, and operative surgeon is a critical adjunct to invasive hemodynamic monitoring to determine the timing and volume of blood and fluid replacement. The blood bank must be notified before a major craniofacial case so that adequate blood may be typed and crossmatched according to the estimated potential loss. This loss varies with the duration and extent of the procedure, as well as the experience of the operating team. There may be a need for intraoperative coagulation studies and blood components. Although the platelet count often dips with large blood loss, platelet transfusion is rarely needed. The use of fresh frozen plasma is often much more useful in coagulopathies related to large losses of blood volume. Because of the potential for large volume shifts associated with extensive craniofacial osteotomies, there is a significant need for comprehensive hemodynamic monitoring.

Adequate perfusion of the brain is of paramount importance throughout a craniofacial procedure. **An arterial line can often provide the best measurement of blood pressure, and it allows immediate access to blood gas samples for the monitoring of acid-base disturbances, as well as oxygen and carbon dioxide tensions.** A urinary catheter is necessary to drain the bladder and to assess renal perfusion. An electrocardiogram and airway pressure gauge are used routinely. A nerve stimulator can be helpful to monitor neuromuscular blockade. Central venous pressure measurement can be useful to determine venous filling pressures, and a precordial stethoscope can help diagnose air embolism by the sound of the beat at the cardiac apex.

The problem of thermoregulation needs to be addressed during lengthy operative procedures and even during shorter operations when an infant is involved. A rectal temperature probe can continuously monitor body temperature, which can vary frequently throughout the case. A heating blanket should be used on the torso, and the extremities should be wrapped with thermal coverings. Other sources of significant heat loss include fluid replacement and the respiratory system. Blood transfusions and intravenous fluids can be run through a blood warmer to help prevent severe dips in body temperature. The normal tracheobronchial system attempts to warm and humidify the cool and dry anesthetic gases administered during an operative case. This thermoregulatory mechanism can lead to a profound depression in body temperature over time. The anesthetic system used can help ameliorate this problem if it is equipped with a mechanism to both warm and humidify inspired gases.

The use of hypotensive anesthetic techniques have been reported to dramatically lower blood loss, associated bleeding problems, and operative time.[4] Sodium nitroprusside infusion or pentolinium tartrate has been used to decrease and maintain the mean arterial pressure to 50 mm Hg, depending on baseline blood pressure measurements. However, tachyphylaxis and cyanide toxicity have been observed when sodium nitroprosside was administered in the pediatric population.

CLEFT LIP

Clefts of the lip and palate (Fig. 15-5) are the most common craniofacial malformations. The incidence varies according to race and is almost 1:750 in Caucasians. At birth, most children with a cleft lip do not show signs of respiratory distress unless the anomaly is part of a syndromic process. Feeding may be difficult, and parents may have to be educated as to the best feeding method available for the child. Problems such as intermittent aspiration may be encountered, however, the child usually can adjust when given a modified feeding regimen. The general rule for repair of the cleft lip is to wait until the child is about 10 weeks of age, weighs about 10 pounds, and has a hemoglobin of about 10.

Preoperative evaluation should focus on approximate gestational age because a preterm infant is at a higher risk for hypoglycemia and hypoxic and apneic spells. Growth, feeding history, and

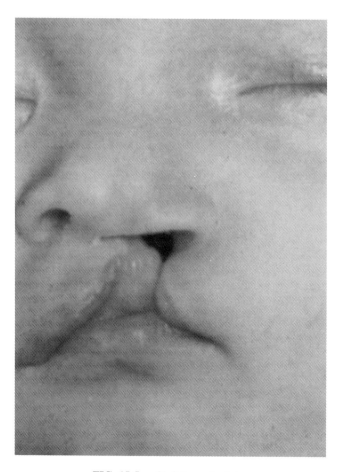

FIG. 15-5 Cleft lip and palate.

medical course since delivery all have a significant bearing on preparation for the operating room. Some centers are doing cleft lip repair in the neonatal period, at which point pertinent questions about the maternal and birth histories become germane. Prematurity, as well as the course of labor and delivery, is an important factor in such cases.

The operation to repair a cleft lip requires that the child's head be placed at the end of an operating table that will be rotated 90 degrees or greater away from the anesthesiologist (Fig. 15-6). Often the head needs to be gently flexed to allow ease of preoperative marking, as well as better technical access to the lip. The need for head flexion during an operative case will change the position of a fixed tube in the trachea, or worse, challenge the security of the tube at the point of fixation. Such problems can often be avoided with adequate communication, forethought, and planning. An uncuffed tube is usually required with a looser fit than normal so as not to traumatize the sensitive upper airway. A small leak is not uncommon. However, this can usually be ameliorated with the use of a well-positioned throat pack. Placement of a throat pack should always be marked separately and the circulating nurse should be aware of placement to assure removal before extubation. Orotracheal intubation is usually not problematic in children with cleft lips, however, proper placement and securing of the tube should be done in concert with the surgeon's input.

Preoperative marking and measurements are the sine qua non of cleft lip surgery, and a fixed tube that alters or deforms the natural landmarks around the mouth can lead to an unfortunate outcome. Careful taping of the tube is a key element to the proper orientation of the lips and often makes the surgeon's job easier. The lower lip and chin should have adequate protection from pressure caused by an endotracheal tube connector. Ulcers and necrosis of soft tissue secondary to misplaced tubing apparatus have been reported and can be prevented with careful attention to detail.

CLEFT PALATE

The surgical and airway management of the cleft palate differs from that of an isolated lip deformity. In this case the nasopharynx and the oral cavity have varying levels of confluence. Infants with cleft palate deformities have as much as a 30% incidence of associated congenital anomalies. A careful

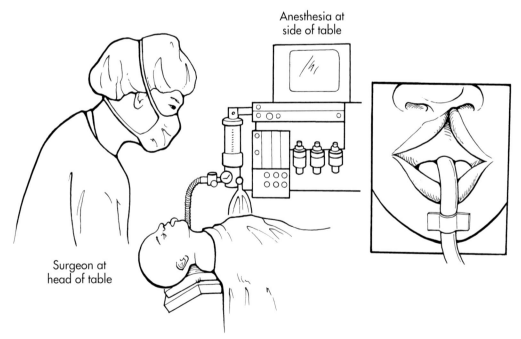

FIG. 15-6   Position of child and fixing of endotracheal tube are of utmost importance for delicate correction of cleft lip.

history and physical examination should ferret out the overall clinical picture and assist in the proper preparation for surgical repair. Surgical intervention to repair the palate often results in restriction of growth of the maxillary arch and midface. However, delay in surgery has a high likelihood of resulting in a speech deficit and nasal regurgitation. In view of these findings, a compromise is usually made so that operative intervention takes place at 9 to 12 months of age.

Children with cleft palates often have copious secretions noted on oral examination. These findings should not delay surgery. However, an upper respiratory tract infection should be carefully ruled out because the sequelae of such an infection would severely compromise the patient during and after surgery. An upper airway infection should be treated aggressively and followed closely, and surgery should be delayed for about a month.

The operative repair of the cleft palate again requires the child's head to be at the top of an operating room table that will be turned about 90 degrees from the anesthesiologist. Repair of the cleft palate requires a specialized, self-retaining retractor (Dingman) to hold the mouth open, to hold the tongue away, and to provide the greatest possible access to an often exceedingly small space (Fig. 15-7). The retractor is placed in the oral cavity after the child has been orally intubated. The device has a notched blade that retracts the tongue, while allowing access for the endotracheal tube. Proper positioning of the retractor to gain full visualization of the operative field can be challenging and may cause kinking of the tube on itself or over any erupting teeth. As the retractor is opened, an increase in the airway resistance will be noted. If this is substantial and persistent, the mouth gag should be released and repositioned.

The use of a Ring-Adair-Elwyn (RAE) or anode (wired) tube often alleviates some of the problems of obstruction by the retractor, however, ingenuity may be necessary to provide a mutually advantageous intraoperative set-up. Because of the depth of the operative field, visualization of the palate often requires more extension at the neck. **Reassessment of the tube after flexion or extension is mandatory to rule out an undiscovered extubation or endobronchial intubation.** Too much extension can also stretch and collapse a soft malleable airway, a caution to note not only in-

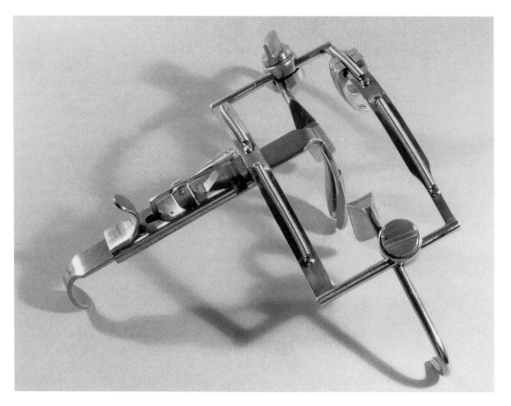

FIG. 15-7   Self-retaining Dingman mouth gag retractor.

traoperatively, but also upon intubation because it could make visualization of the cords and delivery of the tube into the trachea much more difficult. A properly placed throat pack not only effects a seal for the airway, but also, in the case of palate surgery, should prevent the swallowing of copious amounts of blood throughout the operation. A small pediatric suction catheter can be placed through the nose and into the hypopharynx for continuous evacuation of blood, irrigation fluids, and secretions throughout the case (Fig. 15-8). It is advisable to suction the stomach before extubation.

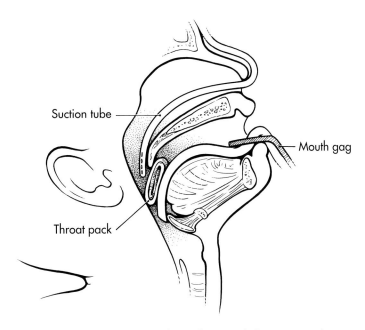

FIG. 15-8   Properly placed throat pack and suction catheter can help prevent copious amounts of swallowed fluid during a case.

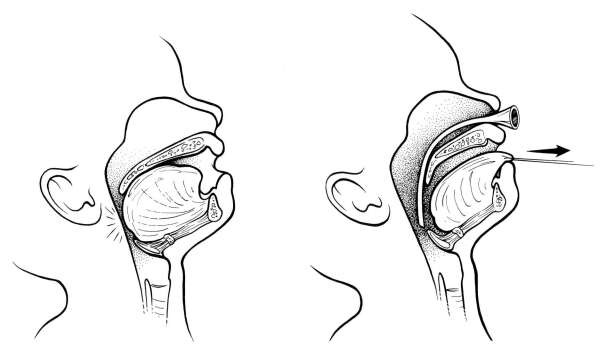

FIG. 15-9   Tongue suture can temporize emergent postoperative airway obstruction caused by edema. Gentle traction can allow careful placement of nasal trumpet, which can be removed once swelling subsides.

Because there is a constant stream of blood into the hypopharynx during this procedure, care must be taken to prevent and treat aspiration both intraoperatively and postoperatively. Many surgeons place a tongue suture at the end of the case to allow a secure handle if the child exhibits respiratory distress after extubation. If necessary, the tongue suture can be pulled gently, then a soft red rubber nasal trumpet can be carefully placed, preferably by the surgeon, so as not to interrupt the repair, bypassing the palate and relieving the obstruction most likely secondary to postoperative edema (Fig. 15-9). The use of nebulized, racemic epinephrine aerosol and systemic steroids has been reported to be helpful in ameliorating postoperative edema. If the postextubation period goes smoothly, the tongue stitch can be removed in the recovery room or, more conservatively, the next morning before discharge.

PIERRE ROBIN SYNDROME

The Pierre Robin syndrome (Fig. 15-10) is a sequence of micrognathia, glossoptosis, and breathing difficulties, afflicting children, many of whom also have an associated cleft palate. At birth these children may present with significant upper airway obstruction and require emergent intubation. Although this alleviates the immediate problem, a long-term solution is needed to allow the patient to be sent home. Some surgeons advocate a tongue-lip adhesion as a first-line strategy. However, the severely obstructed airway may require tracheostomy. The child with borderline or intermittent airway obstruction presents a more difficult airway problem.[5]

Initially, a nasogastric tube and a nasopharyngeal airway may be all that is required to keep the tongue forward and to stabilize the neonate. Positioning the child prone also allows the tongue to fall forward and, in mild cases, may be all that is needed along with a sleep monitor to send the infant home. If there is a question as to the degree of obstruction, a sleep study can be helpful to determine

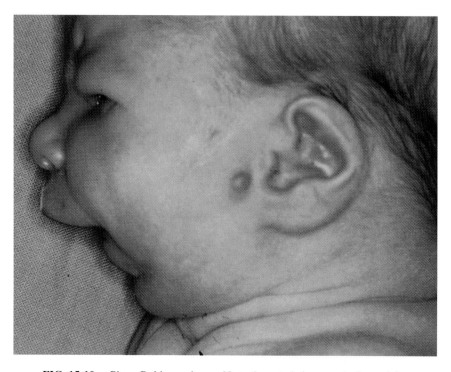

FIG. 15-10   Pierre Robin syndrome. Note characteristic preauricular nodule.

the need for a tongue-lip adhesion. If there is a failure of the tongue-lip adhesion to ameliorate the problem, then a tracheostomy is indicated. Most children with Pierre Robin syndrome show significant improvement in the airway patency as the size of the mandible increases with growth and development. The repair of the cleft palate is usually delayed until the child is about 18 months of age and there are no sleeping or breathing difficulties.

Release of the tongue-lip adhesion and decannulation of the tracheostomy is delayed until after the palate is repaired and when further surgical intervention is not imminent.

Correction of Velopharyngeal Dysfunction

A significant subset of children with repaired clefts of the palate show structural or functional abnormalities that impact on speech. These abnormalities are best picked up early and can often be treated with speech therapy. Despite early intervention and adequate therapy, many children still exhibit speech deficits derived from a short or adynamic soft palate. These children become operative candidates for a pharyngeal flap procedure designed to act as a baffle to the nasopharyngeal airway or a pharyngoplasty designed to construct a dynamic sphincter to improve speech. A mouth gag is placed for access after which, in the case of a pharyngeal flap, soft tissue from the posterior pharyngeal wall is sewn to the free edge of the soft palate (see Fig. 15-4, *A*). This creates a central flap that partially obstructs the nasopharynx, leaving two lateral ports open. Postoperative upper airway obstruction is not uncommon, and a tongue suture is left for safety reasons. A nasal airway may be required for a short time postoperatively but should be placed by the surgeon so as to not disrupt the flap. The pharyngoplasty procedure develops myomucosal flaps from the palatopharyngeus muscles and reorients them in a horizontal position, inserting them in a parallel fashion into the posterior pharyngeal wall. This operation creates a new central port. Precautions for postoperative airway obstruction should still be observed.

Persistent airway problems after these operations could necessitate revision or even takedown of the flaps. These children should be carefully screened for signs of sleep apnea or airway compromise. Reintubation can be challenging in these patients and should be carefully done so as not to destroy the reconstruction and cause the speech dysfunction to recur.

MANDIBULOFACIAL DYSOSTOSIS

Hemifacial microsomia, Goldenhar's syndrome (Fig. 15-11), and Treacher Collins syndrome comprise a group of congenital anomalies, which include sporadic and inherited disorders in the development of the first and second branchial arches. The phenotypic expression in all of these disorders is variable, however, common physical findings include unilateral or bilateral mandibular hypoplasia. The ascending rami and condyle can show mild growth disturbance or be completely absent. This finding is the main reason that these patients have a high incidence of difficulty in airway management.[6] A history of acute neonatal airway compromise may be found in a significant number of these patients.

Other common physical findings include maxillary and zygomatic hypoplasia, macrostomia, microtia, coloboma, and deafness. Facial nerve deficits and neuromuscular hypoplasia can also be found. Children with Goldenhar's syndrome have a high incidence of cervical spine abnormalities (Fig. 15-12). The preoperative assessment of these children is of the utmost importance. The anesthetic record often reveals multiple intubation attempts and gives a clue as to the best plan of action. Radiographs of the nasopharynx and trachea may help better define malalignment and discern the need for fiberoptic endoscopy. An evaluation of the cervical spine may also be worthwhile to determine motion.

Optimizing the medical management of any cardiac or pulmonary anomaly should be assured and assessed concerning tolerance of blood loss and the hemodynamic effect of inducing hypotension. Despite the best preoperative assessment and diligent attention to detail, some of these children cannot be successfully intubated. The possibility of tracheostomy should be discussed with the parents before the operation. This can be performed under local anesthesia, if necessary.

The operative approaches to these disorders vary with the manifestations of the craniofacial deformity. A general operative schedule would include repair of a macrostomia and excision of skin tags in the first year of life. The colobomas are then addressed between the ages of 2 and 4 years. Start-

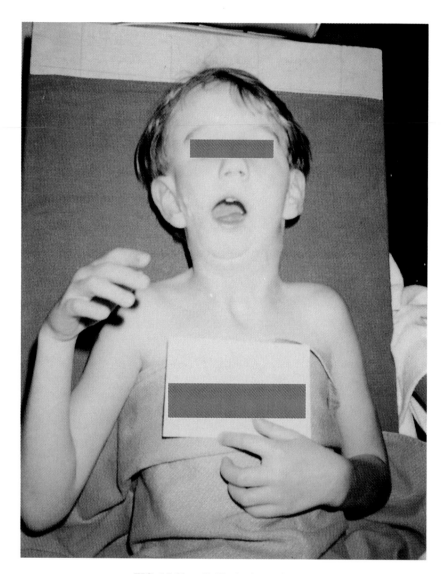

FIG. 15-11 Goldenhar's syndrome.

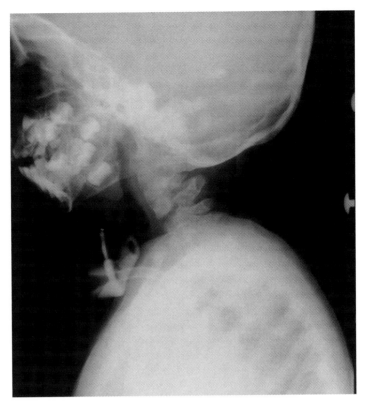

FIG. 15-12   Goldenhar's syndrome (flat plate).

ing at about 5 years of age, a staged ear reconstruction should be undertaken. This is followed by reconstruction of the mandibular ramus and condyle and subsequent rebuilding of the zygoma. An asymmetric genioplasty can be used to camouflage a severe deformity in the early teen years, and finally orthognathic double-jaw surgery and genioplasty are usually required late in adolescence.

CRANIOSYNOSTOSIS

Premature fusion of the cranial sutures results in craniosynostosis (Fig. 15-13). This abnormality causes progressive growth and morphologic disturbances in the affected child. Patients undergoing suture release and cranial vault remodeling usually undergo the operation in the first year of life. The central nervous system should be evaluated preoperatively to determine the likelihood of increased intracranial pressure (ICP). ICP can be found in patients with an isolated suture involved, however, it is a much more common finding when multiple sutures are affected. A computed tomography scan and an ophthalmologic examination can be of great benefit in assessing the effects of increased ICP on the brain. If a shunt is already in place, its functional integrity should also be assured. The cranial vault remodeling and release of the affected sutures are designed to increase the cranial capacity, as well as have a salutary affect on the severity of the deformity. A reduction in ICP is often noted after the operation.[7]

High ICP in craniosynostosis should be managed intraoperatively as would be any pediatric neurosurgical patient with the same problem. Hyperventilation, osmotic diuretics such as mannitol, and a reverse Trendelenburg (head-up) position are mainstays of intraoperative therapeutic intervention. The use of steroids to decrease cerebral swelling has been advocated by some surgical teams. The routine use of lumbar spinal drainage to decrease high ICP and help prevent postoperative cerebrospinal fluid leak has also been reported. An overnight stay in the intensive care unit is usually warranted for close monitoring.

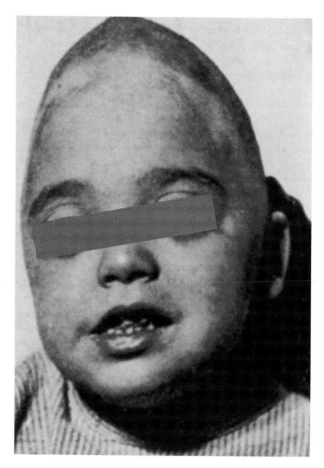

FIG. 15-13   Craniosynostosis.

CRANIOFACIAL DYSOSTOSIS

Certain craniofacial disorders, such as Apert's syndrome and Crouzon's disease, share other growth abnormalities in association with particular patterns of craniosynostosis. Many of these syndromes show a familial tendency, but they are usually sporadic when they occur. Apert's syndrome and Crouzon's disease are important from an airway management point of view because of the severe midface hypoplasia associated with them.[8] In addition, their operative management forms the basis of therapeutic surgical intervention for some of the less common craniofacial dysostoses.

Crouzon's disease is a disorder with a variability in phenotypic expression, most commonly associated with bicoronal craniosynostosis, hypertelorism, exorbitism, and hypoplasia of the maxilla. Patients with this disease have a characteristic appearance and are usually of normal intelligence.

Apert's syndrome is a more severe disorder exhibiting harsher manifestations of the growth disturbances seen in patients with Crouzon's disease. These children also have a dish-face type appearance, brachyturricephaly, acne, syndactyly, and a high incidence of cleft palate and mental retardation. Children born with cranial dysostoses with severe maxillary hypoplasia may show changes in the size and shape of the nasopharynx, pharynx, and the oral cavity. The hypoplasia can be so severe that it does not allow the passage of a nasogastric tube and leads to the erroneous diagnosis of choanal atresia (Fig. 15-14). Because a neonate is an obligate nasal breather, nasal obstruction can lead to significant respiratory distress. Placement of an oral airway should be the first line of treatment, although intubation or even tracheostomy may be required on occasion. Fortunately, respiratory extremis at birth in these children is rare.

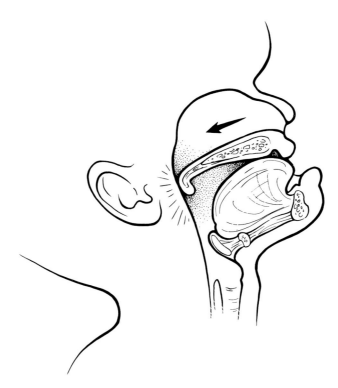

FIG. 15-14   Severe maxillary hypoplasia can cause nasotracheal obstruction, hampering attempts at nasotracheal intubation.

In the case of kleeblattschädel syndrome, a severe pansynostosis, or in other multiple synostotic children, breathing difficulties can be related to compression of the brain stem. Such cases are neurosurgical emergencies. During infancy and the first few years of life, these children may show signs of subtle or overt airway problems. A history of noisy breathing, snoring, or persistent somnolence in the daytime are clinical clues to an obstructed airway. A sleep study can help determine the degree and etiology of the problem. Operations to advance the midface in infancy have been fraught with high morbidity and mortality. Some centers have revisited the early approach to advancement of the midface, touting the use of rigid fixation as a way to cut down on these complications. Early intervention is still risky, however, and the mainstay of treatment in the young age group is tracheotomy. Once these children have reached 5 or 6 years of age, their facial bones have often matured enough to allow predictable and successful surgical mobilization and advancement. These procedures, known as the *monoblock* or *Le Fort III,* are substantial undertakings associated with significant time in the operating room and significant blood loss.

The advances in surgical technique and anesthetic management have given many more children the opportunity to undergo such procedures, thus allowing correction of a small pharyngeal airway, severe prolapse of the eyes secondary to the exorbitism, and a chance of attending school with a reasonably normal appearance. The monoblock and Le Fort III fracture operations deserve some mention as to the management of the airway for these children. In the case of a monoblock, the supraorbital bar and the midface are released and advanced as a unit, requiring an intracranial and extracranial approach. The Le Fort III operation does not include the supraorbital bar and can be performed with or without an intracranial approach, depending on the clinical situation. Rigid fixation has allowed great advances in these operations. There is no longer a need for intermaxillary fixation (IMF) to stabilize advanced bony segments, and the need for a preoperative tracheotomy is rare. Adequate access to the maxilla is best accomplished with a nasotracheal intubation. The tube should be secured with an anchoring heavy silk suture sewn to the membranous nasal septum (Fig. 15-15). The secured tube is most important to help prevent a change in tube po-

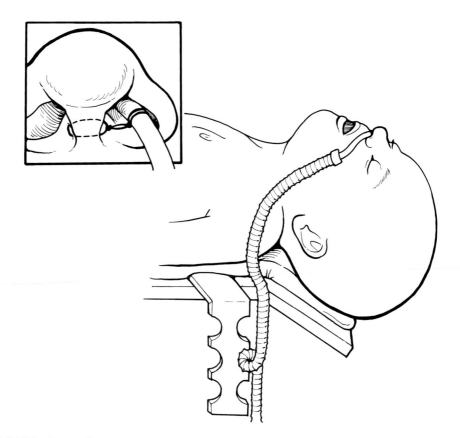

FIG. 15-15   Proper placement of endotracheal tube for monoblock or Le Fort III craniofacial procedure can allow access to a coronal incision and oral cavity and can allow full view of face. *Inset,* Endotracheal tube can be fixed to membranous nasal septum to secure nasotracheal intubation.

sition secondary to the abrupt movements of the face during the procedure. The tube should be brought across the cheek between the lower lid and the commissure to allow equal access to a coronal incision and the oral cavity and to provide the best compromise so as not to obscure the face (see Fig. 15-15). The use of tape along the course of the tubing is discouraged because it restricts the movement of the head and can cause breaks in connections upon mobilizing the midface. Positioning the patient should be done in concert with the surgeons. If a horseshoe headrest is to be used, appropriate precaution is necessary to avoid pressure necrosis of the scalp, as well as adequate padding of the sacrum and other pressure points predisposed to compression during the long operative case. Paralysis can be of great help during the operation, however, neurologic evaluation may be important to evaluate orbital compression by the size and reactivity of the pupils. Operative intervention during or immediately after the case may be required to restore vision loss as a result of compression and to prevent permanent blindness. Occasionally, an ocular-cardiac reflex can be evoked during ocular manipulation. This is manifested by a sudden and significant bradycardia.

   Adequate communication between the anesthesiologist and the surgeon can often prevent overtreatment because simply relieving the pressure often remedies the problem. In extreme circumstances intravenous atropine should successfully treat the bradycardia. Large-bore intravenous lines and multiple lines are mandatory for adequate venous access. Significant blood loss is not uncommon, and getting behind on fluids should be avoided because catching up can be difficult and can lead to hypotensive crisis. Just before craniofacial disimpaction, an osteotome is used to cut the bony septum and a fine osteotomy is made between the tube and the cranial base. On occasion the endotracheal cuff can be ruptured, or worse, the tube itself can be cut (Fig. 15-16). A throat pack should

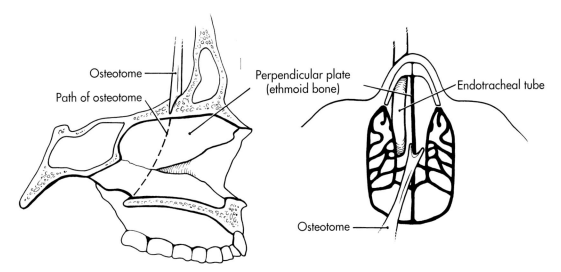

FIG. 15-16   Osteotome is used to separate monoblock facial bones from cranial base. Care is taken to avoid cutting nearby endotracheal tube, but tube is certainly at risk for damage during this portion of procedure.

control a cuff leak, however, a cut tube requires emergent reintubation. A replacement tube of the same caliber and dimension should always be on hand during these procedures in case the one being used is rendered useless.

Postoperatively, these children are managed in the intensive care unit. Conservative airway management is the rule. A traumatic intubation should impact timing of extubation, as well as the length of time the tube has been impinging on the cords. The child should be alert, with no sign of excessive bleeding or laryngeal swelling before removing the endotracheal tube. Rigid fixation and avoiding the need to wire the jaws shut has made the management of the difficult airway in these patients much easier, however, the risk of morbidity or mortality secondary to airway problems is still significant.[9]

CRANIOFACIAL CLEFTS

Encephaloceles and hypertelorism are the two manifestations of craniofacial cleft disorder. A neonate with respiratory distress should be carefully evaluated to discern the etiology. Patients with encephaloceles or gliomas can present in respiratory distress secondary to obstruction of the nasal or even oropharyngeal airway (Fig. 15-17). Physical findings such as a bifid nose, a bulging palate, or hypertelorism can signal the presence of a craniofacial cleft with a congenital herniation of neural tissue obstructing the airway. Management of these infants should consist of careful placement of an oral airway. Although this often decreases the acuity of the situation and allows further investigation, some of these children require intubation or tracheostomy.

FACIAL TRAUMA

Management of acute craniofacial trauma is an area in which the difficult airway is encountered frequently. Often the patient presents in a coma or with a decreased level of consciousness and requires the immediate establishment of an airway. If an oral airway is available, it should be used preferentially. A patient sustaining massive facial trauma can have an adequate airway rapidly deteriorate secondarily to swelling or significant hemorrhage. A low threshold for early intubation should be maintained.

Factures of the mandible or local trauma involving the tongue can cause an acute obstruction of the pharynx. A jaw-thrust maneuver or even direct traction of the tongue with a suture or towel clip can relieve obstruction and allow the oral cavity to be cleared of debris. When an oral airway is pre-

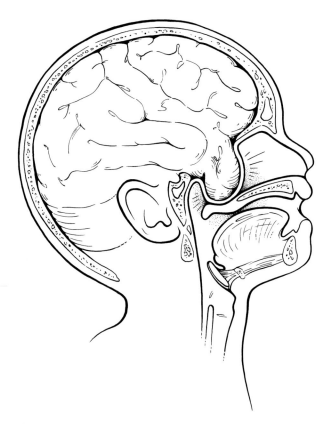

FIG. 15-17 Obstruction of nasotracheal airway or difficulty with oral intubation because bulging palate could be secondary to protruding encephalocele from cranial base.

cluded from use because of local trauma at the mouth, a nasal airway may be attempted. Nasal airways should, however, be approached with caution in the trauma patient because the situation can often require rapid intubation in a patient whose stomach is often filled with blood. In addition, any fractures to the cranial base could allow misdirected tube access to the brain. Unrelieved obstruction or inability to intubate are indications for tracheostomy.

ORTHOGNATHIC SURGERY

Surgery of the jaws is usually reserved for young adulthood or later, after the growth of the facial skeleton has terminated. Although many of these patients routinely had their jaws wired shut postoperatively, the arrival of rigid fixation has changed that considerably. The patient now can often be left with guiding elastic bands that do not significantly inhibit jaw opening postoperatively. This has made management of the airway for these patients much easier and less dangerous.

The most common orthognathic procedures include single or segmental cuts of the maxilla such as in a Le Fort I fracture and vertical or sagittal split osteotomies of the mandible. These operations are usually performed intraorally, with a great deal of retraction. A nasotracheal intubation is required, and a nasal RAE tube can often be helpful to run the tubing easily out of the nose and over the forehead (Fig. 15-18). This tube is best secured with suture to the membranous nasal septum and at the forehead just behind the hairline. The advance of the maxilla may occur rapidly during the case and change the distance from the nares to the tracheal carina. The anesthesiologist should be aware of the sudden advancement and should check the status of the tube position, which may require adjustment. Jaw surgery often elicits marked postoperative swelling and can lead to airway obstruction.

Difficulty handling oral secretions, an edematous tongue, or swelling tracking down into the neck can contribute to airway problems. The situation is compounded in the occasional patient who

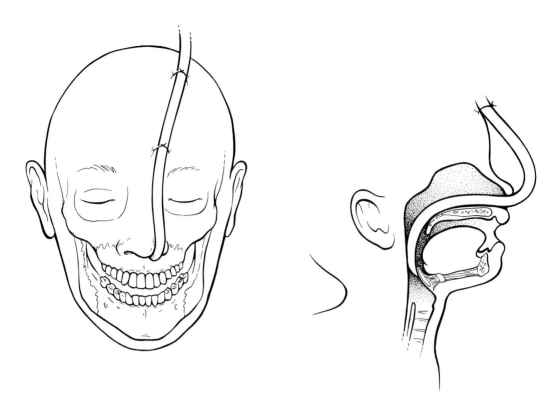

FIG. 15-18   Nasotracheal intubation facilitates extensive procedures that require oral exposure and intraoperative assessment of occlusion. Tube can be fixed to forehead in hairline.

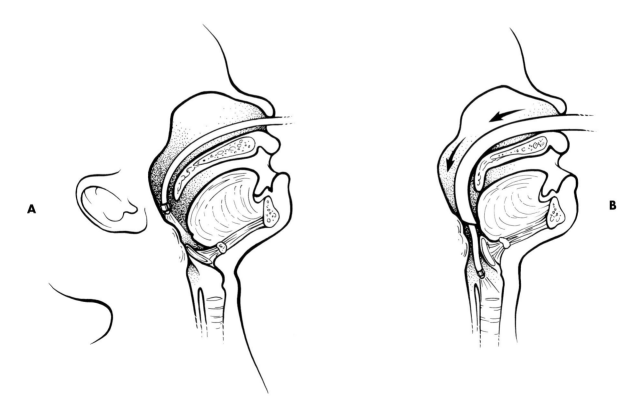

FIG. 15-19   **A,** Nasoendoscopy can be used to evaluate difficult airway. **B,** Endotracheal tube can be passed over a well-positioned endoscope, assuring proper tube placement.

requires a postoperative course of intermaxillary fixation. Peak swelling can occur up to 48 to 72 hours postoperatively, thus a judicious approach to extubation is called for. Patients should be well awake, be able to handle their secretions with a reasonable cough reflex, and show no signs of airway obstruction secondary to swelling. Some centers advocate letting down the cuff to assess the degree of swelling; a leak around the endotracheal tube often signals a patent airway. Perhaps the best way to assess airway patency is to use an endoscope through the endotracheal tube. The tube is guided out of the trachea over the scope, allowing direct visual inspection of the cords. If there are signs of obstruction, the endoscope can serve as a guide by simply slipping the tube back over the scope and into the appropriate position (Fig. 15-19). Extreme caution is warranted when approaching extubation with any patient in intermaxillary fixation. A pair of wire cutters should be readily available to release the jaws in case of emergent need for reintubation.

PLACEMENT AND FIXATION OF THE ANESTHETIC TUBE

The head is often subject to quick and sudden movements during a craniofacial reconstructive procedure, thus taping the anesthetic tube is usually inadequate to the task. Exposure to irrigation, traction, and blood often dislodges the tape and hence puts the tube at risk. The method of suture fixation for nasotracheal intubation has already been described, and the best method to secure an orotracheal tube is to wire it around the teeth. A 24-gauge wire is used around a molar or premolar and then secured to the endotracheal tube, adjusting the tension so as not to kink the tube but to firmly secure it. Liberal use of connection tubing is often necessary to allow the entire face to be prepared for surgical access.

CONCLUSION

Perhaps nowhere is the anesthetic tube as intimate to the operative field as in craniofacial surgery. Accessibility to the face and a nonobscured visual field are of paramount importance to assure correct placement of bone segments and to guard against the devastating disfigurement and dysfunctional consequences associated with a malpositioned facial skeleton. Constant communication and cooperation between the surgeon and the anesthesiologist are keys toward realizing the dual goal of ease of surgical access and successful management of the difficult airway.

REFERENCES

1. Munro IR: Craniofacial surgery: airway problems and management, *Int Anesthesiol Clin* 26(1):72-78, 1988.
2. Freed G, Pearlman MA, Brown AS et al: Polysomnographic indications for surgical intervention in Pierre Robin sequence, *Cleft Palate J* 25(2):151, 1988.
3. Jackson P, Whitaker LA, Randall P: Airway hazards associated with pharyngeal flaps in patients who have Pierre Robin syndrome, *Plast Reconstr Surg* 58(2):184, 1976.
4. Davies DW, Munro IR: The anesthetic management and intraoperative care of patients undergoing major facial osteotomies, *Plast Reconstr Surg* 55:51, 1975.
5. Delegue L, Guilbert M: Management of airway problems during the repair of craniofacial anomalies in children. In Caronni P (ed): *Craniofacial surgery,* Boston, 1985, Little, Brown.
6. Cosman B, Crikelair GF: Mandibular hypoplasia and the late development of glossopharyngeal airway obstruction, *Plast Reconstr Surg* 50:573, 1972.
7. Edgerton MT, Jane JA, Berry FA et al: New surgical concepts resulting from cranio-orbitofacial surgery, *Ann Surg* 182:228, 1975.
8. Whitaker LA, Munro IR, Salyer KE et al: Combined report of problems and complications in 793 craniofacial operations, *Plast Reconstr Surg* 64:198, 1979.
9. Handler SD, Beaugard ME, Whitaker LA et al: Airway management in the repair of craniofacial defects, *Cleft Palate J* 16(1):16, 1978.

CHAPTER **16**

Pediatric Difficult Airways

P. REYNOLDS

Management of the difficult pediatric airway requires some knowledge of developmental anatomy and the differences between the adult and pediatric airway. The skills and techniques used in the management of these patients use many of the principles described for adult patients but with certain modifications and adaptations for pediatric practice.

This chapter describes embryology of the airway and related structures, differences between the pediatric and adult airways, and equipment and techniques available for managing the routine and difficult pediatric airways, particularly when there are differences from adult practice. Many airway problems are associated with congenital syndromes and certain anatomic variants.[1]

AIRWAY EMBRYOLOGY

In fish and larval amphibians the branchial apparatus forms a system of gills.[1] In humans this same apparatus forms the lower face, pharynx, and neck structures. At 4 to 5 weeks postconception the primitive pharynx is bounded laterally by the barlike branchial arches. Each arch contains an artery, a cartilage bar, and a nerve and muscle element. Externally located between the arches are the branchial grooves. Internally, between the arches, are extensions of the pharynx called pharyngeal pouches. The endoderm of each pharyngeal pouch contacts the ectoderm of each branchial groove to form the branchial membrane. The branchial arches, grooves, pouches, and membranes form the branchial apparatus.

Table 16-1 summarizes the origin and fate of the skeletal structures, muscles, cranial nerves, and arch artery of each of the pharyngeal arches. The fifth arch cartilage bar is usually absent. When it is present, the rudimentary sixth arch has no cartilage bar.

The tongue begins to develop around the fourth week postconception when a triangular elevation, the tuberculum impar, and lateral lingual swelling appear in the floor of the pharynx. Originating from the first branchial arch, these structures make up the anterior two thirds of the tongue. The root of the tongue originates from the third branchial arch. As described previously, the innervation of the tongue follows the origins of the branchial arches. Thus the anterior two thirds is supplied by the lingular branch of the mandibular division of the trigeminal nerve (V), whereas the posterior one third of the tongue is innervated by the glossopharyngeal nerve.

The larynx is derived from the fourth and sixth branchial arches. The laryngotracheal groove appears first at 4 weeks postconception. At 5 weeks the epiglottal and arytenoid swellings appear. Between 7 and 10 weeks the entrance to the larynx ends blindly as a result of fusion of the epithelium. As this union breaks down during the tenth week, the laryngeal opening, or additus, enlarges. During this recanalization, a pair of recesses, or laryngeal ventricles, appear. The ventricles are bounded cranially and caudally by folds of mucous membrane, which eventually become the vestibular folds and vocal folds.

Table 16-1   Origin and Fate of Structures of Pharyngeal Arches

Pharyngeal arch	Artery	Cranial nerve	Skeletal structures	Muscles	Ligaments
1	Terminal branch of maxillary artery	Maxillary and mandibular division of trigeminal nerve (V)	Meckels cartilage, malleus, incus	Muscles of mastication (temporalis, masseter, and pterygoids), mylohyoid, anterior belly of the digastric, tensor tympani, and tensor veli palatini muscles	Anterior ligament of malleus Sphereomandibular ligament
2	Caroticotympanic artery	Facial nerve (VII)	Stapes, styloid process, lesser cornu of hyoid, upper rim of hyoid bone	Muscles of facial expression (orbicularis oculi, orbicularis oris, risorius, platysma, auricularis, frontooccipitalis, and buccinator), posterior belly of digastric, styohyoid, and stapedius muscles	Stylohyoid ligament
3	Common carotid artery, root of internal carotid artery	Glossopharyngeal nerve (IX)	Greater cornea of hyoid bone, lower rim of hyoid bone	Stylopharyngeus	—
4	Arch of aorta, right subclavian artery, original sprouts of pulmonary arteries	Superior laryngeal branch of vagus nerve (X)	Thyroid, critical, arytenoid, corniculate, and cuneiform cartilages	Constrictors of pharynx, cricothyroid, and levator veli palatine muscles	—
6	Ductus arteriosus, roots of definitive pulmonary arteries	Recurrent laryngeal branch of vagus nerve (X)	Thyroid, critical, arytenoid, corniculate, and cuneiform cartilages	Intrinsic muscles of larynx	—

PEDIATRIC AND ADULT AIRWAY DIFFERENCES

Not only are children different in overall size than adults, but also the difference in proportion or relative size of body structures in the pediatric age group is less obvious.[2] The box below summarizes the major differences between the pediatric and adult airways. Figs. 16-1 to 16-4 demonstrate major anatomic differences between the pediatric and adult larynxes. Practical application of these differences are detailed in the following sections on equipment and airway management.[3]

DIFFERENCES BETWEEN PEDIATRIC AND ADULT AIRWAY

1. Infants are obligate nasal breathers.
2. Infants have narrow nares.
3. Infants have large heads in relation to their bodies (anteroposterior diameter).
4. An infant's tongue is relatively large and obstructs easily.
5. The infant's larynx is higher in the neck (infant: C3-C4, adult C4-C5).
6. The epiglottis in adults in broad, with its axis parallel to the trachea.
7. The infant's epiglottis is long, narrow, and floppy and angulated away from the axis of the trachea.
8. Vocal folds in the infant have a lower anterior attachment to the glottis than posteriorly.
9. Adult vocal folds are perpendicular to the axis of the trachea.
10. The narrowest portion of the child's larynx is at the cricoid ring.
11. The narrowest portion of the adult's larynx is at the vocal folds.

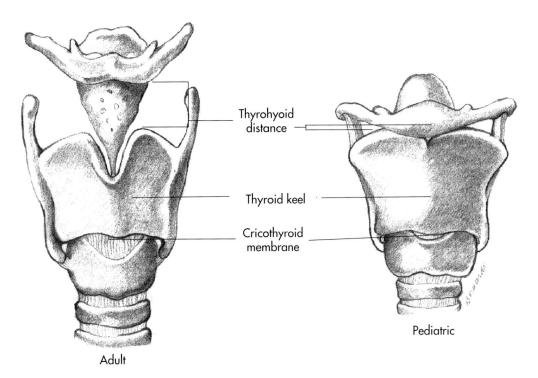

Thyrohyoid distance

Thyroid keel

Cricothyroid membrane

Pediatric

Adult

FIG. 16-1   Anterior view of larynx. Note overlapping of hyoid, thyroid, and cricoid on infant.

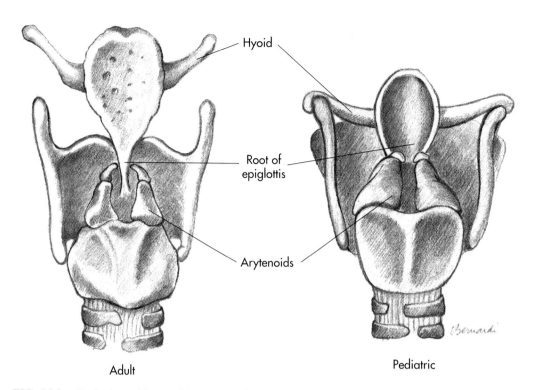

Hyoid

Root of epiglottis

Arytenoids

Adult

Pediatric

FIG. 16-2   Back view of larynx. Note shape of intrinsic laryngeal cartilages (especially arytenoids) and positioning of aryepiglottic folds.

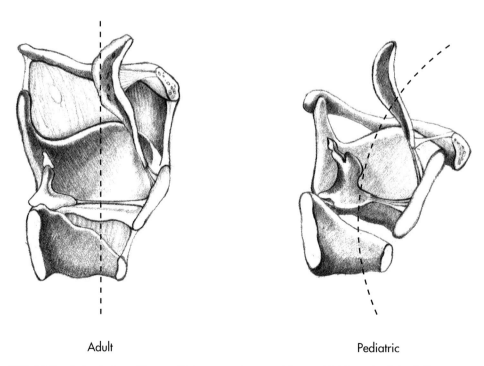

Adult

Pediatric

FIG. 16-3   Lateral view of larynx. Note axes and arytenoids, vocal folds, and epiglottic ligaments.

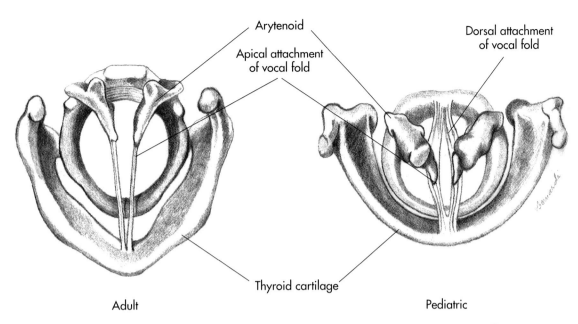

FIG. 16-4   Inferior view of larynx. Compare shape and positioning of intrinsic laryngeal cartilages (arytenoids) and vocal folds.

BASIC EQUIPMENT
Airway Management

Oral airways. Oral airways are designed for several functions. They prevent airway obstruction after induction of anesthesia, facilitate oropharyngeal suctioning, and prevent the patient from biting the endotracheal tube on emergence from anesthesia. To perform these functions, they must be appropriately sized. An airway that is too short may push the base of the tongue posteriorly, causing airway obstruction, whereas one that is too long may push the epiglottis over the laryngeal aperture to produce airway obstruction. The appropriate size airway is one that extends from the corner of the mouth and ends just cephalad to the angle of the mandible.

Nasal airways. Nasopharyngeal airways are sometimes useful in pediatric airway management. Soft, red rubber tubes are available (Rusch, West Germany), or an airway may be fashioned from an endotracheal tube. It is wise to place a safety pin through the end of such an airway to prevent it from being inhaled if it becomes unfastened. The appropriate length can again be estimated by measuring the distance from the nares to just cephalad to the angle of the mandible, allowing for an appropriate curve. The airway should be long enough to bypass obstruction at the level of the base of the tongue. A nasopharyngeal airway that is too long may pass through the hypopharynx into the esophagus, thus although the site of obstruction is bypassed, ventilation is still impossible. In an anesthetized patient it may be appropriate to purposefully advance the airway into the esophagus and then withdraw the airway until breath sounds are heard. The airway should be inserted, directed posteriorly, perpendicular to the patient's face. This is important to ensure that the airway passes through the inferior meatus of the nares under the inferior concha, which is the largest of the three meatus. If resistance to insertion occurs first, the tube should be checked to see that it is directed toward the inferior meatus; then the opposite nostril should be used. If resistance still occurs, a smaller airway should be selected.

Masks. Cushioned masks and noncushioned (Rendell-Baker) masks are available for airway management. A mask that achieves an airtight fit should be chosen. With a cushioned mask this usually requires a fit over the bridge of the nose and seating over the mentum. Some anesthesiologists prefer the noncushioned Rendell-Baker mask. This mask has a lower volume of displacement (dead space) and is designed to fit in the groove of the chin rather than over the mentum (Fig. 16-5). When

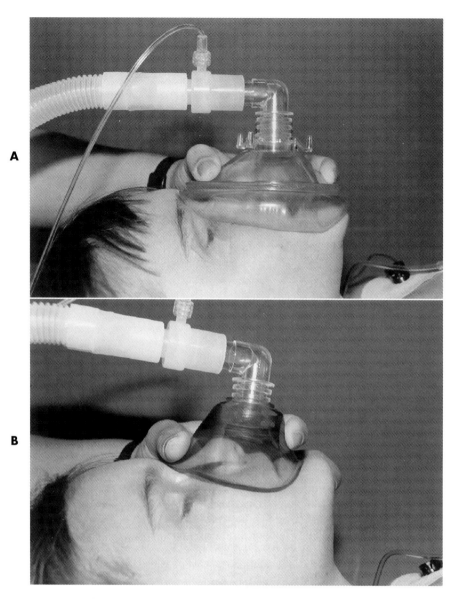

FIG. 16-5 Face masks. **A,** Cushion mask. **B,** Rendell-Baker mask.

properly applied, the mask also forces the user to displace the mandible away from the midface, thus potentially displacing the tongue anteriorly and improving airway management.

Intubation Equipment

Laryngoscope blades. A straight blade is usually used for laryngoscopy in neonates, infants, and young children. The relative macroglossia and cephalad positioning of the larynx (C3-C4 in children vs. C5 in the adult) produce a decrease in space between the base of the tongue and the epiglottis (vallecula), which provides inadequate visualization of the larynx when a curved blade is used. The straight blade is usually passed posterior to the epiglottis, unlike the curved blade laryngoscopes in adults. This is necessary because the epiglottis tends to be angled more posteriorly and lies over the laryngeal aperture, which may then not be visible when the epiglottis is elevated from placement of the tip of the blade in the vallecula. The most commonly used straight blades are the Miller series, and the most commonly used curved blades are the Macintosh series. Also, a straight

Table 16-2   Guide to Sizes of Commonly Used Laryngoscope Blades for Neonates, Infants, and Children

Age	Miller	Wis-Hipple	Seward	Macintosh
Premature	0	—	—	—
Neonate	0	—	—	—
1 month-2 years	1	—	—	—
2-6 years	—	1.5	1	—
6 to 12 years	2	—	2	2
12+ years	3	—	3	3

Table 16-3   Guide to Internal Diameter and Length of Pediatric Endotracheal Tubes

Age	Internal diameter (mm)	Oral length (cm)	Nasal length (cm)
<1000 g	2.5	8-9	10-11
1000 to 2500 g	3.0	9-10	11-12
Neonate to 6 months	3.5	10	13
6 to 18 months	4.0	11	14
18 to 24 months	4.0-4.5	12	15
2+ years	$4.0 + \dfrac{\text{Age (years)}}{4}$	$12 + \dfrac{\text{Age (years)}}{2}$	$15 + \dfrac{\text{Age (years)}}{2}$

blade with a flat cross section that is designed to be placed in the vallecula (the Seward blade) is frequently used for children. A guide for laryngoscope blades commonly used for children can be found in Table 16-2.

Endotracheal tubes.   With the changing diameter and length of the larynx and trachea that comes with age, several different endotracheal tubes of varying diameters and lengths are required. The narrowest part of the upper airway in neonates, infants, and young children is the cricoid cartilage. It is not until 8 to 10 years of age, with the growth of the cricoid cartilage, that the narrowest part of the airway is at the level of the vocal folds (as in adults). This means that, in most children younger than 8 years old, an uncuffed tube should be used. In these patients it is desirable to select an endotracheal tube that produces an audible air leak at 20 to 25 cm H_2O to prevent postintubation edema. The ideal length of an endotracheal tube should leave its distal end lying in the midtrachea. Although visual inspection and auscultation are the surest methods of confirming the appropriate length of insertion of an endotracheal tube, an approximate guide is outlined in Table 16-3.

Technique

Positioning.   The neonate head has a large anteroposterior diameter in relation to the rest of the body, as compared with an adult. This means that the patient's cervical spine is slightly flexed at rest. The optimal position for intubation (i.e., cervical flexion with head extension) is thus produced by extending the patient's head only. This is accomplished by placing a towel under the neonate's shoulders to compensate for the relatively large head. This becomes more important in the premature infant, in whom the difference in relative head size is even more exaggerated. When the child ages and head size decreases relative to body size, the head must be elevated in a manner similar to that of adult patients (i.e., by placing a folded towel or blanket under the occiput to produce cervical spine flexion).

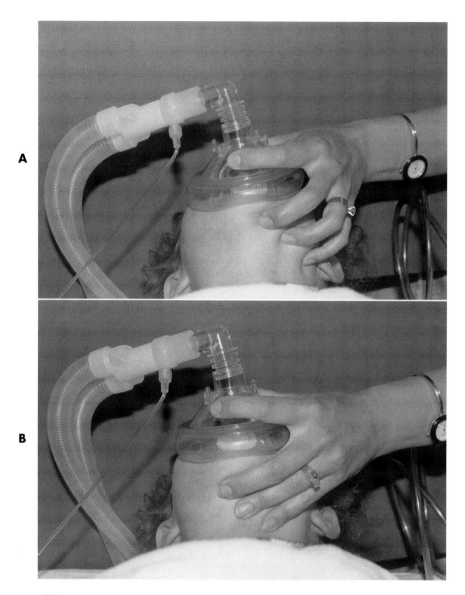

FIG. 16-6   **A,** Correct hand position for holding mask. **B,** Incorrect hand placement.

Holding the mask. It is important that the face mask be applied firmly without compressing the patient's airway (i.e., there should be no pressure applied to the soft tissues of the patient's face or neck). This is achieved by careful placement of the hand so that the thumb and index finger are applied to the mask, the middle finger is applied to the mentum, and the ring or little finger is applied to the bony angle of the mandible (Fig. 16-6).

Laryngoscopy. Visualization of the larynx is achieved using techniques similar to those described for adults. Visualization is frequently improved by posterior displacement of the larynx using cricoid pressure. In neonates this posterior displacement can be achieved with pressure from the little finger (Fig. 16-7). The standard insertion technique of displacing the tongue to the left sometimes causes problems in neonates and infants because of difficulty in controlling the tongue. If this occurs, better visualization may be achieved by inserting the straight blade laryngoscope in the midline and compressing the tongue between the mandible and the laryngoscope blade. If visualization of the larynx is inadequate using the standard insertion technique, insertion of the laryngoscope from the extreme right hand corner of the mouth also may improve visualization of the larynx.

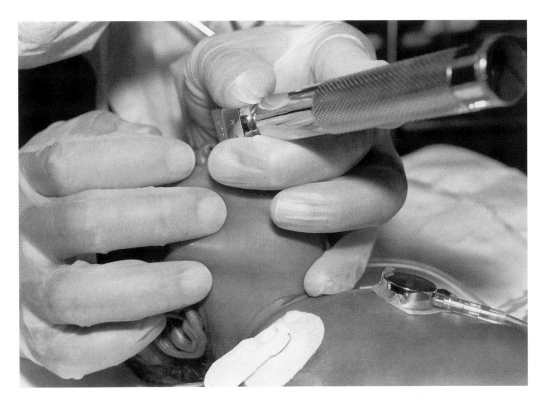

FIG. 16-7   Laryngoscopy in neonate.

Other Techniques of Intubation

Light wand intubation. Placing an endotracheal tube over the light wand may be used to facilitate intubation. The stylet should be bent at a distance from the top that corresponds to the distance from the angle of the mandible to the hyoid. In a low-light environment the stylet can then be advanced over the tongue until a glow is visible. The stylet can then be manipulated, keeping it in the midline. When the glow is visible distal to the hyoid, the endotracheal tube can be advanced into the trachea. Unfortunately there is only one size of light wand currently available, which limits the smallest endotracheal tube to 5.5 mm.

Anterior Commissure Laryngoscope with Optical Stylet

If laryngoscopy proves difficult and endotracheal tube insertion appears impossible in children with mandibular hypoplasia or macroglossia, the use of an otolaryngeal anterior commissure laryngoscope inserted from the extreme right side may improve visualization of the larynx. An endotracheal tube (without a connector) applied over an appropriately sized optical stylet can then be advanced through the anterior commissure laryngoscope and into the trachea (Fig. 16-8). For a neonate, a 9-mm laryngoscope is used, which, with a small optical stylet allows intubation with a 3.0-mm or 3.5-mm endotracheal tube.

Bullard laryngoscope. The pediatric version of the Bullard laryngoscope (Bullard Co. E.D., Cynthiana, Ky.) is a laryngoscope with a fixed, preformed curve of approximately 90 degrees, with an applied fiberoptic light source and image bundle to allow visualization at the tip. The advantage of this laryngoscope is that it can be introduced into the oropharynx with minimal mouth opening. With the patient lying supine, the laryngoscope is placed in the patient's mouth with the handle positioned horizontally and then rotated vertically as the blade is advanced over the patient's tongue to allow visualization of the larynx. In small infants, however, difficulty has been in experienced in displacing the epiglottis sufficiently to allow visualization of the larynx, particularly when tem-

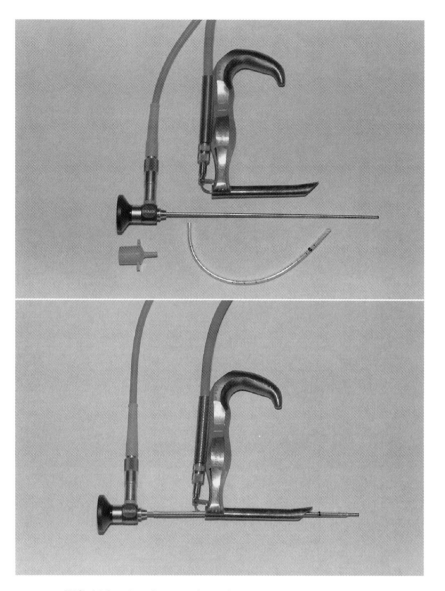

FIG. 16-8 Anterior commissure laryngoscope and optical stylet.

poromandibular joint movement is impaired. The laryngoscope is supplied with an intubating attachment designed to grasp the endotracheal tube through the Murphy eye. Although this device is useful in older children, its lateral offset limits its use as an aid to intubation in neonates and smaller infants.

Fiberoptic endoscopy as an aid to intubation. The fiberscope may be used to aid intubation in both the awake and anesthetized pediatric patient. Awake intubation using the fiberscope is used less frequently than in adult patients because of lack of patient cooperation. At the author's institution, if it is believed that airway management before induction will not be a problem, fiberoptic endoscopy is performed following an inhalational induction of anesthesia. When this is not believed to be appropriate, awake intubation is performed with the patient sedated. It has been found that a combination of midazolam and ketamine following an antisialagogue (atropine or glycopyrrolate) is most effective.

An Olympus LF-1 fiberscope for pediatric patients is routinely used. Instead of using the suction channel to aspirate secretions, it is preferred to pass oxygen at a flow of 2 to 3 L/min through the

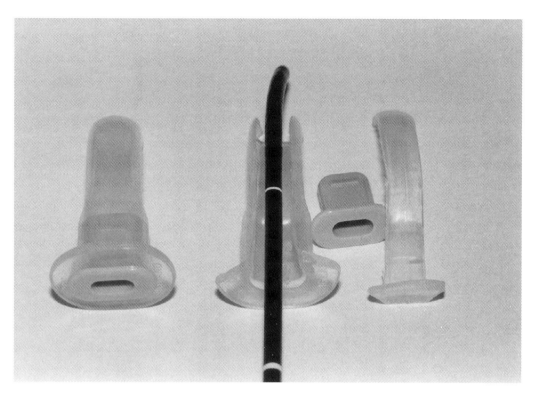

FIG. 16-9   Cutaway oral Guedel airway with fiberscope in place.

channel that serves the dual purpose of maintaining the distal lens clear from secretions and increasing the inspired oxygen concentration.

The technique for awake nasal intubation is essentially the same as that for adults. If the oral route is chosen, the most difficult problem is maintaining the fiberscope in the midline. Unlike adult patients, no specialized oral airways are available. By selecting an oral Guedel airway and cutting away the convex surface, the fiberscope can be kept in the midline (Fig. 16-9). If this technique is used in the awake patient, it is important to ensure that the upper palate and the remainder of the oropharynx are anesthetized and to be aware that, although the airway offers some protection from damage to the fiberscope by teeth, it is not as effective as a bite block.

In anesthetized patients, anesthesia may be maintained using either nasopharyngeal insufflation or a specially adapted face mask (Fig. 16-10). Alternatively, if airway management is trouble free under deep inhalational anesthesia, the patient may be rendered apneic by neuromuscular blockade; then, following preoxygenation, endoscopy can be performed on the paralyzed patient while ensuring adequate oxygenation through continuous measurement of oxygen saturation (SpO_2).

The LF-1 fiberscope does not allow endotracheal tubes of less than 4.5 mm to pass over the insertion tube. Presently, smaller fiberscopes that allow the passage of 3.0-mm endotracheal tubes are available, but these lack a suction port. In children less than 2 years old (or when intubation is required with an endotracheal tube of less than 4.5 mm internal diameter), the LF-1 fiberscope may still be used. It is possible to pass a guide wire (0.35 mm) through the suction port, through the laryngeal aperture, and into the trachea. The wire can be left in place, the fiberscope removed, and an endotracheal tube advanced over the wire. It may be advisable to reinsert the fiberscope through the opposite nostril as a visual aid because in neonates and infants the endotracheal tube may get held up at the laryngeal inlet (frequently the anterior commissure).

Laryngeal mask airway. The laryngeal mask airway (LMA) was invented by Dr. Archie Brain and has been available for use in United States since the beginning of 1993. The LMA provides a clear airway if it is correctly inserted.[4] Protective airway reflexes must be depressed to provide smooth insertion. The inserted mask sits with the tip resting up against the upper esophageal sphinc-

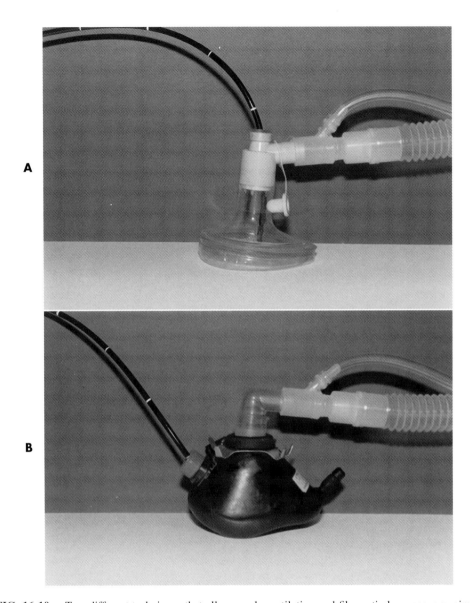

FIG. 16-10   Two different techniques that allow mask ventilation and fiberoptic laryngoscopy simultaneously in small infants. **A,** Portex connector and clear cushion mask. **B,** Patil-Syracuse mask with separate hole and diaphragm for insertion of fiberscope.

ter, the sides facing into the piriform fossea, and the upper border under the base of the tongue. Inflation of the cuff brings the glottic and laryngeal mask apertures in line with each other. In this way the LMA forms a seal around the laryngeal perimeter. If properly sized, the large size of the LMA prevents it from passing through either the glottic opening or the upper esophageal sphincter.

This design has several advantages. There is no danger of mainstem bronchial intubation, and the vocal folds are free to move during respiration. The patient can generate an effective cough with an LMA in place, while providing little stimulation. The LMA can be left in position until protective reflexes return. It must be noted that placement of the LMA is not without complications. Patients with full stomachs may regurgitate through the upper esophageal sphincter, laryngospasm may still occur, and rotation of the LMA may cause total airway obstruction. Also, the mouth opening must be adequate to allow insertion of the bulky LMA.

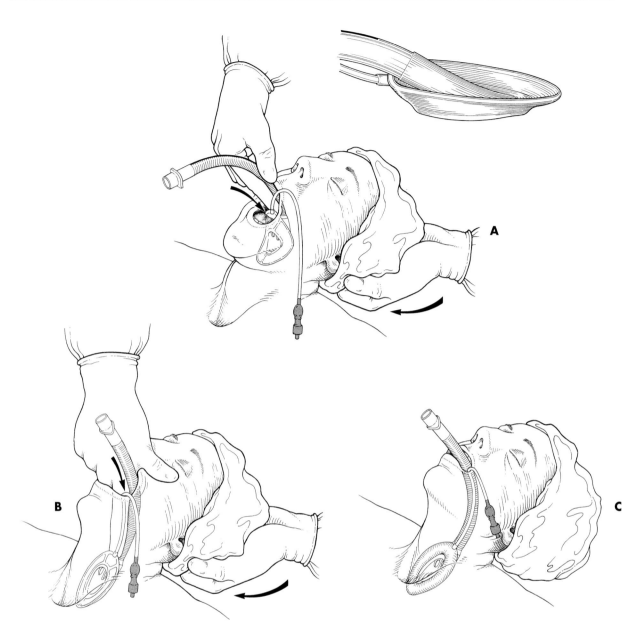

FIG. 16-11　Insertion technique for laryngeal mask airway, starting with **A.** (Courtesy Gensia, Inc., San Diego, Calif.)

INSERTION TECHNIQUE

The cuff should be completely deflated before insertion, with no folds near the distal end and the rim of the LMA facing away from the mask aperture (Fig. 16-11). The back of the LMA should be lubricated. Large globs of lubricant over the laryngeal entrance on the anterior surface must be avoided because this may result in aspiration of lubricant or obstruction of the aperture. For proper insertion of the LMA, correct sizes and cuff inflations must be obtained (Table 16-4).

Anesthesia is induced in the patient either gaseously or intravenously. Airway reflexes must be sufficiently suppressed so patients do not cough or gag upon LMA insertion. Patient anesthetic depth should be at a level at which a direct laryngoscopy could be performed without the use of muscle relaxants. With the head at slight extension, the mouth open, and under direct vision, the mask tip should be passed against the hard palate. Using the index finger of the dominant hand and advanc-

Table 16-4 Laryngeal Mask Airway (LMA) Sizes

LMA size	Suggested patient size	Cuff inflation volumes
1	Up to 6.5 kg	2-4 ml
2	6.5-20 kg	Up to 10 ml
2.5	20-30 kg	Up to 15 ml
3	>30 kg	Up to 20 ml
4	Normal and large adults	Up to 30 ml

ing the mask into the pharynx, the anesthesiologist should press against the hard palate the entire time. Resistance is sometimes met when the mask is being advanced over the base of the tongue at the oral/pharyngeal angle. It is sometimes helpful to pull the tongue forward and position the head with more extension at this point.

The anesthesiologist should continue pushing the mask with the index finger until the mask no longer advances. Grasping the tube with the other hand and withdrawing the index finger from the pharynx, the anesthesiologist should assure that the mask is fully inserted by pressing gently downward on the mask, letting go of the mask and inflating the cuff with recommended volume. The mask rises slightly as it is inflated, finding its own correct position over the laryngeal aperture. A bite block (usually a rolled piece of gauze) is inserted to protect the airway from damage or from compression by the teeth. Correct positioning of the LMA is affirmed by bilateral breath sounds and presence of carbon dioxide on the capnograph. The mask is then fixed with tape to the upper lip. It is important that the black line on the LMA is facing toward the upper lip.

LMAs can also be used in the management of difficult pediatric airways as an emergency airway in a patient in whom airway patency is difficult or impossible to maintain or as a conduit through which an endotracheal tube can be passed either blindly or over an intubating stylet such as a fiberoptic scope. **Perfect positioning of the LMA has been reported to be obtainable only between 40% and 60% of the time, in spite of an adequate airway. If the LMA is to be used as a conduit, endotracheal tube placement should be performed with the use of a fiberoptic endoscope.**

At the author's institution, this procedure is undertaken in the following fashion.[5] After placement of the LMA, the patient is kept breathing spontaneously with 100% oxygen and an adequate concentration of volatile anesthetic. The fiberoptic scope is prepared by placing two endotracheal tubes of the same size over the scope and securing them together with a piece of tape. This is done because of the similarity in length of an endotracheal tube and the LMA, which leads to the inability to maintain endotracheal tube position as the LMA is removed (Fig. 16-12, *A*). The upper and lower endotracheal tube, fiberscope, and LMA must be well lubricated. The fiberscope is then introduced into the LMA. After visualization and intubation of the laryngeal opening with the fiberscope, the upper endotracheal tube is used to advance the lower tube as the LMA is removed (Fig. 16-12, *B*). The adhesive tape is removed and the fiberscope is withdrawn from the patient after proper positioning of the lower endotracheal tube is confirmed.

Pediatric Difficult Airways

Difficult airways in the pediatric population can result from a variety of circumstances. Isolated congenital malformation of the airway, chromosomal abnormalities or syndromes causing airway malformation, deformities of the airway from disease or trauma, inborn errors of metabolism, and infection can all present a challenge to the anesthesiologist involved in the care of these children. Each of these circumstances are reviewed, followed by actual cases performed by the author with intubating techniques previously described.

Isolated congenital malformations. Isolated congenital malformations of the airway often present during the newborn period and can be life-threatening. Examples of isolated congenital malformations can include the Pierre Robin syndrome, hemangiomas, and cystic hygro-

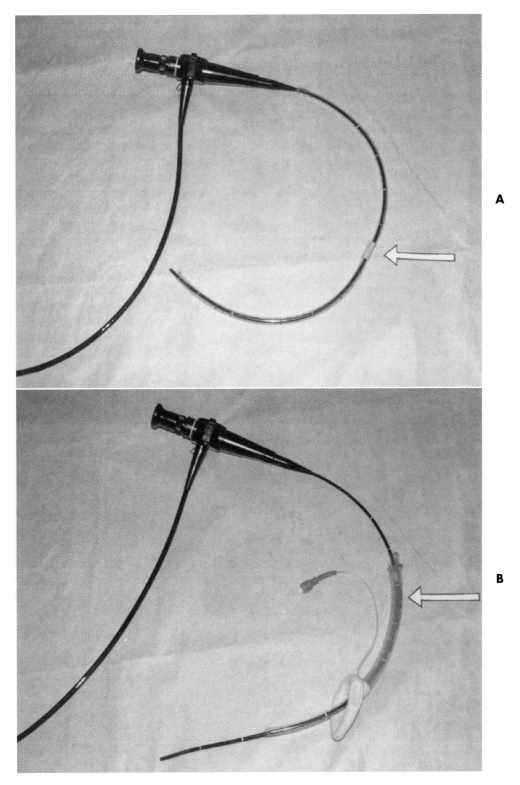

FIG. 16-12 Fiberoptic intubation with aid of laryngeal mask airway (LMA). **A,** Endotracheal tubes positioned on intubating fiberscope. **B,** Advancement of endotracheal tube through LMA.

mas. Cystic hygromas are multilobular, multilocular cystic masses that occur in equal frequency in males and females.[6] About 60% of cystic hygromas appear within the first year of life, and 80% to 90% occur before the second year. Cystic hygromas are thought to develop from the primitive embryonic lymph sacs, occurring more frequently in the posterior triangle of the neck. When presenting in the anterior triangle, they can be associated with intraoral spread. The mass effect of the cystic hygroma in the neck may compromise the neonatal airway by compressing the structures of the pharynx or the trachea, leading to upper airway obstruction, which, if left untreated, could potentially lead to death. The treatment of cystic hygromas is surgical resection; spontaneous regression is rare.

The child in Fig. 16-13 presented on a prenatal ultrasound with a cystic hygroma located in the right side of the neck. Before delivery, it was unknown whether this lesion was compatible with life. The amount of airway compromise was not ascertainable from prenatal studies. Because the diagnosis was made prenatally, airway management of this child was carefully thought out. Before elective cesarean section at 38 weeks' gestation, pediatric anesthesiologists, neonatologists, and pediatric surgeons were all informed as to the child's airway problem and were in attendance in the delivery room. Immediately after cesarean delivery, the newborn was placed on a table next to the delivery table. To continue oxygenating the newborn the umbilical cord was not clamped and the placenta continued to be perfused via the mother's uterus. The infant's airway was quickly examined, and the child was intubated while awake through the right side of the mouth, displacing the tongue away from the cystic hygroma. Continued placental perfusion allowed the anesthesiologist several extra moments in which to secure the airway. Had the anesthesiologist been unable to secure the newborn's airway, personnel and equipment were available to secure a surgical airway. After correct placement of the endotracheal tube the child was brought immediately to the operating room where the cystic hygroma was resected.

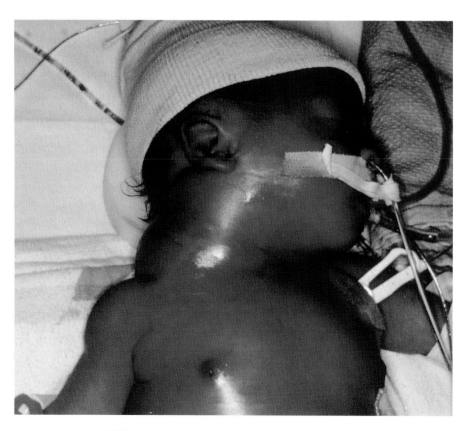

FIG. 16-13 Newborn with cystic hygroma of neck.

Pediatric Airway Syndromes

Syndromes causing airway malformation can include mandibular dysostosis, Beckwith-Wiedemann syndrome, and neurofibromatosis.[7] Mandibular dysostosis is a group of syndromes that has the common findings of micrognathia, retrognathia, and pharyngeal hypotonia. Examples of mandibular dysostosis include the Treacher Collins, Goldenhar's, and Hallermann-Streiff-François syndromes. Treacher Collins syndrome is an autosomal dominant disease (with 60% fresh mutations) with a wide variety of expression. Common findings in this syndrome include malar, mandibular, zygomatic, and maxillary hypoplasia that is bilateral and symmetric. Micrognathia, downward sloping palpebral fissures, external ear deformities, conductive deafness, pharyngeal hypotonia, or cleft palate can also be seen. These patients can develop early respiratory problems as a result of narrowed airways and occasionally require a temporary tracheostomy. Because of their multiple facial malformations, these patients often require multiple anesthetics. As the following case demonstrates, intubation techniques can vary, depending on the age of the child, nature of the surgical procedure, and anatomic variability after surgical repairs.

The child in Fig. 16-14, *A* underwent multiple anesthetics for surgical correction of her facial anomalies caused by Treacher Collins syndrome. As a small child, during an anesthetic for pharyngoplasty to correct pharyngeal hypotonia, she required an emergent tracheostomy because of the inability to intubate her after intravenous induction of anesthesia.

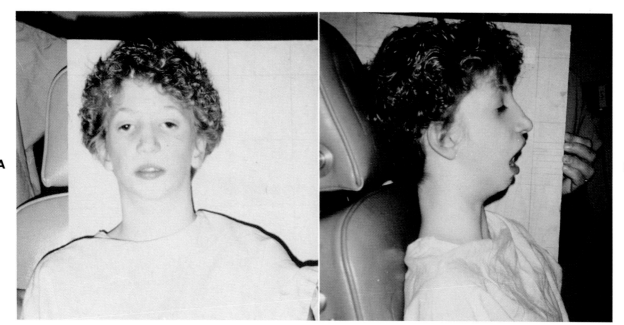

A

B

FIG. 16-14 Frontal, **A,** and lateral, **B,** views of 13-year-old-girl with Treacher Collins syndrome before mandibular surgery. Note downward sloping palpebral fissures, mandibular hypoplasia, and posteriorly rotated, low-set ears.

Continued.

Following the pharyngoplasty, she developed nasopharyngeal stenosis. At 13 years old the patient underwent an oral, awake, fiberoptic intubation for repair of her nasopharyngeal stenosis. At 15 years old the patient was scheduled for a mandibular advancement osteotomy, requiring the presence of a nasotracheal tube. Although her nasopharyngeal stenosis was improved, preoperative evaluation of her airway revealed small posterior nasal passages bilaterally. After the airway was secured with an awake oral fiberoptic intubation, anesthesia was induced and the left nasal passage was dilated with nasal trumpets. The adult fiberscope was advanced through her left naris to the vocal cords, and a wire was placed through the scope along the oral endotracheal tube. The oral endotracheal tube was removed after placing a Teflon tube guide through it into the trachea, and a nasal endotracheal tube was passed over the fiberscope. The patient was breathing spontaneously during the entire procedure. She returned to the operating room when she was 16 years old for bilateral eyelid revisions (Fig. 16-14, *C*). The mandibular advancement had improved her airway both clinically and radiologically. This was evident by airway soft tissue films that revealed the absence of glossoptosis (which had been present on previous studies) and the subjective observations of her parents that she no longer snored at night. After intravenous induction of anesthesia with propofol, the patient was easily ventilated. Spontaneous respirations were maintained. The glottic opening was not visualized with a direct laryngoscopy because of the anterior position of the larynx. An LMA was placed with the patient breathing spontaneously, and then the endotracheal tube was advanced over a fiberoptic scope through the LMA, as previously described.

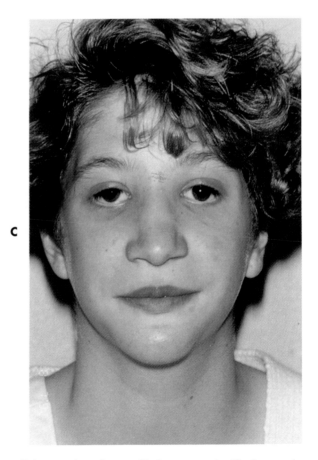

FIG. 16-14, cont'd.   C, Same patient after mandibular osteotomies. Her laryngeal opening was still unable to be visualized during direct laryngoscopy.

Mucopolysaccaridosis. Another cause of pediatric difficult airways can be seen in patients with mucopolysaccharidosis (MPS), a rare group of familial diseases of connective tissue metabolism caused by the absence or deficiency of enzymes that are involved in the metabolism of the main components of connective tissue.[8] These substrates cannot be transformed, and they accumulate in the skin, brain, heart, bone, liver, spleen, blood vessels, cornea, tracheal bronchial trees, and upper airway. The MPSs are classified as true inborn errors of metabolism. There are eight types of MPS, most showing the progressive physical findings of coarse facial features, a short thick neck, macroglossia with tongue protrusion, mouth breathing, and excessive tracheal-bronchial tree secretions. MPS infiltrates can be seen in the upper airway and in the tracheal-bronchial tree. These often appear through the fiberoptic scope as redundant folds of yellowish mucosa. Patients with MPS can also develop stiff joints, with the cervical spine occasionally involved. Two subtypes of MPS, Hurler's and Morquio's syndromes, can present with atlantoaxial subluxation. Progressive involvement of the MPS in the tracheal-bronchial trees, tongue, and upper airway often leads to obstructive sleep apnea and difficulty in airway management after induction of anesthesia. Smaller-than-usual outer diameter endotracheal tubes must be used in children with MPS infiltrates in the tracheal-bronchial tree because of the narrowing of the tracheal lumen.

The child in Fig. 16-15 is an 11-year-old boy with Hunter's syndrome. The coarse facial features and the large protruding tongue should be noted. This child had a history of obstructive sleep apnea and mental retardation, and presented for a repair of an inguinal hernia. After an inhalation induction, the large tongue was pulled forward with a pair of Magill forceps and a nasal airway was carefully placed. Direct laryngoscopy was performed with a Macintosh 3 blade.

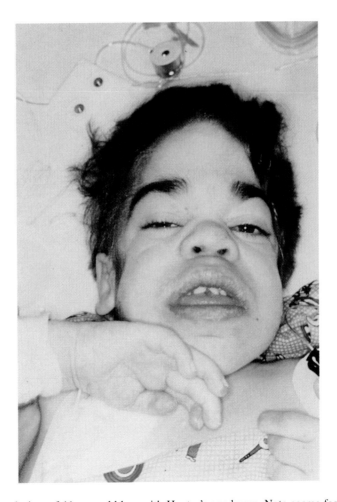

FIG. 16-15   Frontal view of 11-year-old boy with Hunter's syndrome. Note coarse facial features, large tongue, and short neck.

Acquired airway deformities. Airway deformities of children can also be acquired. Examples of this include juvenile rheumatoid arthritis (JRA), obesity, trauma, and tumors. JRA is a chronic, relapsing, systemic disease that is characterized by joint inflammation and extraarticular manifestations.[9] Children with JRA can present airway problems to the anesthetist when the joints involved are in the head and neck. Cervical spine arthritis, seen in 60% to 70% of patients with JRA, can cause restricted neck movements, flexion deformities, loss of extension, and torticollis. Levels affected are usually C2 and C3, but more levels may be involved. Atlantoaxial subluxation is uncommon, but if present, spinal cord compression by the odontoid process of C2 during neck flexion can be disastrous. Temporomandibular joint (TMJ) involvement occurs in about 65% of the patients and may severely limit mouth opening. Of patients with TMJ involvement, 5% have secondary mandibular hypoplasia and retrognathia as a result of retarded mandibular growth. Cricoarytenoid arthritis is uncommon in children but can present with local pain, hoarseness, and stridor and may lead to airway obstruction.

Fig. 16-16 illustrates a 16-year-old boy with JRA. After being scheduled for a mandibular osteotomy, he presented to the clinic for airway evaluation with limited mouth opening (< 2 cm), an immobile, fused, cervical spine, and mandibular hypoplasia secondary to his TMJ disease. There was, however, good air movement through his nasal passages bilaterally. This young man tolerated an awake fiberoptic nasal intubation after topical localization and minimal sedation.

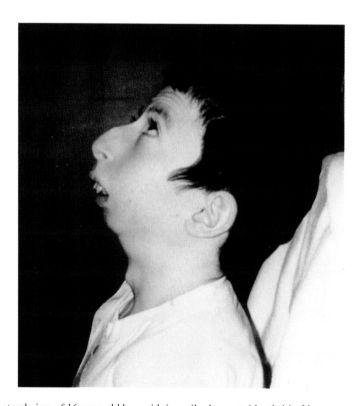

FIG. 16-16   Lateral view of 16-year-old boy with juvenile rheumatoid arthritis. Note severe retrognathia, micrognathia, overbite, and limited mouth opening.

Infection. Finally, a common cause for difficult pediatric airways is infection. The infectious diseases that can lead to difficulty in airway management include croup, epiglottitis, and retropharyngeal and peritonsilar abscesses. Croup (laryngotracheobronchitis) is usually viral in origin, whereas epiglottitis is usually caused by the bacteria *Haemophilus influenzae,* type B.[10] Croup is much more common than epiglottitis; however, it is imperative that the physician make the diagnosis rapidly and accurately. Compounding this dilemma, both croup and epiglottitis can be seen simultaneously in the same patient. At times the differences in the two are striking, but, unfortunately, the differences in presentation may be subtle. Both are diseases of drier temperate zones, and both cluster in winter months when the weather changes (October, November, March, and April). Fortunately, with the advent of *H. influenzae,* type B immunization, the incidence of epiglottitis in children is decreasing. The major differences between croup and epiglottitis are listed in Table 16-5.

Croup usually begins gradually at night, with a barking cough and upper respiratory tract symptoms. Inspiratory stridor is often associated. In severe cases, tachypnea and increased work of breathing may eventually lead to hypercarbia, hypoxemia, and respiratory arrest. Epiglottitis begins acutely, with reduced airflow from inflamed supraglottic tissues producing only muffled stridor and little coughing. Dysphonia and, later, aphonia represent no airflow. Inspiratory stridor can also be heard. Radiographic findings do not correlate with severity, which is diagnosed on an anteroposterior film with the presence of the "steeple sign" (see Chapter 13). Croup usually clears with cold, night air or a misty shower. If symptoms are severe enough for a hospital visit (stridor at rest, severe retractions), racemic epinephrine treatment may be indicated (Table 16-6).

Table 16-5 Comparison of Symptoms of Croup and Epiglottitis

	Laryngotracheobronchitis (croup)	Epiglottitis
Age at onset	Infancy	3-6 years (6 months-6 years)
Fever	<38.5° C	≥38.5° C
Appearance	Anxious, alert (unless impending resp failure)	Toxic, drooling, sitting upright
White blood cell count	7000-10,000	>12,000
Blood cultures	Negative	50% positive for *H. influenzae*
Pathogenesis	Viral, possible bacterial superinfection	90% *H. influenzae* type B obtained
Pathologic condition	Edema and swelling of subglottic tracheobronchial mucosa	Edema and swelling of all supraglottic structures
Onset	Relatively late peak severity after 72° F	Acute onset, hours to peak severity

Table 16-6 Dosage of Racemic Epinephrine

Age (years)	Dose (ml of 2.25% solution)
<1	0.2
1-3	0.3
3-6	0.4
>6	0.5

After treatment, the patient should be monitored for rebound, which can occur up to 7 hours later. If the disease is severe enough to warrant endotracheal intubation, it is acceptable to use muscle relaxants and continuous positive airway pressure (CPAP) by bag and mask. An endotracheal tube *at least* ½ size smaller than would normally be used should be chosen.

Epiglottitis is diagnosed on lateral neck films (done and read first). A positive "thumb sign" (enlarged epiglottis), loss of extension in the neck, and subglottic edema on lateral film may be seen (see Chapter 13). **If the clinician's index of suspicion is high, he or she should avoid further unnecessary diagnostic maneuvers, such as lateral neck x-rays, and proceed directly to the operating suite. The clinician should not look in the patient's mouth or upset the patient. The pediatric patient should be transported and induced with the parent present, in the position most comfortable for the child.** An inhalation induction with 100% oxygen and halothane should be performed, with IV access obtained after the child is asleep. After the child is asleep, he or she should be positioned supine. The degree of airway obstruction with change in position will increase, but this can be partially compensated for by delivery of mask CPAP. When a surgical plane of anesthesia is reached, deft oral intubation should be performed without muscle relaxants, using either a Macintosh or a Miller blade and a smaller-than-expected endotracheal tube. Surgeons should be standing by, ready to provide a surgical airway, if necessary. The epiglottis should then be cultured and the child kept intubated and sedated for 2 to 3 days. Extubation should be considered if an airway leak appears.

REFERENCES

1. William E, Larson J: *Development of the head, neck, eyes and face: human embryology,* New York, 1993, Churchill Livingstone.
2. Cote CJ, Ryan JF, Todres ID et al: *The pediatric airway: a practice of anesthesia for infants and children,* ed 2, Philadelphia, 1993, WB Saunders.
3. Norton ML, Brown ACD: *Atlas of the difficult airway,* St Louis, 1991, Mosby.
4. Brain AIJ: The *intavent laryngeal mask: instruction manual,* San Diego, 1992 Gensia Pharmaceuticals.
5. Reynolds P, O'Kelly S: Fiberoptic intubation and the laryngeal mask airway, *Anesthesiology* 79:1144, 1993.
6. Harrington JF: Cystic hygroma. In Stehling L (ed): *Common problems in pediatric anesthesia,* vol 1, ed 2, St Louis, 1992, Mosby.
7. Smith DW: Recognizable patterns of human malformations, ed 2, Philadelphia, 1976, WB Saunders.
8. Diaz J, Belani K: Perioperative management of children with mucopolysaccharidoses, *Anesth Analg* 77:1261-1270, 1993.
9. Smith M: Rheumatoid arthritis and cervical laminectomy. In Stehling L (ed): *Common problems in pediatric anesthesia,* ed 2, St Louis, 1992, Mosby.
10. Reynolds P: *Croup and epiglottitis,* ed 2, Resident Information Handbook, Ann Arbor, Mich, 1993, University of Michigan, Department of Anesthesiology, Section of Pediatric Anesthesiology.

Anatomic Features of the Airway

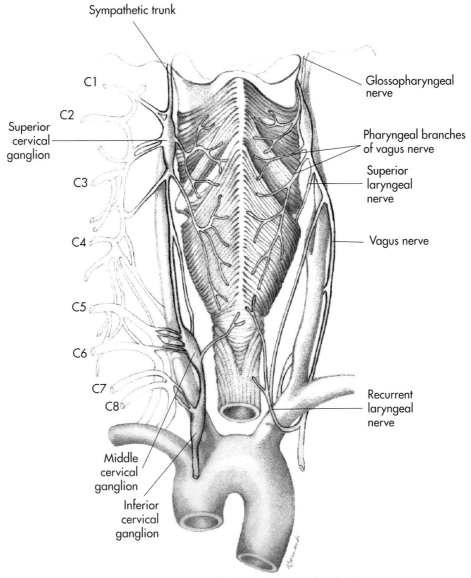

FIG. 1   Innervation of larynx (anteroposterior view).

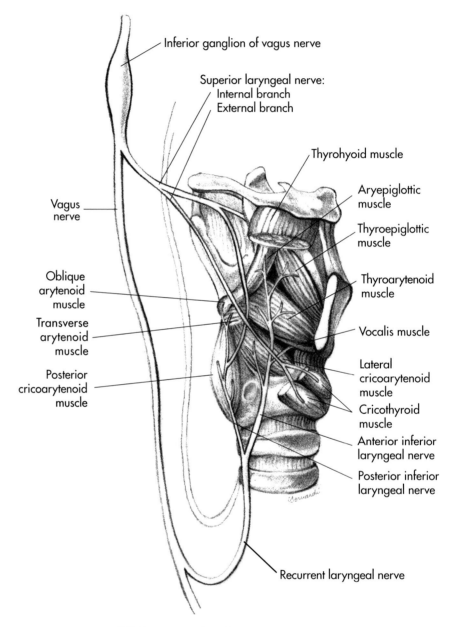

FIG. 2   Innervation of larynx and musculature.

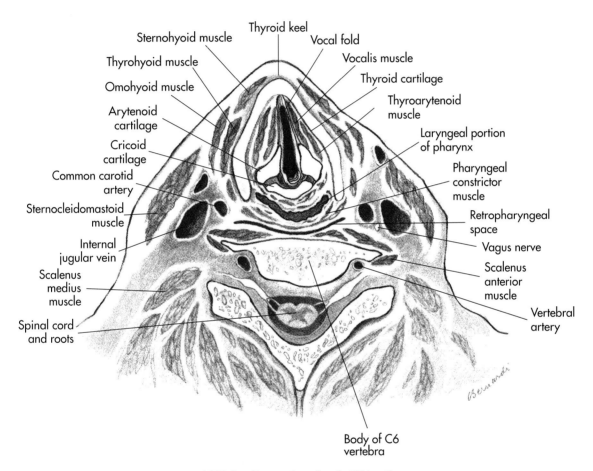

Sternohyoid muscle

Thyroid keel

Vocal fold

Thyrohyoid muscle

Vocalis muscle

Omohyoid muscle

Thyroid cartilage

Arytenoid cartilage

Thyroarytenoid muscle

Cricoid cartilage

Laryngeal portion of pharynx

Common carotid artery

Pharyngeal constrictor muscle

Sternocleidomastoid muscle

Retropharyngeal space

Internal jugular vein

Vagus nerve

Scalenus medius muscle

Scalenus anterior muscle

Spinal cord and roots

Vertebral artery

Body of C6 vertebra

FIG. 3 Transection of neck (C6 level).

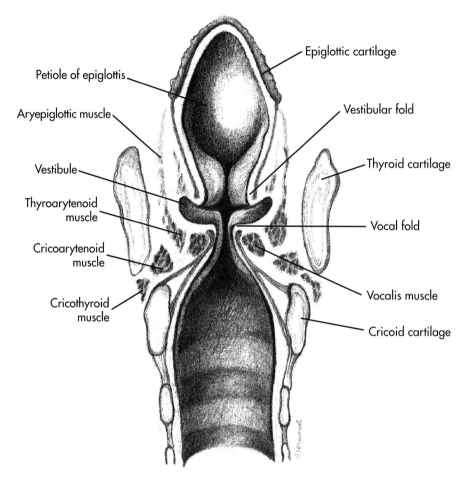

Petiole of epiglottis

Aryepiglottic muscle

Vestibule

Thyroarytenoid
muscle

Cricoarytenoid
muscle

Cricothyroid
muscle

Epiglottic cartilage

Vestibular fold

Thyroid cartilage

Vocal fold

Vocalis muscle

Cricoid cartilage

FIG. 4   Laryngeal structures (dorsal view).

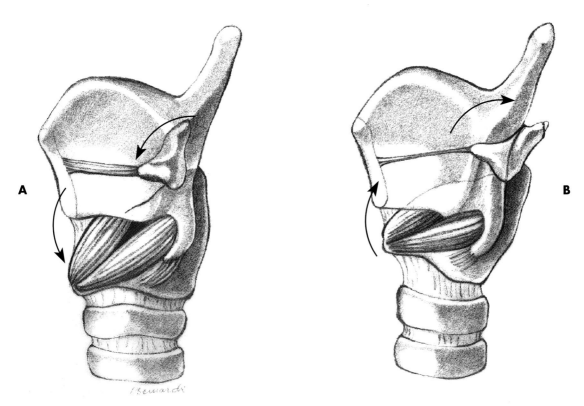

FIG. 5 Vocal fold motion. **A,** Resting. **B,** Phonation.

Adult

Pediatric

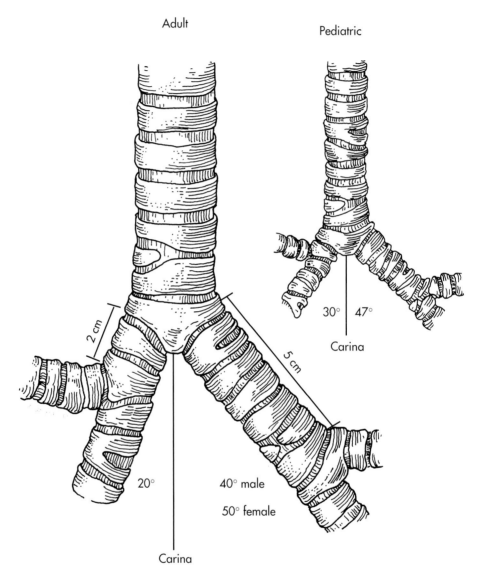

2 cm

5 cm

30° | 47°

Carina

20°

40° male

50° female

Carina

FIG. 6   Tracheobronchus (adult and pediatric).

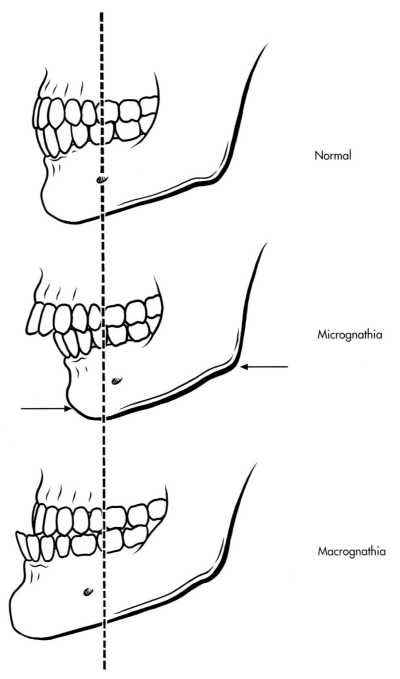

Normal

Micrognathia

Macrognathia

FIG. 7   Mandibular configuration.

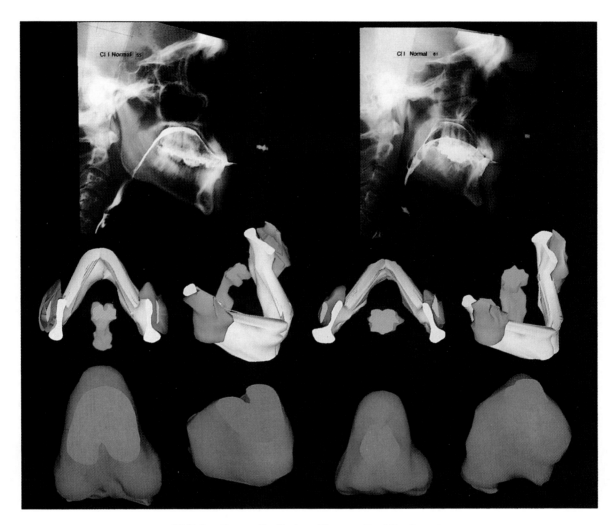

FIG. 8   Tongue distribution. (Courtesy Dr. Allan Lowe.)

Index